Black Americans' Strengths-Based Cultural Practices

||| | ||||||||||||||||| ||| ||| |||
I0131094

Black Americans' Strengths-Based Cultural Practices: Tools for Clinicians to Promote Psychological Well-Being uses historical, social, scientific, and psychological research to detail how mental health professionals can use the cultural practices of Black Americans and communities to promote positive psychosocial health.

Building on experiences of racial oppression and cultural values, Drs. Carter, Pieterse, and Forsyth offer an evidence-based framework for recognizing and enhancing strengths-based cultural practices of Black American clients and families in mental health interventions. This volume will broaden the base of work on the mental health treatment of Black Americans and provide an approach to understanding the unique cultural influences of Black people as they relate to psychological health.

The book is suitable for a wide range of professionals, including social workers, mental health practitioners, nurses, teachers, and sociologists at various levels of education and training.

Robert T. Carter, **Ph.D.,** is professor emeritus of Psychology and Education at Teachers College, Columbia University.

Alex L. Pieterse, Ph.D., is an associate professor and director of the Institute for the Study of Race and Culture at Boston College.

Jessica M. Forsyth, Ph.D., is a licensed psychologist and senior associate at Robert T. Carter & Associates, an expert witness practice specializing in the assessment of racial trauma, where she has consulted on a variety of civil and criminal cases for 15 years.

Black Americans' Strengths-Based Cultural Practices: Tools for Clinicians to Promote Psychological Well-Being is destined to become a must-read for mental health professionals, graduate students, and professors alike. Carter, Pieterse, and Forsyth offer clear definitions of each cultural strength, the research on their historical roots in the African diaspora, as well as the evidence base for their contribution to healthy psychological development and mental health maintenance for Black Americans. Their critical examination of historical and contemporary racial oppression experienced by Black Americans sets the stage well for understanding the vital importance of fostering life-sustaining cultural strengths in mental health care with this population. They also provide an excellent review of the scientific literature on racial identity development, racial socialization, and the intergenerational transmission of Black cultural strengths through familial and community mechanisms.

Clinicians and mental health training professionals will love the practical examples of cultural strength-based case formulation. They will learn about clinical inventories and interview prompts to assess identification with various cultural values, racial identity status, racial socialization, and racism-related coping. The authors also present a model of treatment planning and implementation that centers the voice of Black American clients as well as examples of various evidence-based models of care that incorporate Black cultural strengths into the therapeutic process.

Moreover, they challenge mental health clinicians, educators, and professional organizations to address structural racism as a primary source of psychological distress amongst Black Americans as well as an ever-present obstacle to their utilization of mainstream mental health services. This includes a call to decolonize mental health training curricula, licensing requirements, and best practice protocols to be more inclusive of African-centered theorists and clinical research that will utilize time-proven mental health-promoting strengths of Black Americans.

– Treniece Lewis Harris, Ph.D., *associate professor,*
program director, master in Mental Health Counseling Program,
Department of Counseling, Developmental, and Educational Psychology,
Boston College

Black Americans' Strengths-Based Cultural Practices: Tools for Clinicians to Promote Psychological Well-Being advances our knowledge about the critical role of Black culture in contributing to the psychological well-being and resilience for people of African descent. This book examines how Black racial identity, racial socialization, coping with racism, communalism, and cultural spirituality serve as central positive social and psychological frameworks for Black people and communities. A key emphasis is placed on considering Black cultural values and practices as strength-based strategies in the provision of mental health care, training guidelines for mental health professionals, and emerging issues for mental health policy and services for Black communities. One of the significant strengths of this work involves its interdisciplinary frameworks and evidence-based practice that examine mental disparities and inequalities experienced by Black people in their everyday lives. The book aims to guide mental health practitioners and educators in supporting clients in addressing racism and developing effective coping strategies that align with Black cultural beliefs and practices to promote optimal psychological well-being. This scholarly work offers a superb exploration of culturally grounded prevention strategies that provide a more holistic understanding of Black communities.

– **Leo Wilton, Ph.D., MPH,** *professor, State University of New York at Binghamton, Department of Human Development*

Black psychology experts Robert T. Carter, Alex L. Pieterse, and Jessica M. Forsyth deliver a masterful, deeply researched, and timely exploration of the psychological well-being of Black American clients. Drawing from decades of groundbreaking work, this remarkable volume offers a rare and comprehensive look at the historical, cultural, and structural forces that shape Black American mental health, from the era before slavery to the present day. While acknowledging the profound impact of racial oppression, the authors emphasize the enduring strengths of Black culture—family, spirituality, positive racial identity, and communalism—as central to resilience and healing. This book not only presents rigorous, evidence-based insights but also provides actionable resources for practitioners, policymakers, and scholars alike. A must-read for anyone committed to understanding and promoting the mental health and thriving of Black Americans.

– **Helen A. Neville,** *professor of Educational Psychology and African American Studies, past-president at the Society of Counseling Psychology (APA, Division 17), and past-president at the Society for the Psychological Study of Culture, Ethnicity and Race (APA, Division 45), 2019*

Black Americans' Strengths-Based Cultural Practices

Tools for Clinicians to Promote Psychological Well-Being

Robert T. Carter, Alex L. Pieterse and Jessica M. Forsyth

Routledge
Taylor & Francis Group

NEW YORK AND LONDON

Designed cover image: cienpies © Getty Images

First published 2025
by Routledge
605 Third Avenue, New York, NY 10158

and by Routledge
4 Park Square, Milton Park, Abingdon, Oxon, OX14 4RN

Routledge is an imprint of the Taylor & Francis Group, an informa business

ISBN: 978-0-367-34814-4 (hbk)
ISBN: 978-0-367-34816-8 (pbk)
ISBN: 978-1-003-08322-1 (ebk)

DOI: 10.4324/9781003083221

Typeset in Times New Roman
by codeMantra

08.13.24
We dedicate this book to Black Americans who continue to survive and thrive under the weight of endemic racism within the United States.

Contents

Acknowledgment

We would like to acknowledge Dr. Veronica Johnson for her empirical examinations of Black Cultural Strengths which served as the inspiration for this volume.

Introduction and Overview

The enslavement of Blacks in the North American colonies has left a lasting system of racial oppression in the United States (Feagin, 2006). People of African descent (i.e., Black Americans) have been subjected to harsh treatment and racial oppression in all aspects of life in the United States (Williams & Mohammed, 2013), in part because Blacks were thought to be inferior or culturally deficient, and therefore any shared practices among them were considered to be byproducts of their treatment by and interactions with Whites. Over the course of at least a century, most people, irrespective of race, denied the fact that Africans and their descendants had a past or a distinct culture:

> For most of their stay in ... North America, people of African descent have seen their homeland portrayed as a primitive society in an arrested state of development and themselves as a congenitally backward people. In, 1835, the governor of South Carolina asserted what would become conventional wisdom for most white Americans during the century that followed. "The African negro is destined by Providence to occupy a condition of servile dependency ... it is marked on the face, stamped on the skin, and evinced by intellectual inferiority and natural improvidence of the race...They are in all respects – physical, moral, and political – inferior to millions of the human race ... [and] are doomed to this hopeless condition by the very qualities which unfit them for a better life."
>
> (Berlin, 2010, p. 3)

From a mental health perspective, similar notions have been promulgated. The authors of the well-received and popular book *The Mark of Oppression* about Blacks Americans, mental health noted that the Black personality arose from the stigma of their condition in America. The authors' idea was that oppression created an unerasable mark that damaged the psyche of Blacks. They stated that "there is not one personality trait of the Negro the source of which cannot be traced to the difficult living conditions. There is no exception to this rule. The final result is a wretched internal life" (Kardiner & Ovesey, 1951, p. 3).

DOI: 10.4324/9781003083221-1

These authors believed that Blacks had no basis for a healthy sense of self nor any foundation for their culture other than to mimic Whites. They argued that Blacks must adapt to the White culture but inherently fail to do so, since for Kardiner and Ovesey Blacks exhibited self-contempt. However, other psychologists pointed to the variations in responses that Blacks had available to them. Clark (1965) states:

> Human beings who are forced to live under ghetto conditions and whose daily experiences tells them that almost nowhere in society are they respected and granted the ordinary dignity and courtesy accorded others will as a matter of course (…) begin to doubt their worth. But the threat to self-esteem does not have uniform consequences. Some individuals may be overwhelmed. Others become aware of the source of the threat, develop appropriate anger at the injustices they suffer and focus their energies on the struggle against oppression. Still others may show a mixture of healthy and unhealthy responses which manifest differently in different situations.
>
> (pp. 63–64)

Therefore it is possible that Black Americans were able to adapt to their situation in a range of ways, suggesting that there may be a set of complex reactions and responses that were not fully identified or understood. In terms of culture, Carter (1995) observes that Black culture was grounded in beliefs in cooperative group relations, sharing a present time sense, harmony with nature or spirituality, and that the Black family was organized in terms of flexible roles and extended networks and strong kinship (blood- and non-blood-based) bonds, with a high value placed on religion, education, and work. There were/are also clear and distinct language forms and behavioral preferences, that were shared by many but not all, thus again emphasizing the wide range of variation within the racial group and culture or the multidimensional nature of Black cultural practices. Most scholars and researchers that focus on Black Americans document their low levels of social and political participation in U.S. society, their poor physical and mental health, their low levels of educational achievement, and their high levels of criminal justice involvement (Griffith, Jones, & Stewart, 2019), as well as the myriad social-psychological issues and challenges they experience as a consequence of their social status:

> the poorer health of (…) racial minority populations is evident in higher rates of mortality, earlier onset of disease, greater severity and progression of disease, and higher levels of comorbidity and impairment. In addition, disadvantaged racial populations tend to have both lower levels of access to medical care and to receive care that is poorer in quality. In U.S. data, these patterns tend to be evident for African Americans (or Blacks).
>
> (Williams & Mohammed, 2013, p. 1153)

The health and social disparities are persistent over time and exist at all levels of income and education (Williams, 2012). But at the same time, Blacks have also shown personal and cultural strengths, and engage in behaviors that counter the various forms of racial oppression, and hold values that contribute to their survival both as individuals and as a racial group.

Social scientists and historians have identified cultural values that originated in African communities and remain present in Black American people, families, and communities (Belgrave & Allison, 2019). Scholars have argued that there needs to be a shift from perspectives of Black culture as deficient to one that recognizes its strengths (Marshall, Thorpe, & Szanton, 2017). Even further, contemporary work has identified aspects of Black culture that both enabled Blacks to survive constant racial oppression in the United States, and maintain for many psychosocial health. The current work documents how this process has occurred, presents evidence of strength-based aspects of Black American culture, and shows how these cultural strengths can be used in mental health treatment and interventions.

It is important to note that we use the term Black American to refer to all people of African descent who reside in the United States. We prefer the term Black American rather than African American in recognition of the fact that any person who has immigrated to the United States from the continent of Africa, regardless of race, may identify as African American, while Black refers to the racial group that descends from Africa. We recognize the significant historical and current contributions of Black people who immigrated from Africa and the Caribbean to Black American culture across generations. In this book we describe primarily the culture that has emerged over centuries out of the experiences of Black people of African descent who experienced the middle passage arriving on North American shores, and survived slavery and racialized terror in the United States.

Culture is defined as a system of meaning with values, norms, behaviors, language, and history that is passed from one generation to the next through socialization and participation in the group's families, organizations, and traditions (Stewart & Bennett, 2011). This includes familial roles, communication patterns, affective styles, and beliefs about how to function best while being subjected to racial oppression and held as property. We argue that some cultural practices of their African ancestors have come to be practices and traditions of Blacks in America (Nobles, 2013). Some of these practices appear to have a positive influence on Black Americans' psychological and social functioning (Jagers & Mock, 1993). We argue, as do others, that Black Americans have retained African cultural beliefs and practices. These African cultural beliefs and practices are reflected in forms of self-expression, such as one's psychological orientation to their racial group membership or racial identity, social and family relationships (e.g., communalism, racial socialization), and their connection to nature and their ancestors which is reflected in and has been defined as "cultural spirituality." An important element of Black culture, these practices are also sources of Black cultural strength, which allows for continued growth and progression for many Black Americans. Each aspect of Black culture is multi-dimensional and as such some parts contribute to well-being more than others.

For instance, Black people have had and continue to have a sense of group connection, as Africans and as captives brought to the new world, and currently as people put upon due to their race. Berlin (2010) describes it this way:

> Much of the collective conscious of black people in mainland North America and then the United States – the belief of individual men and women that their fate was linked to that of the group – has long been articulated through a common history, indeed a particular history; centuries of enslavement, freedom in the course of Civil War, a great promise made amid the political turmoil of Reconstruction and a promise broken, followed by disfranchisement, segregation, and finally the long struggle for equality capped by a speech on the steps of the Lincoln Memorial, a celebration in the Oval Office, a heart-stopping moment on the balcony of a Memphis motel, and the euphoria of the elevation of a black man to the American presidency.
>
> (p. 2)

Thus, communalism or a group-oriented cultural value is evident as having been present over the sweep of time and is still present today. We contend that there are at least five cultural practices that can be identified that contribute to Black cultural beliefs and practices that promote psychosocial well-being. These include the belief in cultural spirituality, in communalism, in racial socialization (i.e., passing on how to deal with racism and racism-related coping), racial identity (i.e., psychological orientation to one's racial group membership), and racism-related coping. We argue that some of these cultural practices and beliefs evolved due to the circumstances associated with American racism directed at Black Americans and others are cultural values passed down from their African ancestors.

We argue that it is essential that mental health professionals, and in fact all people and professionals who work with Black people, grasp these critical aspects of Black culture. It is imperative that these cultural practices and beliefs, rather than social and cultural deficits, be comprehended to effectively deliver care and mental health treatment. It is well established that Black people in the United States have been subjected to centuries of racial oppression of different forms. What is less well established are what the people who were racially oppressed did to survive and what cultural patterns, beliefs, and values they possess.

We contend that Black people held on to beliefs and values that reflected their ancestors, that they altered them to fit their circumstances, and that they contributed to their survival. We show how this occurred and present evidence to support the position that cultural practices contribute to the psychosocial health of Black Americans.

We see that Africans and their decedents were isolated in their communities and were/are able to pass on lessons to their offspring about the value of community, about the strength of spirit, the wisdom of their ancestors, and about how to deal with racial oppression. This is not to say that there was/is not variation among Black Americans regarding these beliefs and practices. There are variations in how best to cope and survive, or even to decide if survival was/is warranted. Blacks did find ways to reclaim portions of their lives little by little.

> slaves established the right to control a portion of their lives. When permitted to do so, they used small grants of time to cultivate gardens, hunt, and fish; raise poultry, pigs and cattle; make baskets, weave clothes, and practice other handicrafts (Berlin, Favreau, & Miller, 1998, p. xxxvi). They also lobbied and [were] granted the ability to deliver and name their offspring, who more often than not, were named after their parents. In the 1800's the center of slave life was the family which was enmeshed in a dense network of kin relationships (Berlin et al., 1998, p. xxxviii). It was typical that they would marry and maintain long-term relationships. A web of distinctive customs and beliefs sustained those lifelong relationships and separated the family life of African American slaves from that of other Southerners.
>
> (Berlin et al., 1998, p. xxxviii)

In addition, their religion also stood apart from that of the slaveowners:

> Scarcely less important than the family was the slaves' religion…the dense network of kinship that knit together the slave communities of the 17th and 18th centuries, the religion of the quarter emerged…the slaves' religious beliefs and practices nevertheless stood apart.
>
> (Berlin et al., 1998, pp. xxxix–xii)

What was passed on were how to cope with racism, the value of family, however defined the power of the spirits of the ancestors, and how to believe in one's own people (racial identity). The transmission of the essential messages and ways of living were critical to the group's survival and were/are aspects of Black cultural practices that contribute(d) to the people's psychosocial well-being.

We draw on some contemporary constructs to illustrate some aspects of Black cultural practices and beliefs that operate today and account for Blacks' psychosocial health. We think elements of racial identity, racial socialization, racism-related coping, cultural spirituality, and communalism capture some parts of the essential constellation of cultural values present today.

Black Cultural Values: An Overview

Several theories of racial identity have been posited: Cross' Model of Black Nigrescence (Cross, 1991; Vandiver, Fhagen, Cokley, Cross, & Worrell, 2001); Sellers, Smith, Shelton, Rowley, and Chavous, (1998) Multidimensional model of Black identity, and Helms' (1990) theory of Black Racial Identity Statuses. Cross (1991) and Vandiver et al. (2001) updated and modified to include the Cross Racial Identity Scale (CRIS) in their model of Nigrescence, in which a Black person moved through five stages from Pre-encounter, where a person's worldview is Euro-American, to Internalization, where a person resolves conflict between previous Euro-American worldview to confidence in ones self as a Black person. At each stage or schema, the person experiences changes in worldview and affect.

Sellers and colleagues' (1998) multidimensional theory of racial identity includes the qualitative aspects of being Black American and the properties of racial and ethnic identity that comprise four dimensions: salience, centrality, regard, and ideology. Salience refers to how relevant an individual's race is to their self-concept at any given time. It is thought to be person and situation specific. Centrality is a person's normative perception of racial self and is believed to remain relatively constant. Regard is feelings of negativity or positivity associated with being Black. It consists of both public (i.e., how one believes others view Blacks) and private (i.e., how one feels about Blacks) domains. Ideology refers to one's beliefs and opinions about how Blacks should interact and be in society. These dimensions represent manifestations of racial identity. Helms (1990) proposed a stage, then status model of Black racial identity, where all statuses exist together and some have more influence than others. She proposed that with each racial identity status came a new cognitive, emotional, and behavioral template which a person used to organize racial information about themselves and others. Further, she posited that maturation accompanied movement from one status to another (Helms, 1990). These statuses ranged from Pre-Encounter, rejections of one's own racial group, to Internalization, acceptance and investment in one's race and culture.

From theory, measures have been developed to assess Black racial identity (Vandiver, Cross, Worrell, & Fhagen-Smith, 2002; Parham & Helms, 1981). Despite theoretical differences in Black racial identity theories, empirical findings suggest some consistency in understanding how Black people vary in their thinking, affect, and behavior as a result of their membership in the racial group. And yet, few studies to date have examined two or more measures of Black racial identity simultaneously. Further, while many schemas, statuses, or dimensions exist to understand Black racial identity, only some of them have been positively associated with psychological health.

Investigators have found that psychosocial well-being was associated with racial identity that reflected Black pride and investment in Black culture, in addition to tolerance for other racial groups (Sellers, Copeland-Linder, Martin, & Lewis, 2006; Heads & Castillo, 2014). For instance, scholars have reported that Internalization status attitudes, high centrality, and high private regard were positively related to psychological well-being (Sellers et al., 2006). Psychological health reflects a general sense of wellness rather than specific psychological symptoms (e.g., positive affect, self-esteem). Measures used to assess psychological health (e.g. psychological well-being, life satisfaction) have been negatively associated with the presence of affective disorders, and psychological distress (Ryff & Keyes, 1995). However, to fully understand how one develops a health-promoting racial identity orientation, we must understand how it is transferred from person to person and from generation to generation. This process is best described as *racial socialization* (Belgrave & Allison, 2019).

Racial Socialization

Racial socialization involves the transmission of direct and indirect messages about race, being aware of oppression, and having racial-cultural pride typically transmitted by parents, family, and members of the community (Barr & Neville, 2014; Lesane-Brown, 2006). Researchers have found that racial socialization messages are intertwined with racial identity status attitudes, presenting a cyclical pattern between the two. Studies show that parental racial identity influences the degree to which parents talk or care about race, what types of racial messages they transmit, and the resulting racial identities of recipients (Tang, McLloyd, & Hallman, 2016; Cooper, Smalls-Glover, Metzger, & Griffin, 2015).

Studies show that racial socialization occurs more frequently when the receiver has high Internalization status attitudes and racial pride (Thomas & Speight, 1999; Thomas, Speight, & Witherspoon, 2010). Further, higher salience and centrality, private regard, and Internalization attitudes are positively related to transmitting messages of racial pride, cultural socialization, and preparation for bias (Demo & Hughes, 1990). These messages are then positively related to better psychological and social functioning including better college adjustment and academic achievement, increased family and peer self-esteem, increased anger management, and decreased behavioral problems (Anglin & Wade, 2007; Scott, 2003). Therefore, mature Black racial identity is enhanced when racial socialization messages are received that prepare the person for racial bias and that promote racial pride.

Despite multiple investigations into the linkages between racial identity and racial socialization, very few researchers have added other constructs into these queries. In broadening the breadth of cultural values in our investigation, we examined constructs that were usually studied in isolation, not as interdependent aspects of Black culture (i.e., cultural spirituality, racism-related coping; Johnson & Carter, 2020). We contend these are related to socialization and racial identity, and are aspects of Black cultural practices which promote psychological well-being in the face of racial oppression. Key elements of racial socialization and racial identity are communalism and spirituality, which bind the group together.

Communalism and Cultural Spirituality

As one can imagine, Black cultural values could have only been maintained in a context that placed value on the interconnectedness of Black Americans. This quality of Black American culture is defined as communalism, the overarching belief that the success of the Black individual and the Black group are inseparable (Boykin, Jagers, Ellison, & Albury, 1997). The belief is expressed in Black cultural customs such as preserving extended family systems (defined broadly, not just by blood), and the practice of shared child-rearing beyond family members. Scholars have found communalism to be positively related to positive emotions and a sense of purpose (Gooden, 2013; Abdou et al., 2010). Communalism is also manifested in the achievements of Blacks that occurs in cooperative settings, such as the Black church. And while the influence of the Black church on the social and economic survival of the Black community is significant (Blank, Mahmood, Fox, & Guterbock, 2002), there are other cultural ties that bind Black Americans (Mattis & Jagers, 2001).

Often conflated with religiosity, Jagers and Smith (1996) contend that Black American spirituality is a cultural value which encompasses a sense of connection with one's ancestors and contains the idea that things in nature have a life force that directs life events. This value exists in tandem or separate from one's religious practices. Spirituality, as a cultural belief, has been found to be positively associated with quality of life and optimism (Underwood & Teresi, 2002) and negatively associated with depression and posttraumatic stress disorder (Watlington & Murphy, 2006). Africultural spirituality has been found to be positively associated with both psychological well-being and life satisfaction (Reed & Neville, 2014). Some scholars have recognized spirituality as an important aspect of racial socialization (Stevenson, 1998; Anglin & Wade, 2007). Others believe spirituality is an important part of coping with racism (Forsyth & Carter, 2014). Therefore, spirituality appears to be an important cultural factor that may converge with other values such as racial identity and communalism.

Along with evidence of their positive impact on psychosocial functioning, both communalism and cultural spirituality have been positively associated with mature Black racial identity and other African cultural values. Specifically, Brown et al. (2013) found positive correlations between communalism and mature Black racial identity status attitudes. These authors also found communalism to be predictive of empathy, when combined with spirituality and affect. Cultural spirituality has been explored less often than other Black cultural values; however, it has been associated with a communalistic orientation (Jagers et al., 1997), along with mature racial identity development. We suspect that group behavior and spiritual beliefs are also related to how Blacks handled racism and are implicated in their unique manner of coping. We think the way that Black Americans cope is not generic but particular to their lived experiences with racism. While they may use methods to deal with general life stressors, racism demanded its own set of ways to adapt.

Racism-Related Coping

As posited, Black cultural values emerged and were maintained not because of Black Americans' contact with Whites, but rather despite it. However, Blacks had to develop ways to cope with the oppression they faced. Scholars have found seeking social support and engaging in confrontation and/or anger expression mitigated the negative impact of racism. Collective (i.e., group-centered activities) and spiritual coping styles were also positively associated with private regard (Belgrave & Allison, 2019). Forsyth and Carter (2014), using the only known measure of coping specific to racism for Blacks, found four distinct cluster groups for racial identity status attitudes and racism-related coping strategies demonstrating the interrelatedness of these two constructs. These authors found that confrontation, followed by empowered action, spiritual coping, and constrained resistance coping tactics were associated with mature Black racial identity (e.g., Internalization status attitudes). Further, these strategies coupled with mature racial identity (i.e., Internalization status attitudes) were associated with decreased depression, anxiety, hostility, somatization, and interpersonal sensitivity. Their findings demonstrate the interrelatedness of racism-related coping within the larger constellation of Black cultural practices, particularly those that promote psychological health.

Blacks have not only survived but also thrived through centuries of social and economic oppression in the United States. Scholars and researchers in the social sciences have not, in general, sought to understand the cultural practices of Black Americans in lieu of their harsh reality in the United States. (Boykin et al., 1997; Mattis & Jagers, 2001; Jagers & Smith, 1996; Helms, 1990; Gutman, 1976). There is evidence that aspects of racial identity, racial socialization, communalism, cultural spirituality, and racism-related coping have protective properties that have contributed to Black survival. Most of the evidence has resulted from analysis of these cultural values apart from one another with only a few instances of researchers attempting to understand how they might intersect.

The central aim of this book is to present the relationships between these aspects of Black culture, with the goal of further understanding the factors that have enabled survival and progress for Blacks in the United States. The positive and affirming components of Black racial identity, racial socialization, and racism-related coping, along with communalism and cultural spirituality have been associated with positive social and psychological outcomes in Blacks.

We think that the cultural values of Blacks should be promoted and reinforced for Black American clients in therapy. Clients may be facing pressures to conform to White cultural values and norms in a variety of settings (e.g., academic institutions, the workplace) and clinicians should consider ways in which the person may regain their sense of communalism, even within an institution which does not reflect their own cultural values. A therapist may suggest the person consider joining Black organizations or a historically Black religious organization.

Clinicians may serve the role of additional racial socializers and suggest racism-related coping strategies that have been empirically proven to be effective. For instance, a clinician may find that a client relies heavily on cognitive racism-related coping. The clinician may suggest that the client "get out of their head" and confront the parties involved. Further, a clinician can rely on their knowledge of the client's spirituality to suggest they also utilize spiritual coping strategies as well (e.g., praying). Even if the individual does not regularly engage in formalized religious practices, clinicians should be aware they may endorse high levels of spiritual coping.

Future research would be enhanced by examining the role of additional Black cultural factors in relation to the psychosocial health of Black Americans. For example, Grills and Longshore (1996) posited other Africultural values (e.g., cooperative economics, self-determination) that may be important to understand in the examination of Black cultural and psychosocial health. Additionally, it will be important to determine if there is a benefit of Black cultural constructs over and above culturally non-specific factors such as degree of social support, cognitive ability, and family system functioning as others have done. We feel that these ideas about positive Black cultural behavior and research evidence that supports it are novel and important findings in the areas of cultural values for Black Americans. Black cultural values are interdependent and should be examined as a complex set of factors, rather than as separate variables that are disconnected. Clinicians should be aware of the ways in which cultural values interact to impact the psychological functioning and overall life satisfaction of Black Americans and their clients. Specifically, we show evidence for the relationships of these cultural beliefs and practices and we provide recommendations for working from a Black cultural strengths-based approach to mental health interventions with Black clients.

Outline of the Book

The book is organized into 12 chapters. In Chapter 1, we present the social status of Black America, historically and presently, and include discussions of the concepts of race and racism and the various justifications used to oppress Black Americans. In Chapter 2, we focus on the mental health of Black Americans. It was believed for many centuries that Blacks suffered from poor mental health and lacked any semblance of distinct culture. As such we provide estimations about how many Black Americans appear to be suffering with psychological symptoms (e.g., depression), as well as literature on their well-being. Chapter 3 introduces the debate about Black American culture and its implications for Black Americans' mental health. Chapter 4 highlights and documents aspects of Black American culture, the manner in which Black American culture was shaped by racial oppression, and introduces the concept of racial identity. Chapter 5 continues the focus on the transmission of Black American culture through the process of racial socialization, that is, ways in which cultural values and practices are learned and taught among Black Americans. Chapter 6 introduces the role of communalism as a cultural value among Black Americans. It documents the cultural origins of communalism and the role collectivism plays within Black American culture. In Chapter 7, we review dimensions of the various Black cultural beliefs associated with spirituality and how spirituality as a cultural value has played an important role in racism-related coping among Black Americans. Chapter 8 provides a review of the research literature that outlines the clinical relevance and benefit of Black American cultural practices. Chapter 9 addresses the application of Black American cultural strengths within counseling and psychotherapy. Chapter 10 presents a clinical case to illustrate the application of Black American cultural strengths in the process of counseling and psychotherapy. Chapter 11 discusses the training of psychological practitioners and outlines approaches to incorporate Black American cultural strengths. We conclude with Chapter 12 in which we provide suggestions for future directions for mental health policy, practice, and research as it pertains to the Black American population.

References

Abdou, C. M., Dunkel Schetter, C., Campos, B., Hilmert, C. J., Dominguez, T. P., Hobel, C. J., Glynn, L. M., & Sandman, C. (2010). Communalism predicts prenatal affect, stress, and physiology better than ethnicity and socioeconomic status. *Cultural Diversity & Ethnic Minority Psychology, 16*(3), 395–403. https://doi.org/10.1037/a0019808

Anglin, D. M., & Wade, J. C. (2007). Racial socialization, racial identity, and Black students' adjustment to college. *Cultural Diversity and Ethnic Minority Psychology, 13*(3), 207–215. doi: 10.1037/1099-9809.13.3.207

Barr, S. C., & Neville, H. A. (2014). Racial socialization, color-blind racial ideology, and mental health among Black college students: An examination of an ecological model. *Journal of Black Psychology, 40*(2), 138–165. doi: 10.1177/0095798412475084.

Belgrave, F. Z., & Allison, K. W., (2019). *African American psychology: From Africa to America* (4th ed.). Thousand Oaks, CA: Sage.

Berlin, I. (2010). *The making of African America: The four great migrations*. London: Penguin Group.

Berlin, I., Favreau, M., & Miller, S. F. (1998). *Remembering slavery*. New York, NY: The New Press.

Blank, M. B., Mahmood, M., Fox, J. C., & Guterbock, T. (2002). Alternative mental health services: The role of the Black church in the South. *American Journal of Public Health, 92*(1), 1668–1672. doi: 10.2105/AJPH.92.10.1668.

Brown, C. L., Love, K. M., Tyler, K. M., Garriot, P. O., Thomas, D., & Roan-Belle, C. (2013). Parental attachment, family communalism, and racial identity among African American college students. *Journal of Multicultural Counseling and Development, 41*(2), 108–122. doi: 10.1002/j.2161-1912.2013.00031.x.

Carter, R. T. (1995). *The influence of race and racial identity in the psychotherapy process: Toward a racially inclusive model.* New York, NY: Wiley.

Clark, K. B. (1965). *Dark ghetto.* New York, NY: Harper & Row.

Cooper, S. M., Smalls-Glover, C., Metzger, I., & Griffin, C. (2015). African American fathers' racial socialization patterns: Associations with racial identity beliefs and discrimination experiences. *Family Relations, 64*(1), 278–290. doi: 10.1111/fare.12115.

Cross, W. E., Jr. (1991). *Shades of Black: Diversity in African American identity.* Philadelphia, PA: Temple University Press.

Demo, D. H., & Hughes, M. (1990). Socialization and racial identity among Black Americans. *Social Psychology Quarterly, 53*(1), 364–374. doi: 10.2307/2786741.

Feagin, J. R. (2006). *Systemic racism.* New York, NY: Routledge.

Forsyth, J. M., & Carter, R. T. (2014). Development and preliminary validation of the Racism- Related Coping Scale. *Psychological Trauma: Theory, Research, Practice, and Policy, 6*(6), 632–643.

Gooden, A. S. (2013). *Individual and community factors associated with thriving among African American adolescents in the context of stressors.* Chicago, IL: DePaul University.

Griffith, E. E. H., Jones, B. E., & Stewart, A. J. (2019). *Black mental health.* Washington, DC: American Psychiatric Association.

Grills, L., & Longshore, D. (1996). Africentrism: Psychometric analyses of a self-report measure. *Journal of Black Psychology, 22*(1), 86–106. doi: 10.1177/00957984960221007.

Gutman, H. G. (1976). *The Black family in slavery and freedom, 1750–1925* (p. 385). New York, NY: Blackwell.

Heads, A. M., & Castillo, L. G. (2014). Perfectionism and racial identity as predictors of life satisfaction in African American female college students. *Interamerican Journal of Psychology, 48*(3), 269–275.

Helms, J. E. (1990). *Black and White racial identity: Theory, research, and practice.* New York, NY: Greenwood Press.

Jagers, R. J., & Mock, L. O. (1993). Culture and social outcomes among inner-city African-American children: An Afro-graphic exploration *Journal of Black Psychology, 19*(4), 391–405.

Jagers, R. J., & Mock, L. O. (1995). The Communalism Scale and collectivistic-individualistic tendencies: some preliminary findings. *Journal of Black Psychology, 21*(2), 153–167.

Jagers, R. J., & Smith, P. (1996). Further examination of the Spirituality Scale. *Journal of Black Psychology, 22*(4), 429–442.

Jagers, R. J., Smith, P., Mock, L. O., & Dill, E. (1997). An Afrocultural social ethos: Component orientations and some social implications. *Journal of Black Psychology, 23*(4), 328–343.

Johnson, V., & Carter, R. T. (2020) Black cultural strengths and psychological well-being: An empirical analysis with Black American adults *Journal of Black Psychology*, *46*(1), 55–89.

Kardiner, A., & Ovesey, L. (1951). *The mark of oppression.* New York, NY.: Norton.

Lesane-Brown, C. L. (2006). A review of race socialization within Black families. *Developmental Review*, *26*(4), 400–426.

Marshall, G. L., Thorpe, R. J., & Szanton, S. L. (2017). Material hardship and self-rated mental health among older Black Americans in the National Survey of American Life. *Health and Social Work*, *42*(2), 87–94. doi: 10.1093/hsw/hlx008.

Mattis, J. S., & Jagers, R. J. (2001). A relational framework for the study of religiosity and spirituality in the lives of African Americans. *Journal of Community Psychology*, *29*(5), 519–539. doi: 10.1002/jcop.1034.

Nobles, W. W. (2013). The fundamental task and challenge of Black psychology. *Journal of Black Psychology*, *39(3)*, 292–299.

Parham, T. A., & Helms, J. E. (1981). The influence of Black students' racial identity attitudes on preferences for counselor's race. *Journal of Counseling Psychology*, *28*(3), 250–257.

Reed, T. D., & Neville, H. A. (2014). The influence of religiosity and spirituality on psychological well-being among Black women. *Journal of Black Psychology*, *40*(4), 384–401. doi: 10.1177/0095798413490956.

Ryff, C. D., & Keyes, C. L. M. (1995). The structure of psychological well-being revisited. *Journal of Personality and Social Psychology*, 69, 719–727. doi: 10.1037/0022-3514.69.4.719.

Scott, L. J. (2003). The relation of racial identity and racial socialization to coping with discrimination among African American adolescents. *Journal of Black Studies*, *33*(4), 520–538. doi: 10.1177/0021934702250035.

Sellers, R. M., Copeland-Linder, N., Martin, P. P., & Lewis, R. L. (2006). Racial identity matters: The relationship between racial discrimination and psychological functioning in African American adolescents. *Journal of Research on Adolescence*, *16*(2), 187–216. doi: 10.1111/j.1532-7795.2006.00128.x.

Sellers, R. M., Smith, M. A., Shelton, J. N., Rowley, S. A. J., & Chavous, T. M. (1998). Multidimensional model of racial identity: A reconceptualization of African American racial identity. *Personality and Social Psychology Review*, *2*(1), 18–38.

Stevenson, H. C. (1998). Theoretical considerations in measuring racial identity and socialization: Extending the self-further. In R. Jones (Ed.), *African American identity development: Theory, research, and intervention* (pp. 227–263). Hampton, VA: Cobb & Henry.

Stewart, E. C., & Bennett M. J. (2011). *American cultural patterns: A cross-cultural perspective*. Hachette: Nicholas Brealey.

Tang, S., McLoyd, V. C., & Hallman, S. K. (2016). Racial socialization, racial identity, and academic attitudes among African American adolescents: Examining the moderating influence of parent–adolescent communication. *Journal of Youth and Adolescence, 45*(1), 1141–1155. doi: 10.1007/s10964-015-0351-8.

Thomas, A. J., & Speight, S. L. (1999). Racial identity and racial socialization attitudes of African American parents. *Journal of Black Psychology*, *25*(2), 152–170.

Thomas, A. J., Speight, S. L., & Witherspoon, K. (2010). Racial socialization, racial identity, and race-related stress of African American parents. *Family Journal, 18*(4), 407–412. doi: 10.1177/1066480710372913.

Underwood, L. G., & Teresi, J. A. (2002). The daily spiritual experience scale. *Annals of Behavioral Medicine, 24*(1), 1, 22–33. doi: 10.1037/t01587-000.

Vandiver, B. J., Fhagen, P. E., Cokley, K. O., Cross, W. E., & Worrell, F. C. (2001). Cross's Nigrescence model: From theory to scale to theory. *Journal of Multicultural Counseling and Development, 29*(3), 174–200. doi: 10.1002/j2161-1912.2001.tb00561x.

Vandiver, B., J., Cross, W. E., Worrell, F. C., & Fhagen-Smith, P. E. (2002). Validating the cross racial identity scale. *Journal of Counseling Psychology, 49*(1), 71–85.

Watlington, C. G., & Murphy, C. M. (2006) The roles of religion and spirituality among African American survivors of domestic violence. *Journal of Clinical Psychology, 62*(1), 837–857. doi: 10.1002/jclp.20268.

Williams, D. R. (2012). Miles to go before we sleep: Racial inequities in health. *Journal of Health and Social Behavior, 53*(3), 279–295.

Williams, D. R., & Mohammed, S. A. (2013). Racism and health I: Pathways and scientific evidence. *American Behavioral Scientist, 57*(8), 1152–1173. doi: 10.1177/0002764213487340.

Chapter 1

The State of Black America

The history of the United States captures the enduring and powerful narrative of race. Although the colonial encounter that began with the Jamestown settlement in 1607 had the colonists initially viewing Native Americans as positive, it quickly devolved into Natives being viewed as not better than animals (Horsman, 1982). Here we have the American version of Whiteness with all things of European origin, be it people, ideas, culture etc., viewed as normative, setting the standard by which all others would be judged (Fredrickson, 1988). In turn, the normative began to be equated with superiority, laying the seeds of White supremacy that would later account for the racialized nature of American society. It is within this context that America began to be populated by individuals of African descent, primarily through forced relocation which was the hallmark or bedrock of the institution of Slavery (Smedley, 2018). As such, what initially began as a "suspicion" of inferiority evolved to be a social-scientific construct, which, at both an ideological and empirical level, branded Africans and African-descended individuals as less than human. The manner by which Africans were introduced into the Americas through the vehicle of slavery has significantly shaped Black American involvement in society across many domains, including wealth accumulation, educational access and attainment, employment and income, civic engagement, mass incarceration, access to health care, and health status (Feagin, 2006).

Given the enduring practice of inequality to which Black Americans have been subjected, and the ideological perceptions that have contributed to their dehumanization, we believe that there are cultural patterns which are particularly relevant in an understanding of the psychological processes that have allowed Black Americans to survive and, in some cases, even thrive (Span, 2015; Walters, 2012; Wilkins, Whiting, Watson, Russon, & Moncrief, 2013). As such, in this chapter, we review the status of Black America in regard to a number of social indicators, including wealth, education, criminal justice, and health. We provide a socio-historical context to understand the current status, and focus on important historical markers that have influenced and framed the current State of Black America.

DOI: 10.4324/9781003083221-2

Black American Participation in Society

The history of Black American involvement in American society is varied based on migration status, genealogy including ancestry tracing back to either enslaved or free Blacks, geographical location within the United States, and social class status (Copeland, 2013; Johnson, Michael, & Roark, 1984; Litwack, 1961; Green, 1981; Ogbu, 2004). Access to education, participation in the political system, accumulation of wealth, and access to effective healthcare have all been influenced by the variations in Black Americans' social location, however there is one constant that has affected all Black Americans irrespective of social location – the enduring presence of anti-Black racism. Consider the following illustration. While in a therapy session, a Black American elder relays the following information from their ancestry – on the maternal side, the genealogy goes back to enslaved Africans located in one of the southern states. Beyond that, their African homeland is unclear. After enduring slavery, emancipation, reconstruction, and Jim Crow, the family migrates north to the State of New York. The paternal side represents free Blacks living in a mid-Atlantic state. The paternal genealogy includes a level of social participation as educators and involvement in local/city politics. The family however is forced to relocate after a family member is murdered, property is seized, and no one is held accountable. The murder is viewed as racially motivated indicating that even for free Blacks, freedom has been illusory and full participation in society has been conditional. A review of the status of Black America provides an important reminder of the enduring nature and consequences of racial categorization and racism within the United States (Smedley, 2018).

As a measure of how well Black Americans are participating in society, the National Urban League's annual Equality Index uses nationally representative statistics to compare Black and White Americans on a variety of indices, including economics, health, education, social justice, and civic engagement and reflects the extent to which Black Americans experience full equality with White Americans in these areas (National Urban League, NUL, 2024). White Americans are chosen as the comparison group, given the history of unearned advantage in American society associated with assumptions of White supremacy and accompanying institutionalized racism (Embrick & Moore, 2000; Liu, Liu, & Shin, 2023). In 2024, the National Urban League found that Black Americans had 75.7% overall equity with White Americans, for an overall improvement of 2.8% since 2005. Black equity in 2024 was 65.6% in economics, 74.8% in education, 55.7% in social justice, 88.6% in health, and 95.6% in civic engagement. Together, these indices underscore the way Black Americans continue to experience inequality and inequity within American society (NUL, 2024). At the core of this continued inequity is structural racism or the interlocking set of historical and current laws, and institutional policies, procedures, and practices that perpetuate the legacy of racial inequity that began with slavery and persists to this day.

It has been widely understood that racism has had an indelible impact on the experience of Black populations within the United States. As noted by Bailey, Feldman, and Bassett (2021),

> Structural racism reaches back to the beginnings of U.S. history, stretches across its institutions and economy, and dwells within our culture. Its durability contributes to the perception that Black disadvantage is intrinsic, permanent, and therefore normal.
>
> (p. 771)

Historical aspects of anti-Black racism include the institution of slavery; the legalized discrimination, violence, and terrorism of Jim Crow; economic deprivation through the government policies of red-lining and racial residential segregation (Mensah et al., 2011); and the withholding of adequate health care as evidenced by the Tuskegee experiment (Bailey et al., 2021; Yearby, Clark, & Figueroa, 2022). Although the Civil Rights Acts of the 1960s made illegal some of the deprivations associated with historical racism, enforcement mechanisms have always been contested and minimized (Massey, 2011), and contemporary aspects of anti-Black racism continue to be evidenced within the United States. These include the surveillance and hyper-incarceration of Black Americans; racial disproportionality in the educational system where Black youth are more likely to experience the application of disciplinary procedures and less likely to graduate than their White counterparts; disproportionality in child welfare with Black children being over-represented in the child welfare system; higher rates of police violence directed at Black Americans; and disproportionately lower levels of Black representation among elected officials (Tate, 2004; Dettlaff & Boyd, 2024; Hines, King, & Ford, 2018; DeAngelis, 2024). To fully understand the current state of Black America, one must understand the socio-historical context, which created the circumstances experienced today.

A Brief History of the Fight for Civil Rights in the United States

The fight for racial justice and civil rights in the United States has been characterized by periods of Black resistance and civil rights progress, followed by periods of significant White backlash, and regression. Scholars frame each period of progress as a reconstruction (Glickman, 2020; Joseph, 2022), and each period of backlash is characterized by the evolution of the previous racial caste system and its associated forms of racialized social control (Alexander, 2020). The first and original Reconstruction period stretched from the Emancipation Proclamation in 1863, including: the end of the Civil War, abolition of slavery via the Thirteenth Amendment, and establishing of the Freedmen's Bureau in 1865; passage of the

Civil Rights Act of 1866, declaring Black Americans citizens entitled to civil rights; granting of citizenship to Blacks via the Fourteenth Amendment in 1868; granting Black men the right to vote via the Fifteenth Amendment in 1870; and passing of the Civil Rights Act of 1875 prohibiting discrimination in public places and facilities (Alexander, 2020; Equal Justice Initiative, EJI, 2017; Glickman, 2020; Hannah-Jones, 2024; Joseph, 2022). The first reconstruction period consisted of significant political and economic progress for Black Americans during which the majority of Black people voted, 2000 Black men from former confederate states held public office at all levels from local to federal, and interracial governments were established in a number of former Confederate states (Alexander, 2020; EJI, 2017; Joseph, 2022).

This period of progress was by no means peaceful and was persistently aggressively and violently contested, including: formation of the Ku Klux Klan in 1865; President Andrew Johnson's attempt to veto the Civil Rights Act of 1866; initial refusal of most former confederate states to ratify the Thirteenth Amendment; the 1883 Supreme Court decision declaring the Civil Rights Act of 1866 unconstitutional; campaigns of racial mob violence and suppression starting in 1866; and the withdrawal of federal troops from former confederate states in 1877, which had held back some of the political suppression and violence used in attempts to reestablish White supremacist rule. The final blow was the 1896 *Plessy v. Ferguson* decision wherein the Supreme Court held that racial segregation laws did not violate the Constitution (Alexander, 2020; EJI, 2017; Joseph, 2022), ushering in six decades of American apartheid constructed of "an entire code of race law and policies designed to segregate, marginalize, exclude and subjugate descendants of slavery across every realm of American life" (Hannah-Jones, 2024, n.p.).

The end of the first Reconstruction was followed by an unabated period of White backlash, including: the establishment of Black Codes leading to the mass arrest, conviction, and criminalization of Black people for newly devised crimes such as loitering and vagrancy; convict leasing laws starting in 1866, which permitted the sale of the forced labor of state and local prisoners to private interests and created a second slavery for criminalized Black people; and the rewriting of southern states' constitutions from 1885 to 1908 and establishing of Jim Crow laws, which created a racial caste system of subordination, disenfranchisement, segregation, and exclusion in all areas of life enforced through state and local laws, custom, and violence (Alexander, 2020; EJI, 2017).

During this period of White backlash vicious, brutal racial violence and terror escalated significantly and Jim Crow laws and customs were enforced through race riots, destruction of Black property, and massacres of Black people by angry White mobs, as well as a 70-year campaign of terror from 1877 to 1950 during which more than 4,400 Black Americans were tortured and murdered in racial terror lynchings (EJI, 2017). These lynchings, which were usually public spectacles including the torture, mutilation, dismemberment, and burning of victims, were a tool of racial terror and control. Though White people were also lynched, the ratio of Black to White victims of lynching had reached 17 to 1 by 1900 (EJI, 2017). Over the next 50 years, Black people would be systematically and legally excluded from sweeping public policy designed to establish economic benefits and social protections (Massey, 2011). Though Black people did benefit from the New Deal, the social programs of the New Deal were intentionally racialized, thereby accommodating racial segregation throughout the country, and perpetuating and enshrining the social and spatial isolation of Black people:

> Traditionally black occupations were not covered by the Social Security Act; labor legislation was written to allow segregated unions; states were delegated authority to exclude African Americans from receiving veterans benefits; and bureaucratic rules were written to prohibit black families and black neighborhoods from receiving Federal Housing Association and Veterans Administration loans.
>
> (Massey, 2011, p. 41)

The second period of reconstruction started with the 1948 desegregation of the Armed Forces and Supreme Court ruling against restrictive racial covenants in real estate (Massey, 2011), and the 1954 *Brown v. Board of Education* ruling finding that the racial segregation of public schools was unconstitutional (Alexander, 2020; Joseph, 2022; Massey, 2011). It shifted from legal to political strategies with the Civil Rights Act of 1957, which established the Commission on Civil Rights and the Civil Rights Division of the Department of Justice and authorized prosecution of those violating citizens' right to vote (Massey, 2011), and spanned the Civil Rights movement of the 1950s and 1960s through the enacting of the 1964 Civil Rights Act, which dismantled Jim Crow, the 1965 Voting Rights Act, and the 1968 Fair Housing Act (Joseph, 2022; Massey, 2011).

As with the backlash to Reconstruction, the progress of the Civil Rights movement was fought persistently and aggressively through excessive and repressive state force against protestors; "law and order" rhetoric employed primarily by segregationists fighting against the dismantling of Jim Crow; counterprotest, mob violence, bombings of Black churches and homes, assassinations, and lynchings, which continued into the late 1960s (Alexander, 2020). The formal political backlash to Civil Rights and the economic advances of Johnson's War on Poverty came in the form of the Southern Strategy, a conscious effort leveraged by conservative political strategists, initially during Nixon's 1968 presidential campaign, to galvanize the "silent majority" of working class White people by stoking intense anti-Black racial resentment, mostly subliminally via coded language focusing on antibusing and law and order (Alexander, 2020; Massey, 2011; Patterson et al., 2021).

The rhetoric of the Southern Strategy was leveraged effectively by Nixon and was arguably mastered by Ronald Reagan, who exploited racial resentment and hostility, while completely removing explicit references to race, and relying instead on colorblind, race neutral language to attack social welfare policies, and advance racialized social control via criminal justice (Alexander, 2020). Nixon declared a War on Crime in 1970, initiating the racialization of the criminal justice system, which was further cemented by Ronald Reagan's War on Drugs (Alexander, 2020; Bailey et al., 2021; Massey, 2011), through which:

> former state-level crimes were federalized and mandatory minimum sentences and strict sentencing guidelines were imposed. Particularly severe penalties were enacted for nonviolent drug offenses, most notably for the use and sale of crack cocaine… Criminal possession of a controlled substance became the principal legal instrument used by white authorities to regulate the behavior of poor African Americans, despite the fact that rates of drug use are much lower in the black community compared to the white… legal infractions were more likely to result in arrests; arrests were more likely to result in imprisonment; imprisonment was likely to involve a long sentence; and long sentences were less likely to be shortened by parole… By imposing harsher penalties on crimes committed by socially marginal groups, such as young black males, Congress effectively racialized the criminal justice system.
>
> (Massey, 2011, p. 46)

Simultaneous with the War on Drugs, over the period from 1980 to 2008, enforcement mechanisms for the Civil Rights legislation of the 1960s and 1970s were stripped, removing any ability of the federal government to uncover or sanction racial discrimination, and budgets for urban development, public housing, public assistance, and unemployment insurance were slashed (Massey, 2011). The rhetoric of the Southern Strategy continued to be used effectively by subsequent presidents including George H.W. Bush, George W. Bush, and Donald Trump (Patterson et al., 2021), but was also embraced by Bill Clinton who oversaw further expansion of state and federal prisons, significant restrictions on access to welfare, and the redirection of funding from public housing to prison construction (Alexander, 2020). By the 1980s, mass incarceration had become the *New Jim Crow*, a means of "sweep[ing] people of color off the streets, lock[ing] them in cages, and then release[ing] them into an inferior second-class status" (Alexander, 2020, p. 130). Once labeled felons or criminals, they are permanently marginalized and stigmatized, remaining under state surveillance (via probation or parole) often for years, are no longer permitted to vote, and can be subjected to legal discrimination in employment and access to food stamps, public benefits, housing, credit, and financial aid to further their education (Alexander, 2020). In essence,

> Systems constructed and enforced over centuries to subjugate enslaved people and their descendants based on race no longer needed race-based laws to

sustain them. Racial caste was so entrenched, so intertwined with American institutions, that without race-based *counteraction*, it would inevitably self-replicate.

(Hannah-Jones, 2024, n.p.)

Some scholars argue that the period from the election of Barack Obama in 2008 (Massey, 2011) to the rise of the Black Lives Matter movement and the racial justice protests following the murder of George Floyd in 2020 is a third period of reconstruction (Joseph, 2022). This third reconstruction has been followed predictably by White backlash in the form of the Tea Party and birtherism; increases in White nationalist militias; the Supreme Court ruling in *Shelby County v. Holder* that eliminated critical protections of the 1965 Voting Rights Act; the election of Donald Trump; the January 6th, 2021, insurrection; the 2023 Supreme Court reversal of affirmative action in college admissions (Joseph, 2022), and the re-election of Donald Trump in 2024. It has also included a sweeping attack on racial justice initiatives and programs from the banning of books and prohibition of curricula focused on racism and Black American history that allows people to better understand the roots of racial inequality; and legal efforts to end programs designed to address racial inequality from corporate Diversity Equity and Inclusion (DEI) programs and diversity fellowships at law firms to race-conscious programs intended to support small businesses run by Black business owners, and programs meant to prevent the death of Black women in childbirth (Hannah-Jones, 2024; Alexander, Baldwin Clark, Reinhard, & Zatz, 2023). Hannah-Jones (2024) argues that conservative groups have co-opted the legal legacy of Black civil rights activism and the rhetoric of colorblindness to dismantle the constitutional tools used to attempt to undo the racial caste system, and are now actively leveraging them to reverse racial progress

for the last 30 years, the court has almost exclusively ruled in favor of white people in so-called reverse-discrimination cases while severely narrowing the possibility for racial redress for Black Americans. Often, in these decisions, the court has used colorblindness as a rationale that dismisses both the particular history of racial disadvantage and its continuing disparities.

(Hannah-Jones, 2024, n.p.)

An important, but often underappreciated lynchpin in the history of racial disadvantage, which remains at the root of continuing racial disparities in virtually all areas of life is racial residential segregation.

Racial Residential Segregation

At the root of most enduring present day structural racial inequity in wealth, education, employment, exposure to criminal justice and mass incarceration, and health is the historical legacy of de jure (by law) and de facto (by practice) racial residential segregation. Racial residential segregation created and continues to perpetuate a level of social and economic stratification of Black Americans by spatially isolating large segments of the Black population and significantly and systematically limiting access to resources and opportunities (Massey, 2020). In a comprehensive review of the research on the harmful effects of racial residential segregation, Menendian and colleagues (2021) outline links with poor outcomes in all areas of life. They report that racial residential segregation is linked to a variety of poor health outcomes, including cardiovascular disease, diabetes, obesity, hypertension, asthma, infant mortality, and COVID-19 infections. It has also been linked to increased exposure to environmental pollutants, and proximity to hazardous waste facilities, reduced access to childcare facilities, recreational spaces, grocery stores and healthy food, as well as clinics, hospitals, and pharmacies. Racial residential segregation necessarily leads to segregated schools and has been associated with the concentration of high-poverty schools, lower test scores, achievement gaps, larger class sizes, poor teacher quality and high teacher turnover, and lower graduation rates. It is associated with lower median and per capita incomes, unemployment, and access to credit (Menendian, Gailes, & Gambhir, 2021).

Residential segregation was initially achieved through attempts by city councils to legally designate separate neighborhoods by race during the Great Migration of Blacks to northern cities in the first few decades of the 20th century (Massey, 2020; Massey & Denton, 1993). When these laws were struck down by the Supreme Court in 1917, racial violence ensued against Black people attempting to move out of Black neighborhoods, but was eventually replaced and perpetuated through the institutionalization of racial discrimination in housing markets via development of restrictive deeds (prohibiting transfer of deeds in particular neighborhoods to Black people) and racial covenants (wherein property owners in a defined area agree not to rent or sell homes to Black people; Massey & Denton, 1993; Rothstein, 2017). Racial covenants were further cemented by the federal government via the requirement that home loans from the Veterans Administration (VA) and the Federal Housing Administration (FHA) only be provided to mortgage properties covered by racially restrictive covenants. Both the VA and the FHA also recommended the use of red-lining maps that designated the creditworthiness, or lack thereof, of specific neighborhoods, coding Black neighborhoods as red and therefore ineligible for VA or FHA loans (Massey & Denton, 1993; Massey, 2020; Rothstein, 2017).

The segregation and isolation of Black urban neighborhoods was further perpetuated and entrenched throughout the postwar period with the mass migration of White people from cities to the suburbs, and the destruction and redevelopment of neighborhoods through federal public housing and urban renewal projects (Massey, 2020; Rothstein, 2017). The development of public housing and urban renewal projects blocked the expansion of Black neighborhoods, concentrating low-income Black residents in newly built high-rise racially segregated public housing, ultimately leading to increasing segregation from 1940 to 1970, which along with White flight to the surrounding suburbs, led to the hyper-segregation of Black metropolitan residents in neighborhoods with high concentrations of poverty by 1980 (Massey & Denton, 1993; Massey, 2020). A third of all Black metropolitan residents continued to live in conditions of hyper-segregation in 2010 (Massey, 2020). Hyper-segregated neighborhoods typically have higher levels of poverty, joblessness, crime, and criminal justice exposure, and fewer educational and economic opportunities and public services (Hess, 2021; Massey, 2020).

While legal (de jure) racial residential segregation was outlawed via federal legislation between 1968 and 1977, de facto discrimination in the banking industry via racial disparities in mortgages, and racial steering in the real estate industry have persisted, along with exclusionary zoning policies that restrict the development of low- and moderate-income housing, and policies impacting the location of subsidized housing (Weinstein, 2017). There have been modest reductions in racial residential segregation over time, which are mostly accounted for by increases in Latinx populations in Black neighborhoods (Jargowsky, 2020). Some research estimates that 81% of metropolitan regions with populations greater than 200,000 were more segregated as of 2019 than they were in 1990 (Menendian et al., 2021). Furthermore, increases in economic segregation between low-income, middle class, and affluent neighborhoods have only exacerbated the impact of racial segregation, with low-income Black and Latinx immigrant communities continuing to be highly isolated from middle class and affluent White neighborhoods where access to resources and opportunity is hoarded (Hess, 2021; Jargowsky, 2020). Furthermore, rates of racial residential segregation among school age children, and the schools they attend, are on average as high as they were in 1970 (Jargowsky, 2020).

Since 1980, there has been increasing movement of lower- and middle-income Black Americans to the suburbs (Hess, 2021; Jargowsky, 2020). From 1990 to 2020, the percentage of Black people living in the suburbs increased from 37% to 51%, the greatest increase for all racial groups, but they continue to be highly segregated from White people (Johnson, 2014; Lichter, Thiede, & Brooks, 2023). As Black populations in older inner-ring suburbs (those closest to cities and often to Black urban neighborhoods) have increased, White flight to outer-ring suburbs and exurbs and movement back into gentrified cities has also increased (Jargowsky, 2020). The rate of poverty in suburbs has increased overall for all races since 1990, but Black people are about twice as likely as White people to be exposed to suburban poverty (Hess, 2021). Significant increases in suburban poverty between 2000 and 2008 due to the Great Recession in particular, resulted in the continued concentration of lower-income Black people in highly segregated low-income suburbs that don't have the social service, economic, or physical infrastructure to support high-need populations (Hess, 2021; Johnson, 2014).

One consequence of racial residential segregation is significant racial disparities in income and wealth. Given the importance of wealth within American society, we briefly review the current status of Black America with respect to wealth, followed by related indices of educational attainment, exposure to the criminal justice system, and health status.

Racism and Wealth

Conley, (2010) has documented the persistent disparity in wealth, the accumulation of past and present income, across White and Black Americans. As of 2022, data indicates that White Americans hold 10 times more wealth than Black Americans (Urban Institute, 2024). Furthermore, there is no evidence to suggest that the wealth gap could close, and in fact over the past 30 years, the wealth gap has widened (Herring & Henderson, 2016). It has been long established that level of wealth is associated with health status; however, more recent research provides evidence of how nuanced and intractable this relationship is. Boen, Keister, and Aronson (2020) document ways in which specific types of wealth are associated with greater health status, and debt is associated with lower levels of health. Most Black families hold their wealth in home equity, which is not as strongly associated with positive health outcomes as is wealth in the form of investments. Furthermore, for Black Americans, debt does not translate to financial products as it does for White Americans (Seamster, 2019), and the disparity in wealth across Black and White Americans has been directly tied to the institution of slavery, legalized discrimination, and continued racial residential segregation. As the noted Conservative commentator Charles Krauthammer has stated: "The American people owe a special debt to Black Americans...There is nothing to compare with centuries of state-sponsored slavery followed by a century of state-sponsored discrimination" (see Craemer et al., 2020).

> Wealth affords the most useful economic indicator of a social group's subaltern status. It is a far superior indicator of economic well-being than income. Greater wealth or net worth – in general, the larger the difference between the value of what you own and what you owe – enables households to meet emergencies without extreme stress. Emergencies can include loss of employment, collapse of a small business, or a catastrophic illness.
>
> Wealthier households also can ensure that their children receive high quality schooling, including access to tutors that enable them to pass the requisite examinations. Wealthier households have the capacity to live in more upscale neighborhoods, to live in neighborhoods with desirable amenities, to leave bequests, to exercise political influence, and to largely be free of anxiety over their financial condition.
>
> (Darity, 2020)

The currency of wealth in American society goes beyond one's financial status, but indeed is directly correlated with power, position and influence (Conley, 2010). The wealth gap in the United States therefore serves as a mechanism for maintaining racial oppression and also contributes to other societal outcomes such as the nature of, and outcomes associated with participation in the educational system.

Racism and Education

"Education and racial oppression are inextricably linked" (Diamond & Gomez, 2023, p. 1). Because school districts are determined by residential neighborhoods, schools remain racially segregated, and in fact have resegregated over the last 30 years despite 20 years of efforts to desegregate schools following the *Brown v. Board of Ed* decision. The manner in which withholding education has been used in the service of racial oppression is well documented in the social science literature. The effect of such oppression is clearly evidenced in lower school completion rates, lower levels of engagement in higher education, and lower rates of attainment of professional credentials along a range of disciplines (Lee, Cornell, Gregory, & Fan, 2011; Hechinger Report, 2022). Merolla and Jackson (2019) outline a range of factors implicated in the "academic achievement gap" between White and Black Americans, including socioeconomic status, school quality, family cultural resources, and racial composition of schools; however, they believe that the fundamental cause of this achievement disparity is structural racism, i.e., "a system of social organization that privileges White Americans" (p. 1). To illustrate:

> In 2021, approximately 32,000 PhDs were awarded to U.S. citizens in the United States. Although the U.S. population is 12% Black and 19% Hispanic, only 8% and 9% of the PhDs were awarded to Black and Hispanic researchers, respectively. When limiting PhDs to Science, Technology, Engineering, and Mathematics (STEM) fields, disparities are even more stark, with only 5% and 8% of STEM PhDs awarded to Black and Hispanic researchers in 2021.
>
> (Velez & Heuer, 2023, p. 3)

An additional and startling aspect of racism within the educational system is the school-to-prison pipeline, a phenomenon that outlines the relationship between racial disproportionality in school discipline, increased rates of school incompletion, and higher likelihood of incarceration, in particular as it relates to communities of Color in the US (Barnes et al., 2018). National data demonstrates that Black males are exposed to more frequent and more severe school disciplinary measures than their White counterparts with the pattern existing even within the preschool and kindergarten populations (Wright & Ford, 2016). Furthermore, the phenomenon of racial disproportionality does not only impact Black males. Data indicates that Black girls are also disciplined more frequently and more harshly for the same offense as their White counterparts. Indeed, the phenomenon of treating Black girls as young adults has been noted by scholars such as Bettina Love (2019). Many scholars have identified with urgent concern the relationship between racial disproportionality in school discipline, lower academic performance, increased law enforcement surveillance in the public school system, and higher rates on incarceration among Black Americans, the phenomenon known as the school-to-prison pipeline that we have already addressed (Pieterse, 2016; Welsh et al., 2022). Indeed, what criminal justice scholars and legal professionals now to refer to as hyper-incarceration is another ongoing aspect of the history of racial oppression within the United States (Bell, 2017; Cloud et al., 2023)

Racism and Criminal Justice

Racial inequality has been noted to be the "foundational feature of the criminal justice system within the United States" (Rucker & Richeson, 2021, p. 1). This practice of inequality is seen through the history of policing in the United States with the precursor of modern policing being the slave patrols that were established to capture enslaved Black people pursuing their freedom (Brown, 2019), to the current state of hyper-incarceration within the United States and the disproportionate representation of People of Color within U.S prisons and jails. To illustrate, current data indicates that for every adult White male, there are six adult Black males incarcerated. When you compare that to the representation in the larger population (67 and 13% respectively), one gets a sense of the pervasiveness of this inequality (Hinton & Cook, 2021).

It is important to note that the effects of racial inequality in the criminal justice system go beyond the racially disproportionate nature of incarceration however, as it has a larger impact on the social location of Black Americans including participation in the political process, opportunities for employment, impact on families (Western & Wildeman, 2009), fragmentation of Black communities, and increased levels of violence (Western and Sirois, 2019). Here it is also important to note the intersectional nature of the effects of racism as noted by the data presented by Wacquant (2014), indicating that the lifetime probability of incarceration for Black males who did not complete a high school education is 12 times greater than for Black men who attended college.

For Black Americans, the disparities in housing, wealth, education, and exposure to the criminal justice system represent the ubiquity of racism and racial discrimination, which are associated with a range of adverse health outcomes (Bleich et al., 2019).

Racism and Health

It is widely understood that racism has both direct and indirect effects on the health status of Black Americans. David Williams, a leading sociologist who specializes in understanding the health-related effects of racism states

> The persistence of racial inequities in health should be understood in the context of relatively stable racialized social structures that determine differential access to risks, opportunities, and resources that drive health. We conceptualize this system of racism, chiefly operating through institutional and cultural domains, as a basic or fundamental cause of racial health inequalities... Understanding and effectively addressing how racism affects health is critical to improving population health and to making progress in reducing large and often intractable racial inequities in health.
>
> (Williams et al., 2019, p. 107)

The observed findings outlining the impact of racism on health include direct and positive associations between reports of racism and hypertension, obesity, diabetes, cardiovascular disease, anxiety, depression, trauma symptoms, suicidal ideation, low self-esteem, and general psychological distress (Paradies et al., 2015; Carter et al., 2019; Pieterse, Todd, Neville, & Carter, 2012; Kirkinis, Pieterse, Martin, Agiliga, & Brownell, 2021; Williams et al., 2019). In addition to direct negative health effects are the indirect effects where outcomes are noted to be as a function of structural racial inequalities. Race-related health disparities are noted to be a phenomenon in which Black Americans experience higher rates of morbidity and mortality associated with a range of diseases including cancers such as breast and lung, cardiovascular disease, diabetes, obesity, and HIV/AIDS. It is thought that a combination of structural racism resulting in unequal access to quality health care and provider racial bias that influences treatment-related decisions partly contribute to the health disparities phenomenon (Neblett, 2019). Additionally, the ways in which the fields of medicine, psychiatry, and psychology have endorsed racist ideology and racist practice is also thought to influence the levels of trust that Black Americans exhibit in regard to health care (Jaiswal, 2019; Fernando, 2017; Washington, 2006; Sabshin, Diesenhaus, & Wilkerson, 1970).

It is clear that Black America is profoundly impacted by the role of racism and racial categorization in American society. Still, Black America has also played an active role in American society with multiple contributions across a range of domains including medicine, the sciences, education, arts and entertainment, and sports (Hannah-Jones, 2021). Additionally, research in the social sciences have established multiple factors associated with Black American well-being and psychological health.

Black Americans' Well-Being

Given the increased interest in the psychosocial impact of racism on Black Americans, multiple systematic reviews of the literature have noted an interesting pattern. Although the relationship between experiences of racism and psychological distress has been clearly established, the relationship between racism and psychological well-being is not that clear. Positive and statistically significant relationships have been found for racism and depression, suicidal ideation, anxiety, trauma symptoms, substance use, and general psychological distress (Carter et al., 2019; Britt-Spells, Slebodnik, Sands, & Rollock, 2018; Kirkinis et al., 2021; Goodwill, Taylor, & Watkins, 2021; Pieterse et al., 2012). When looking at racism and well-being, however, the findings are less conclusive with some studies indicating no relationship with well-being and others documenting an inverse relationship; however, the effect sizes are typically considerably smaller than that of the effects for racism and psychological distress (Paradies et al., 2015; Pieterse & Carter, 2007; Pieterse, Carter, & Rays, 2013; Seaton, Neblett, Upton, Hammond, & Sellers , 2011). These findings suggest that in spite of the ubiquitous experience of racism, Black Americans have developed cultural strengths that allow for a certain level of well-being irrespective of the pain and distress associated with racism, a phenomenon that becomes clearer as we turn to an examination of Black Americans' mental health.

References

Alexander, M. (2020). *The New Jim Crow: Mass incarceration in the age of colorblindness*. New York, NY: The New Press.

Alexander, T., Baldwin Clark, L., Reinhard, K. & Zatz, N. (2023). *Tracking the attack on Critical Race Theory*. Los Angeles, CA: CRT Forward, UCLA School of Law Critical Race Studies Program.

Bailey, Z. D., Feldman, J. M., & Bassett, M. T. (2021). How structural racism works—racist policies as a root cause of US racial health inequities. *New England Journal of Medicine*, *384*(8), 768–773.

Barnes, J. C., & Motz, R. T. (2018). Reducing racial inequalities in adulthood arrest by reducing inequalities in school discipline: Evidence from the school-to-prison pipeline. *Developmental Psychology*, *54*(12), 2328–2340. doi: 10.1037/dev0000613.

Bell, M. (2017). Criminalization of blackness: Systemic racism and the reproduction of racial inequality in the US Criminal Justice System. In R. Thompson-Miller & K. Ducey (Eds.), *Systemic Racism: Making Liberty, Justice, and Democracy Real* (pp. 163–183). Palgrave Macmillan US. https://doi. org/10.1057/978-1-137-59410-5_7

Bleich, S. N., Findling, M. G., Casey, L. S., Blendon, R. J., Benson, J. M., SteelFisher, G. K., ... & Miller, C. (2019). Discrimination in the United States: Experiences of black Americans. *Health Services Research*, *54*, 1399–1408.

Boen, C., Keister, L., & Aronson, B. (2020). Beyond net worth: Racial differences in wealth portfolios and black–white health inequality across the life course. *Journal of Health and Social Behavior*, *61*(2), 153–169.

Britt-Spells, A. M., Slebodnik, M., Sands, L. P., & Rollock, D. (2018). Effects of perceived discrimination on depressive symptoms among Black men residing in the United States: A meta-analysis. *American Journal of Men's Health, 12*(1), 52–63.

Brown, R. A. (2019). Policing in American history. *Du Bois Review: Social Science Research on Race, 16*(1), 189–195.

Carter, R. T., Johnson, V. E., Kirkinis, K., Roberson, K., Muchow, C., & Galgay, C. (2019). A meta-analytic review of racial discrimination: Relationships to health and culture. *Race and Social Problems, 11*, 15–32.

Cloud, D. H., Garcia-Grossman, I. R., Armstrong, A., & Williams, B. (2023). Public health and prisons: priorities in the age of mass incarceration. *Annual Review of Public Health, 44*(1), 407–428. https://doi.org/10.1146/annurev-publhealth-071521-034016

Conley, D. (2010). *Being black, living in the red: Race, wealth, and social policy in America.* Berkley, CA: University of California Press.

Copeland, R. W. (2013). In the beginning: Origins of African American real property ownership in the United States. *Journal of Black Studies, 44*(6), 646–664.

Craemer, T., Smith, T., Harrison, B., Logan, T., Bellamy, W., & Darity Jr, W. (2020). Wealth implications of slavery and racial discrimination for African American descendants of the enslaved. *The Review of Black Political Economy, 47*(3), 218–254.

Darity, W., Jr. (2020) Understanding the subaltern native middle class. In: W. Dolsma, W. Hands & R. McMaster (Eds.) *History, Methodology, and Identity: Essays in Honor of John B. Davis.* London: Routledge, pp. 89–98.

DeAngelis, R. (2024). Systemic racism in police killings: New evidence from the mapping police volence database, 2013–2021. *Race and Justice, 14*(3) 413–432. https://doi.org/10.1177/21533687211047943

Dettlaff, A. J., & Boyd, R. (2022). The causes and consequences of racial disproportionality and disparities. In R. D. Krugman & J. E. Korbin (Eds.), *Handbook of Child Maltreatment* (2nd ed. pp. 221–239). Springer Nature.

Diamond, J. B., & Gomez, L. M. (2023). Disrupting white supremacy and anti-black racism in educational organizations. *Educational Researcher, 0*(0). https://doi.org/10.3102/0013189X231161054

Embrick, D. G., & Moore, W. L. (2020). White space (s) and the reproduction of white supremacy. *American Behavioral Scientist, 64*(14), 1935–1945.

Equal Justice Initiative (2017). Lynching in america: Confronting the legacy of racial terror. *Montgomery: Equal Justice Initiative.*

Feagin, J. R. (2006). *Systemic Racism.* Routledge: New York, NY.

Fernando, S. (2017). Institutional *racism in psychiatry and clinical psychology* (Vol. 17517893, No. 0). London: Palgrave Macmillan.

Fredrickson, G.M., (1988). *The Arrorance of Race: Historical Perspetives on Slavery, Racism and Social Inequality.* Middletoem CT.: Wesleyan University Press.

Glickman, L. (May 21, 2020). *How White Backlash Conrols American Progress.* The Atlantic, retrieved from https://www.theatlantic.com/ideas/archive/2020/05/white-backlash-nothing-new/611914/

Goodwill, J. R., Taylor, R. J., & Watkins, D. C. (2021). Everyday discrimination, depressive symptoms, and suicide ideation among African American men. *Archives of Suicide Research, 25*(1), 74–93.

Green, V. M. (1981). Blacks in the United States: The creation of an enduring people. In G. P. Castile & G. Kusher (Eds.), *Persistence peoples: Cultural enclaves in perspective* (pp. 69–77). Tucson: University of Arizona Press.

Hannah-Jones, N. (2021). The 1619 *project: A new american origin story*. New York: New York, NY: Random House.

Hannah-Jones, N. (March 13, 2024). *The Colorblind Campaign to Undo Civil Rights progress*. The New York Times Magazine. Retreived from https://www.nytimes.com/2024/03/13/magazine/civil-rights-affi rmative-action-colorblind.html

HechingerReport(2022).Retrievedfromhttps://hechingerreport.org/%E2%80%8B%E2%80%8Bwhy-white-students-are-250-more-likely-to-graduate-than-black-students-at-public-universities/. July 6, 2023.

Herring, C., & Henderson, L. (2016). Wealth inequality in black and white: Cultural and structural sources of the racial wealth gap. *Race and Social Problems, 8*(1), 4–17. https://doi.org/10.1007/s12552-016-9159-8

Hess, C. (2021). Residential segregation by race and ethnicity and the changing geography of neighborhood poverty. *Spatial Demography, 9*, 57–106.

Hines, D. E., King Jr, R., & Ford, D. Y. (2018). Black students in handcuffs: Addressing racial disproportionality in school discipline for students with dis/abilities. *Teachers College Record, 120*(13), 1–24.

Hinton, E., & Cook, D. (2021). The mass criminalization of Black Americans: A historical overview. *Annual Review of Criminology, 4*, 261–286.

Horsman, R. (1982). Well-Trodden Paths and Fresh Byways: Recent Writing on Native American History. *Reviews in American History, 10*(4), 234–244.

Jaiswal, J. (2019). Whose responsibility is it to dismantle medical mistrust? Future directions for researchers and health care providers. *Behavioral Medicine, 45*(2), 188–196.

Jargowsky, P. A. (2020). Racial and economic segregation in the US: overlapping and reinforcing dimensions. In Sako Musterd (Ed.). Handbook of Urban Segregation, pp. 151–168. Cheltenham, UK: Edward Elgar Publishing, Inc.

Johnson, K. S. (June 24, 2014). *'Black' suburbanization: American dream or the new banlieue?*. Items. Retrieved from https://items.ssrc.org/the-cities-papers/black-suburbanization-american-dream-or-the-new-banlieue/

Johnson, Michael P., & Roark, James, L. (1984). *Black masters: A free family of color in the old south*. New York: Norton.

Joseph, P.E., (2022). *The third reconstruction: America's struggle for racial justice in the 21st century*. New York: Basic Books.

Kirkinis, K., Pieterse, A. L., Martin, C., Agiliga, A., & Brownell, A. (2021). Racism, racial discrimination, and trauma: A systematic review of the social science literature. *Ethnicity & Health, 26*(3), 392–412.

Lee T., Cornell D., Gregory A., Fan X. (2011). High suspension schools and drop-out rates for Black and White students. *Education and Treatment of Children*, 34, 167–192.

Lichter, D. T., Thiede, B. C., & Brooks, M. M. (2023). Racial diversity and segregation: Comparing principal cities, inner-ring suburbs, outlying suburbs, and the suburban fringe. *The Russell Sage Foundation Journal of the Social Sciences*, 9(1), 26–51.

Litwack, Leon F. (1961) *North of slavery: The Negro in the free states, 1790–1860*. Chicago: University of Chicago Press.

Liu, W. M., Liu, R. Z., & Shin, R. Q. (2023). Understanding systemic racism: Anti-Blackness, white supremacy, racial capitalism, and the re/creation of white space and time. *Journal of Counseling Psychology, 70*(3), 244–257. doi: 10.1037/cou0000605.

Love, B. L. (2019). *We want to do more than survive: Abolitionist teaching and the pursuit of educational freedom.* Beacon press.

Massey, D.S., (2011). The past and future of American civil rights. *Dædalus, the Journal of the American Academy of Arts & Sciences, 140(2),* 37–54.

Massey, D.S. (2020). Still the linchpin: Segregation and stratification in the USA. *Race and Social Problems, 12,* 1–12.

Massey, D.S. & Denton, N.A. (1993). *American apartheid: Segregation and the making of the underclass.* Cambridge, MA: Harvard University Press.

Menendian, S., Gailes, A., & Gambhir, S. (2021). *The roots of structural racism: Twenty-first century racial residential segregation in the United States.* Berkeley, CA: Othering & Belonging Institute. Retrieved from https://belonging.berkeley.edu/roots-structural-racism.

Mensah, M., Ogbu-Nwobodo, L., & Shim, R. S. (2021). Racism and mental health equity: History repeating itself. *Psychiatric Services, 72*(9), 1091–1094.

Merolla, D. M., & Jackson, O. (2019). Structural racism as the fundamental cause of the academic achievement gap. *Sociology Compass, 13*(6), e12696.

National Urban League (2024). *2024 State of Black America: The Civil Rights Act of 1964: 60 Years Later.* New York, NY: National Urban League.

Neblett, E. W., Jr. (2019). Racism and health: Challenges and future directions in behavioral and psychological research. *Cultural Diversity & Ethnic Minority Psychology, 25*(1), 12–20. https://doi.org/10.1037/cdp0000253

Ogbu, J. U. (2004). Collective identity and the burden of "acting White" in Black history, community, and education. *The Urban Review, 36*(1), 1–35.

Paradies, Y., Ben, J., Denson, N., Elias, A., Priest, N., Pieterse, A., ... & Gee, G. (2015). Racism as a determinant of health: A systematic review and meta-analysis. *PloS One, 10*(9), e0138511.

Patterson, K., Santiago, A.M., & Silverman, R.M. (2021). The enduring backlash against racial justice in the United States: mobilizing strategies for institutional change. *Journal of Community Practice, 29*(4), 334–344.

Pieterse, A. L. (2016). Racialized perspectives on the prison industrial complex. In E. L. Short, L. Wilton, E. L. Short, L. Wilton (Eds.), Talking about structural inequalities in everyday life: New politics of race in groups, organizations, and social systems (pp. 205-223). Charlotte, NC: Information Age Publishing.

Pieterse, A. L., & Carter, R. T. (2007). An examination of the relationship between general life stress, racism-related stress, and psychological health among black men. *Journal of Counseling Psychology, 54*(1), 101–109. doi: 10.1037/0022-0167.54.1.101.

Pieterse, A. L., Carter, R. T., & Ray, K. V. (2013). Racism-related stress, general life stress, and psychological functioning among Black American women. *Journal of Multicultural Counseling and Development, 41*(1), 36–46.

Pieterse, A. L., Todd, N. R., Neville, H. A., & Carter, R. T. (2012). Perceived racism and mental health among Black American adults: A meta-analytic review. *Journal of Counseling Psychology, 59*(1), 1–9. doi: 10.1037/a0026208.

Rothstein, R. (2017). *The color of law: A Forgotten History of How Our Government Segregated America.* New York: Liveright Publishing Company.

Rucker, J. M., & Richeson, J. A. (2021). Toward an understanding of structural racism: Implications for criminal justice. *Science*, *374*(6565), 286–290.

Sabshin, M., Diesenhaus, H., & Wilkerson, R. (1970). Dimensions of institutional racism in psychiatry. *American Journal of Psychiatry*, *127*(6), 787–793.

Seamster, L. (2019). Black debt, white debt. *Contexts*, *18*(1), 30–35.

Seaton, E. K., Neblett, E. W., Upton, R. D., Hammond, W. P., & Sellers, R. M. (2011). The moderating capacity of racial identity between perceived discrimination and psychological well-being over time among African American youth. *Child Development*, *82*(6), 1850–1867. doi: 10.1111/j.1467-8624.2011.01651.x

Smedley, A. (2018). *Race in North America: Origin and evolution of a worldview*. Oxfordshire, UK: Routledge.

Span, C. M. (2015). Post-slavery? Post-segregation? Post-racial? A history of the impact of slavery, segregation, and racism on the education of African Americans. *Teachers College Record*, *117*(14), 53–74.

Tate, K. (2004). *Black faces in the mirror: African Americans and their representatives in the US Congress*. Princeton: Princeton University Press.

Urban Institute (2024). Nine charts about Wealth Inequality in America. https://apps.urban.org/features/wealth-inequality-charts/

Velez, E. D. & Heuer, R. (2023). *Exploring the Educational Experiences of Black and Hispanic PhDs in STEM*. Retrieved from https://www.rti.org/sites/default/files/documents/2023

Wacquant, L. (2014). Class, race and hyperincarceration in revanchist america. *Socialism and Democracy*, *28*(3), 35–56. https://doi.org/10.1080/08854300.2014.954926

Washington, H. A. (2006). *Medical Apartheid: The Dark History of Medical Experimentation on Black Americans from Colonial Times to the Present*. New York, NY: Doubleday Books.

Weinstein, A. C., (2017). Reflections on the persistence of racial segregation in housing. *Capital Law Review*. *45*, 59–77. https://engagedscholarship.csuohio.edu/fac_articles/1052

Welch, K., Lehmann, P. S., Chouhy, C., & Chiricos, T. (2022). Cumulative Racial and Ethnic Disparities Along the School-to-Prison Pipeline. Journal of Research in Crime and Delinquency, 59(5), 574-626. https://doi.org/10.1177/00224278211070501

Western, B., & Sirois, C. (2019). Racialized re-entry: Labor market inequality after incarceration. *Social Forces*, *97*(4), 1517–1542.

Western, B., & Wildeman, C. (2009). The Black family and mass incarceration. *The ANNALS of the American Academy of Political and Social Science*, *621*(1), 221–242. https://doi.org/10.1177/0002716208324850

Wilkins, E. J., Whiting, J. B., Watson, M. F., Russon, J. M., & Moncrief, A. M. (2013). Residual effects of slavery: What clinicians need to know. *Contemporary Family Therapy*, *35*, 14–28.

Williams, D. R., Lawrence, J. A., & Davis, B. A. (2019). Racism and health: evidence and needed research. *Annual Review of Public Health*, *40*(1), 105–125. https://doi.org/10.1146/annurev-publhealth-040218-043750

Wright, B. L., & Ford, D. Y. (2016). "This little light of mine": Creating early childhood education classroom experiences for African American boys PreK-3. *Journal of African American Males in Education (JAAME)*, *7*(1), 5–19.

Yearby, R., Clark, B., & Figueroa, J. F. (2022). Structural racism in historical and modern US health care policy: Study examines structural racism in historical and modern US health care policy. *Health Affairs*, *41*(2), 187–194.

Chapter 2

The State of Black Americans' Mental Health

Historical Context

In 2021, the American Psychological Association (APA) issued a formal apology to People of Color for its "role in promoting, perpetuating, and failing to challenge racism, racial discrimination, and human hierarchy" in the United States (APA, 2021), based in part on a chronological cataloguing of the history of racism in the discipline of psychology (Cummings Center, 2021). This catalogue provided historical evidence and confirmation that structural and systemic racism, as well as paradigms of racial inferiority and deficiency, were woven into the development of the research, profession, and practice of psychology in the United States in a manner that has fomented, propagated, and is inextricably tied to the racial mental health disparities evident today. From the earliest precursors and origins of the discipline in the United States in the 18th century to the present, psychology has been complicit in promoting and providing pseudo-scientific evidence to support the belief in an innate biologically based racial hierarchy, with Black people as the inferior race and White people as the superior race.

There is a consistent history of pathologizing Black people in psychology that started even before the development of a formal mainstream discipline of psychology in the United States. Justifications for the maintenance of slavery in the United States in the 1800s relied in part on a belief that Black people were more like animals than people, were happiest when held in subjugation, and that servitude and dependence on White slave owners was a natural and beneficial state for them. With the rise in the abolition movement and increases in runaway slaves in the second half of the 19th century, supporters of slavery sought to explain why happy slaves would seek to escape (Guthrie, 1998). In 1851, Samuel Cartwright, a southern physician, slave owner, and leader in plantation and racial medicine who specialized in Black inferiority and slave diseases, published "Report on the Diseases and Physical Peculiarities of the Negro Race" (Willoughby, 2018). In this report, he described *drapetomania*, a mental disorder which caused slaves to run away, and *dyaesthesia Aethiopis*, which afflicted

DOI: 10.4324/9781003083221-3

free Black people more than slaves and caused them to behave in a careless and mischievous way, destroying property and refusing to work (Guthrie, 1998). The notion that freedom caused insanity among Black Americans was further supported by the 1840 census, which found that the rate of insanity among Black people in the north was 11 times higher than that in the south (Grossi, 2021; Warren, 2016). This finding, which was based on erroneous and statistically inconsistent data, was the source of significant controversy and disagreement. It shaped political discourse and debate around slavery and the sanity of free Black people over the next few decades leading up to, during, and after the Civil War (Grossi, 2021), just as the scientific discipline and profession of psychology was being formalized in the United States (Cummings Center, 2021).

Much of the early leadership of the APA, founded in 1892, who were instrumental in establishing the first psychology research programs and journals, had significant involvement in, leadership, and advocacy roles in the eugenics movement (Cummings Center, 2021), which focused on providing scientific evidence of biological differences between racial groups and the inferiority of People of Color. The racist pseudoscience of eugenics had a central role in the development of psychometric intelligence and ability testing, and was used to justify segregation, anti-miscegenation laws, race-based immigration policies, and even sterilization of those deemed feeble-minded (APA, 2021; Cummings Center, 2021). For example, although Black psychologists Mamie Phipps Clark and Kenneth Clark provided expert testimony in *Brown v. Board of Education*, prominent White psychologists, including former APA president Henry E. Garrett, provided research evidence and testimony in favor of maintaining segregation in 1952; to challenge the Brown decision in 1963; to support anti-miscegenation laws in 1967; and in opposition to passage of the Civil Rights Act in 1967 (Cummings Center, 2021).

The paradigm of racial inferiority predominated in psychology well into the first half of the 20th century, but as more People of Color began to earn PhDs in psychology, they began to challenge this prevailing paradigm. Along with the civil rights activism that characterized the era, there was a shift in the 1950s and 1960s from the predominance of the racial inferiority paradigm to a cultural deprivation paradigm, which focused on explaining psychological differences between Black and White Americans as the result of the impact of oppression in Black communities and environments rather than their inherent genetic or biological inferiority (Carter, 1995). The 1965 Moynihan Report, written by then Assistant Secretary of Labor and focusing on poverty and the Black family (Geary, 2015), made cultural deprivation synonymous with the inherent deficiency of Black urban communities and culture. The concept of cultural deprivation combined the social meaning of race (i.e., Blacks are culturally deficient) with the biological meaning (i.e., Blacks are genetically inferior), to create a criterion whereby Black people were compared to a White middle-class normative standard. Within this comparison, Black people lacked cultural values separate from the "culture of poverty," and disparities in economic, social, and cultural experiences were responsible for the apparent psychosocial, behavioral, and personality differences between Black people and middle-class White people. As a result, Black people were characterized by this construct as lacking, deprived, or deviant. The positioning of Whiteness and White culture in psychological research and practice as a standard and norm against which all other races and cultures are unfavorably compared and viewed as marginal or deficient is a common thread that persists to this day (Cummings Center, 2021).

While the cultural deprivation paradigm for understanding differences between White and Black Americans provided acknowledgment of the destructive influence of systems of oppression on Black people, there was an overwhelming emphasis on negative aspects of Black adaptation to oppression, racial discrimination, and poverty. Much of the research in this era focused on crime, poverty, juvenile delinquency, and discrimination, and assumed that all Black people were permanently psychologically damaged (Carter, 1995). As with the work of the 1800s and the first half of the 1900s, rather than exploring positive Black cultural practices that promoted psychological well-being and health, the focus in mainstream psychology was on pathologizing Black people's ostensibly maladaptive behaviors and personalities (Carter, 1995).

Even as the predominant paradigm shifted from one of cultural deprivation to one that emphasized cultural difference with the significant increase in Black psychologists in the late 1960s and 1970s, deficit models of the Black family, youth development, and pathology continued to predominate in mainstream psychology (Tyrell, Neville, Causadias, Cokley & Adams-Wiggins, 2023). It is important to note that there were Black people in the field of psychology from the early 20th century, with the first Black American earning a doctoral degree in psychology in 1920 (Guthrie, 1998). Black psychologists have persisted in regularly producing research challenging the inferiority and cultural deprivation paradigms, critiquing mainstream research supporting these paradigms, and promoting a strength-based perspective on the Black experience since the 1930s and continuing to the present, but their work has been consistently marginalized from mainstream psychology publications and is rarely taught in psychology training programs (Cummings Center, 2021; Tyrell et al., 2023).

The Black-White Mental Health Paradox

Despite the failure of mainstream psychology to integrate the work of Black psychologists, and to tend to pathologize Black people, certain patterns in mental health epidemiology have perplexed researchers for decades. Although mid-20th-century research suggested that Black Americans suffered from an inescapably poor self-image (e.g., Kardiner & Ovesey, 1951), research starting in the 1970s consistently demonstrated that Black Americans have higher self-esteem than White Americans (Gray-Little & Hafdahl, 2000; Twenge &

Crocker, 2002), and that there was significant growth in self-esteem within the Black community that emerged with the Black is Beautiful and Black Power movements of the 1970s (Twenge & Crocker, 2002). Additionally, despite the marked racial disparities in virtually all areas of life, and the significantly greater exposure to stress associated with these disparities, both contemporaneously and intergenerationally across time, three decades of research has consistently found that Black Americans report the same or better mental health than White Americans, defined as lower rates of mental disorder. This phenomenon, known as the Black-White Mental Health Paradox, has been most studied in rates of major depression, but has been found in 16 different mental health disorders, including mood, anxiety, and substance use disorders, measured both in the past year and across the lifetime, with the relative advantage to Blacks intensifying when socioeconomic status and age were controlled (Erving, Thomas, & Frazier, 2019; Gibbs et al., 2013).

Even more confounding, the research literature has simultaneously found that rates of psychological distress remain equal or significantly higher among Black as compared to White people, even as rates of symptoms and disorder remain equal or lower (Barnes & Bates, 2017). Research has focused on nationally representative stably housed and noninstitutionalized populations, thereby not accounting for rates of mental illness in incarcerated and homeless populations, as well as those housed on military bases, all of which have been found to have higher rates of depression and to be disproportionately Black (Pamplin & Bates, 2021). Still, at least one study adjusting for this artifact has found that these differences do not account for the Black-White paradox when it comes to depression (Barnes, Keyes, & Bates, 2013).

Research has found evidence suggesting that the Black-White mental health paradox may be explained at least in part by higher rates of flourishing or overall positive mental health among Black as compared to White people (Keyes, 2009). Flourishing was assessed as having: generally positive affect (i.e., feeling happy, calm, peaceful, satisfied, and full of life); interest in and satisfaction with life; self-acceptance (i.e., positive attitudes toward self, including accepting both positive and negative aspects of oneself); social acceptance (i.e., positive attitudes toward others while accepting differences and complexity); personal growth (i.e., understanding of one's own potential and openness to challenging experiences); social actualization (i.e., belief that people, social groups and society have the potential to grow in a positive direction); purpose in life (i.e., belief that life has purpose and direction); social contribution (i.e., perception of one's life as useful to society and valued/valuable to society); environmental mastery (i.e., ability to manage a complex environment and mold the environment to suit ones' needs); social coherence (i.e., an interest in society and social life and belief that society and culture are meaningful); autonomy (i.e., self-direction guided by internal standards and resisting negative social pressures); positive relations with others (i.e., warm and trusting interpersonal relations and capacity for empathy and intimacy); and social integration (i.e., sense of belonging to, comfort in, and support from community). In examining the Black-White mental health paradox, Keyes (2009) found that 27% more Black than White people were found to be flourishing and free of mental disorder, and when racial discrimination was controlled for, rates of flourishing increased for Black people. This research suggests that Black Americans have developed a number of strengths in their perception of self, community, and ways of dealing with adversity and racial discrimination that significantly promote psychological health and well-being.

A recent study found that self-esteem and church attendance were found to explain racial differences in depressive symptoms and disorder, with self-esteem contributing to about 80% of the observed variance in depressive symptoms between Black and White Americans (Louie, Upeneiks, Erving, & Tobin, 2022). There is also evidence that racial identity contributes to increased self-esteem and mastery for Black as compared to White people, and that Black people who had a stronger racial identity were less likely to have mental health and substance use disorders than White people (Hughes, Kiecolt, & Keith, 2022). With respect to religiosity and spirituality, Louie and colleagues (2022) found that divine control contributed to about 51% of the variance in depression disorder for Black as compared to White people. Upeneiks and colleagues (2023) also found that Black people experience less religious and spiritual struggles than White people and that these struggles contributed to greater distress among White people (Upeneiks, Louie, & Hill, 2023). They suggested that Black people may experience greater spiritual support from their religious congregations than do White people, providing them with greater strength and less conflict. Research has also found that there are protective effects on mental health for Black people living in predominantly Black neighborhoods with up to 84% Black residents (Becares, Nazroo, & Jackson, 2014), suggesting that the social cohesion, sense of community, and social support of predominantly Black, though not racially segregated and isolated neighborhoods, may help reduce rates of depression. Taken together, the results of these studies on flourishing, self-esteem and racial identity, religiosity and spirituality, and ethnic density provide strong support for the notion that the Black cultural strengths we describe in this book, including racial identity, racial socialization, communalism, cultural spirituality, and racism-related coping, may contribute to the ability of Black Americans to thrive in the face of centuries of significant and unrelenting adversity.

Notably, there are two major exceptions found to the Black-White mental health paradox: Black people have higher rates of posttraumatic stress disorder (PTSD) and are significantly more likely to be diagnosed with schizophrenia. Over the last 20 years, suicide appears to be yet another emerging exception to the Black-White mental health paradox. These three trends tell a story about the stunningly severe impact of the interaction between structural racism, interpersonal racism, and unconscionably poor access to mental health care in Black communities.

Exceptions to the Black-White Mental Health Paradox: Posttraumatic Stress Disorder

Research has found higher lifetime prevalence and conditional risk of PTSD among Black as compared to White people in the general population (Alegría et al., 2013; Erving et al., 2019; Himle, Baser, Taylor, Campbell, & Jackson, 2009; McLaughlin et al., 2019; Roberts, Gilman, Breslau, Breslau, & Koenen, 2011), and greater prevalence and chronicity among Black war veterans (Dohrenwend, Turner, Turse, Lewis-Fernandez, & Yager, 2008). Studies have found that Black people are more likely than Whites to be exposed to physical and sexual violence, both of which have a stronger association with trauma-related disorders (McLaughlin et al., 2019; Roberts et al., 2011). Yet, Black people remained less likely than White people to develop anxiety, depression, and substance use disorders as a result of their greater exposure to physical and sexual violence (McLaughlin et al., 2019).

There is evidence that the higher prevalence rates of PTSD among Black Americans are explained by greater exposure to racial discrimination and harassment, which makes them more vulnerable to developing PTSD or exacerbates the impact of other traumatic experiences. Racial discrimination was significantly associated with trauma-related symptoms in Black college students (Pieterse, Carter, Evans, and Walter, 2010) and significantly predicted PTSD, and exposure to frequent racial discrimination has been found to reduce rates of recovery among Black Americans, even with high rates of treatment (Sibrava et al., 2019). These studies suggest that cumulative exposure to racism exacerbates the severity of PTSD symptoms, prolongs chronicity of the disorder, and may contribute to re-traumatization. Further, existing treatments for trauma appear to be significantly less effective for Black people than they are for White populations. This is likely because these treatments are executed by predominantly White clinicians who do not explicitly address the role of race and cumulative lifetime exposure to racial discrimination and structural racism in the etiology, maintenance, and chronicity of the disorder. Further, it is likely that the use of PTSD symptoms in existing epidemiological research, rather than the more broad and varied symptoms of complex trauma reactions, which fall outside of the narrow criteria required for a PTSD diagnosis and are more common in reactions to experiences of race-based traumatic stress (Carter & Pieterse, 2020), significantly underestimates the true prevalence of traumatic stress reactions experienced by Black Americans.

Exceptions to the Black-White Mental Health Paradox: Schizophrenia Diagnoses

The remarkably high rates of schizophrenia-spectrum disorders among Black as compared to White people provides a particularly apt illustration of the history and persistence of pathologizing Black people in America. More than 30 years of research has found that Black people are between 2 and 4 times more likely to be diagnosed with schizophrenia than Whites (Barnes, 2013; Eack, Bahorik, Newhill, Neighbors, & Davis, 2012; Olbert, Nagendra, & Buck, 2018; Schwartz & Blankenship, 2014), and were nearly 2.5 times more likely to be diagnosed with schizophrenia-paranoid subtype (Olbert et al., 2018).

Metzl (2009) identifies the origin of racial disparities in the diagnosis of schizophrenia in the late 1960s and 1970s with the convergence of anxieties around racial and social change, and the perception of uncontrollable urban uprising and unrest, along with advancing pharmacological technology that allowed for the possibility of using psychotropic medication and institutionalization in inpatient facilities to maintain social control. During this time, he documents the evolution of the diagnostic criteria and public perception of schizophrenia from that of a predominantly White, female, docile, and harmless disorder, to a disorder with a paranoid subtype characterized by volatility, rage, and aggression that was predominantly Black and male. He cites a 1968 article in *Archives of General Psychiatry* where schizophrenia is described as

a "protest psychosis" whereby black men developed "hostile and aggressive feelings" and "delusional anti-whiteness" after listening to the words of Malcolm X, joining the Black Muslims, or joining groups that preached militant resistance to white society.

(Metzl, 2009, p. xiv)

Along with the evolving criteria for schizophrenia diagnosis, significantly higher rates of schizophrenia among Black men, in particular, began to be evident in the late 1960s, just as their civil rights activism threatened the racial order. By the 1980s and 1990s, Black men were up to seven times more likely to be diagnosed with paranoid schizophrenia than White men (Metzl, 2009). Metzl's work highlights a direct historical thread from the pathologizing of Black people who rose up against slavery, through the diagnosis of drapetomania, to the pathologizing of Black people who fought for civil rights through the overdiagnosis of schizophrenia. Tragically, the increase in the diagnosis of schizophrenia in Black people in the 1960s was further exacerbated by the deinstitutionalization of mental health care between 1963 and 1965, forcing many people diagnosed with serious mental illness into the streets and prisons, which ultimately led to the racialized criminalization of mental illness (Faber, Khanna Roy, Michaels & Williams, 2023; Misra, Etkins, Yang, & Williams, 2022), and the carceral system becoming the largest provider of mental health care in the United States (Ford, 2015).

Two main explanations proposed for the observed high prevalence of schizophrenia diagnoses of Black Americans are: (1) misdiagnosis and overdiagnosis driven by clinician bias; and (2) the contribution of the cumulative stress of structural racism to proximal risk factors, which accumulate across the life course and intergenerationally, increasing the risk for the development of psychotic symptomology (Faber et al, 2023; Anglin et al., 2021; Misra et al., 2022). Faber and colleagues (2023) describe four reasons, supported by research, why misdiagnosis may occur. First, mental health professionals may misinterpret Black patients' healthy suspicion and cultural mistrust, which are adaptive responses to racial discrimination, as clinical paranoia and delusion. Second, implicit bias may lead mental health professionals to misperceive Black patients, through the prism of prevailing stereotypes, as violent, aggressive, noncommunicative, and poorly educated, negatively impacting their ability to conduct an accurate clinical assessment, and making them more likely to attribute their behaviors and manner of interacting to psychotic symptoms. Third, mental health professionals may misinterpret Black patients' nonmainstream (i.e., spiritual or paranormal) religious experiences as psychotic symptoms.

Fourth, clinicians may overemphasize psychotic symptoms and underemphasize mood-related symptoms in Black patients, thereby misdiagnosing them as having a schizophrenia-spectrum disorder when a more appropriate diagnosis would be a mood disorder (Gara, Minsky, Silverstein, Miskimen, & Strakowski, 2019; Gara et al., 2012). Black patients are more likely to be diagnosed with schizophrenia rather than a mood disorder than White patients, even when presenting with the same symptoms (Schwartz & Blankenship, 2014). Research has found that Black people with bipolar disorder have symptom expression very different from White people, possibly contributing to misdiagnoses of schizophrenia (Li, Richards, & Goes, 2023). There are high rates of undocumented PTSD among Black clients with serious mental illness (i.e., schizophrenia-spectrum disorders, major depressive disorder, bipolar disorder) receiving outpatient community mental health services (Lu et al., 2022). Research has also found that Black people are more than three times more likely to be exposed to police violence than White people, and that exposure to police violence is significantly associated with psychological distress, suicidal ideation, suicide attempts, and psychotic symptoms, with severe assaultive violence associated most significantly with psychotic symptoms and suicide attempts (DeVylder et al., 2018). This research suggests the possibility that the expression of severe trauma symptoms for Black people may fall outside the bounds of existing diagnostic criteria.

Misra and colleagues (2022) argue that the stress of structural racism can lead to alterations in physiological, neurological, and psychological systems, contributing to an increased risk for and incidence of psychotic disorders among Black people over and above the influence of misdiagnosis alone. They provide evidence that structural racism, expressed through racialized policing and incarceration, and economic exploitation and disinvestment contribute to the unique risk, incidence, and consequences of schizophrenia-spectrum disorders among Black Americans. They argue that as a result of racialized policing, Black people witness and experience greater police violence, which is associated with increased mental health symptoms, including psychotic symptoms. As a result of racialized policing and racial bias in the criminal justice system, they are more likely to experience negative interactions with the criminal justice system, and to be incarcerated. Black people's negative contact with the criminal justice system, and harsher treatment once incarcerated, increase the likelihood of developing mental illness and exacerbate existing conditions. Furthermore, Black people with psychotic symptoms are at a far greater risk of contact with police and involuntary and coercive admission into inpatient care, which leads to worse outcomes including avoidance of necessary care, longer and more frequent hospitalizations (Misra et al., 2022), and death at the hands of police (Faber et al, 2023). Racialized police violence against Black people with schizophrenia is the most acute example of the intersection of structural racism and interpersonal racism with mental health disparities in access to care.

Due to the confluence of various forces of structural racism on housing, employment opportunity, wealth accumulation, and neighborhood deprivation, Black people are more likely to live in high-poverty racially segregated neighborhoods with fewer resources, greater exposure to violence, and poor access to mental health care, all of which are associated with higher rates of psychosis (Misra et al., 2022). Additionally, because of greater exposure to trauma across the life course, higher rates of incarceration, and lower income, Black people are more likely to be homeless or unhoused, and homeless people are 50 times more likely to have a psychotic disorder than the general population.

Faber and colleagues (2023) argue that Black people may have increased vulnerability to, and therefore risk of, developing schizophrenia-spectrum disorders due to their higher prevalence of PTSD and trauma, exposure to structural racism, including neighborhood factors, collective stress and trauma, and exposure to various life traumas, including racial discrimination and racism. Black people suffering from other mental disorders who are misdiagnosed as schizophrenic receive inappropriate and often harmful treatment, including antipsychotic medications that can negatively impact their health, that further exacerbates their existing disorder, and can lead to lifelong negative consequences. Black people are also more likely to be prescribed first-generation antipsychotics, which have greater and more severe and damaging side effects, at higher doses than White people.

Exceptions to the Black-White Mental Health Paradox: Suicide

Despite the persistence of overall lower rates of mental disorder among Black as compared to White populations in the United States, and historically low rates of suicide, an alarmingly drastic upward trend in suicide among Black children, adolescents, and young adults has begun to emerge over the last two decades

(Marcotte & Hansen, 2023). The most prominent increase was observed in the last decade: suicide rates for Black people increased by four times the rate of increase among White people between 2010 and 2020 (Panchal, Saunders, & Ndugga, 2022). Death by suicide for Black children age 10–14 increased by 131.5% between 2000 and 2020 (Meza, Patel, & Bath, 2022). While White and First Nation people continue to have the highest rates of suicide overall, from 2003 to 2017, Black children age 5–12 were twice as likely to die by suicide as White children (Bridge, Horowitz, & Fontanella, 2018). The increase in rates of suicide among Black girls between 2003 and 2017 was nearly twice that among Black boys (Sheftall et al., 2022), and suicide among Black adolescent girls increased by 182% from 2001 to 2017 (Price & Kubchandani, 2019).

The trend has continued since the COVID-19 pandemic. Suicide death rates increased for Black adolescents by 129% from 2012 to 2022 (Panchal, 2024). Overall suicide rates for Black Americans increased by 19.2% as compared to a decline of 3.9% among White people from 2018 to 2021, with suicide among Black children, teenagers, and young adults age 10-24 increasing by nearly 37% in the same time period, which was the largest proportional increase of any demographic group (Stone, Mack, & Qualters, 2023). Black teenagers were also found to be more likely to attempt suicide than White teenagers in 2021 (Centers for Disease Control, 2023).

There is some indication that the suicide rates for Black people, and Black adolescents in particular, may be underestimated due to the misclassification of deaths by overdose and other causes as undetermined rather than as suicide (Ali, Rockett, Miller, & Leonardo, 2022; Panchal, Saunders, & Ndugga, 2022; Rockett et al., 2010). Suicide classifications have stringent corroborating evidence requirements including a documented history of mental health issues and treatment (Ali et al., 2022). Research indicates that Black youth are more likely to attempt suicide without traditional risk factors (Robinson, Whipple, Keenan, Flack, & Wingate, 2022). For example, at least one study found that Black youth were over four times more likely than White youth to attempt suicide without prior suicidal thoughts or plan (Romanelli, Sheftall, Irsheid, Lindsey, & Grogan, 2022). They were also found to endorse suicidal ideation without a previous mental health diagnosis or history of reporting symptoms of depression (Goodwill, 2024; Robinson et al., 2022; Sheftall et al., 2022; Talley et al., 2021).

Talley and colleagues (2021) argue that suicide rates for Black youth and young adults are likely underestimated as the significant stigma around mental illness and cultural pressure to be strong may increase the likelihood that Black people would end their lives in ways that would not be immediately identifiable as suicide, such as drug overdose or victim-precipitated suicide, wherein a person unconsciously or consciously and intentionally encourages their own death through violent confrontation. They note that, particularly in hyper-segregated urban environments, the hopelessness, fatalistic view of the future, rage, and aggression that result from exposure to racial discrimination, stress, and poor neighborhood conditions likely increase risky, antisocial, violent behavior that is itself a predictor of suicide. Given that rates of death by homicide for Black men has remained persistently and disproportionately high over the last 50 years (Council on Criminal Justice, 2023), and rates of death by overdose among Black adolescents increased by more than four times from prior to the pandemic to 2022 (Panchal, 2024), it is indeed likely that the suicide rates for Black youth are underestimated.

A number of scholars have argued that the risk factors for and pathways to suicide for Black youth differ from those found through decades of suicide research, in which Black people are underrepresented (Congressional Black Caucus, 2020; Meza et al., 2022; Opara et al., 2020). There is evidence that precipitating behaviors or symptoms that differ from traditional warning signs may be more common among Black boys than girls. Sheftall and colleagues (2022) found that Black girls who committed suicide were more likely than Black boys to have been diagnosed with depression or dysthymia and anxiety; to have a history of receiving mental health treatment; to have been receiving mental health treatment at the time of suicide; to have had a history of suicidal ideation, plans, and attempts; and to have left a suicide note. Black boys were more likely to have had a recent criminal or legal problem and to have been diagnosed with attention deficit hyperactivity disorder (ADHD). Research indicates that depression in Black children and adolescents is often masked by anger and is more likely to manifest as externalizing behaviors and be expressed as aggression (Assari, Gibbons, & Simons, 2018; Lu, Lindsey, Irsheid, & Nebbitt, 2017).

Scholars have argued that in addition to poverty and related neighborhood context, lack of adequate access to mental health services, sexual and gender minority status, and witnessing violence, exposure to racism and discrimination is an important risk factor for suicide among Black youth, which has empirical support. Walker and colleagues (2017) found that racial discrimination contributes to symptoms of depression and anxiety as well as subsequent suicide ideation and morbid ideation among African American youth. The effect of racism was mediated by symptoms of depression. Another meta-analysis involving Blacks found that racial discrimination was related to depression, anxiety, and suicidal ideation (Britt-Spells, Slebodnik, Sands, & Rollock, 2016). A study on a national sample of Black youth (age 13–17) found significant associations between increased racial discrimination and suicidal ideation that was consistent regardless of age, gender, or ethnicity (African American vs. Caribbean American; Assari, Lankarani, & Caldwell, 2017). Elisha and Collins (2022) found that increased incidents of racial discrimination were associated with higher rates of suicidal ideation and psychological distress among Black youth. Similar results have been found in longitudinal studies of national probability samples for experiences of major discriminatory events among Black adults (Oh, Waldman, Koyanagi, Anderson, & DeVylder, 2020). Another study found that exposure to subtle (e.g., being treated as inferior or less capable), but not overt, racial discrimination by their peers was associated with suicidal ideation for Black youth, and that suicidal ideation related to discrimination increased over time, controlling for depressive symptoms (Madubata, Spivey, Alvarez, Neblett, & Prinstein, 2022).

Despite the growing rates of suicide among Black youth, it is important to highlight that their overall rates remain comparatively low, suggesting that there are a number of protective factors that buffer the relationship between racial discrimination and suicide among Black youth. These include racial identity, racial socialization, and spirituality/religiosity (Robinson et al., 2022).

Racial Disparities in Mental Health Access and Care

Despite the evidence of generally good mental health among Black people as compared to White people in America, there are significant racial disparities in mental health that are not driven or explained by the high rates of PTSD and schizophrenia diagnosis. These disparities lead to a disproportionate impact of mental illness on the lives of Black individuals, families, and communities. Although Black people are statistically less likely to have mood, substance, and anxiety disorders, when they do, the disorders are more likely to be chronic, severe, and persistent (Alang, 2019; Cook et al., 2014; Guerra, 2022). These disparities are driven primarily by racially driven social determinants that have their roots in the socio-historical racial context of the United States, such as under/poor employment, income inequality, housing instability, racial residential segregation in high-poverty neighborhoods, and educational inequality, that increase exposure to adverse childhood experiences while simultaneously reducing access to mental health care (Shim et al., 2014).

As a result of reduced access to care, Black people are less likely to receive mental health treatment. According to the Substance Abuse and Mental Health Services Administration (SAMHSA), the majority (62.1%) of Black adults with any mental illness and 47.7% of Black people with serious mental illness received no treatment at all in 2022, and 77.5% of Black people over age 12 with substance use disorder did not receive any treatment at all (Substance Abuse and Mental Health Services Administration, 2023). Although the Affordable Care Act led to an increase in health insurance for people of all races, as of 2021, Black people remain less likely to be insured than White people (Hill, Ndugga, & Artiga, 2023). For those who are insured, regardless of race, mental health care is costly and difficult to access (Davenport, Darby, Gray, & Spear, 2023; Lopez, Kirzinger, Sparks, Stokes & Brodie, 2022). Furthermore, Black people are seven times more likely to live in high-poverty neighborhoods with limited or no access to mental health services (Guerra, 2022), are more likely to use the Emergency Room for mental health care than long-term supportive mental health services (Peters, Santo, Davis, & DeFrances, 2023), and are more likely to be in inpatient care (SAMHSA, 2023). When they do receive care, Black patients are less likely to receive treatment that is aligned with guidelines for care, and they are less likely to be included in research that determines guidelines and best practices for care (American Psychiatric Association, 2017).

The criminal justice system is the largest provider of mental health care in the United States (Ford, 2015). Black people with serious mental illnesses, specifically those with psychotic disorders, as well as those diagnosed with bipolar disorders, are more likely to be incarcerated than people of other races (APA, 2017). Given the extremely high rates of incarceration among Black populations, Black people are more likely to receive mental health care in a jail or prison than any other race, which is itself a source of significant trauma and increased mental illness.

Given the history of racism in the development of psychology, the associated lack of predominantly White psychologists with adequate training in providing racially culturally sensitive care, the dearth of licensed Black psychologists, as well as the significant disparities in the quality of the care Black people have access to, it is not surprising that Black people are reluctant to seek mental health treatment.

The State of Black Mental Health and Black Cultural Strengths

Perhaps the Black-White mental health paradox and the higher incidences of PTSD and schizophrenia, as opposed to other psychological disorders among Black people, is evidence that the stress and distress that Black people experience does not fit into the diagnostic criteria of disorder. Rather, it is a normal reaction to significant exposure to abnormal levels of racial insult, injury, and terror both currently and intergenerationally. Despite similar or lower rates of mental illness, Black people consistently endorse greater psychological distress (Barnes & Bates, 2017), as well as more feelings of hopelessness, sadness, and worthlessness than White people (Villarroel, Blackwell, & Jen, 2018). Barnes and Bates (2017) argued that it is possible that the comparably low rates of depression symptoms and disorder among Black people despite higher rates of psychological distress suggest that psychological distress better characterizes Black people's experiences than disorder. Psychological distress may be perceived as a normal response to stressors and adversity one faces in one's environment, whereas disorder implies dysfunction in the individual, assumed to be intrapsychic in nature.

Although PTSD is characterized as a mental disorder, it is one of the only disorders in the DSM that requires the identification of a specific precursor that causes symptoms. Similarly, we have argued elsewhere that the trauma Black people experience because of racial discrimination and harassment is better characterized as an injury rather than as a disorder (Carter & Pieterse, 2020).

The fact that paranoid symptoms along with clinicians' biased misperceptions of Black people's symptoms are some of the drivers of racial differences in schizophrenia diagnoses further suggests that there is a fundamental mismatch between Black people's experiences and the diagnostic system that exists to label and understand them. Few psychological disorders are biologically based diseases. Rather, most mental disorders are socially and culturally constructed by those who have historically dominated the development of mainstream psychology and psychiatry (Horowitz, 2002). As such, the definitions of normal vs. abnormal psychological functioning have consistently been determined by those with racial and social power who equate normal functioning as aligned with White, western cultural and social norms. The experiences of Black people in America fall well outside the bounds of what the mainstream predominantly White psychological institutions have been able to comprehend, let alone effectively address or treat. As a result, behaviors and symptoms that represent normal reactions to the extraordinary experiences, stressors, strains, and circumstances that result from structural racism have been systematically pathologized.

A recent clinical encounter provides an illustration of this phenomenon. A middle-aged Black man participating in a mandated psychological evaluation described a variety of experiences and exposures to explicit interpersonal racism over the last year and explained his hypervigilant reactions and behaviors in response. When asked to describe any symptoms he experienced as a result of these experiences, he denied symptoms. He reported being afraid for his life at times, experiencing healthy paranoia, and struggling to persevere in the face of such significant adversity and explicit threats to his well-being. Yet, he didn't feel that characterizing his reactions and responses as symptoms of depression or anxiety was appropriate. He remarked that, a White person would probably "throw themselves out a window" if they experienced everything he'd been through, but that as a Black man these experiences were just a part of life and were something he had learned to be strong enough to deal with. He described his family's history of significant achievement which placed them in positions where they had a close view of White power and corruption. This history provided him simultaneously with a keen awareness of acts of physical, psychological, and economic violence against Black people that are often kept out of view, as well as a sense of strength in being part of a family legacy of resisting, persevering, and achieving in the face of this violence. A psychologist with limited meaningful exposure to Black people outside of a public clinical setting, and minimal racial-cultural training that is decontextualized from the history of race in the United States, might have dismissed the man's experiences as fanciful, conspiracy-laden stories that were delusional and paranoid. Given this interpretation of the client's statements, along with the absence of mood disorder symptoms, the clinician would have likely diagnosed him as having a schizophrenia spectrum disorder.

The mental health of Black people in America is a complex story consisting of devastating examples of the consequences of structural racism, bias in institutions and systems, and significant disparities in access to care, along with remarkable strength in the face of unimaginable and intergenerational trauma and adversity. We argue that this remarkable strength takes the form of specific aspects of Black culture that have allowed Black Americans to survive and thrive over centuries.

Over the next few chapters, we will present the relationships between these aspects of Black culture, with the goal of further understanding the factors that have enabled survival and progress for Blacks in the United States. The positive and affirming components of Black racial identity, racial socialization, and racism-related coping, along with communalism and cultural spirituality have been associated with positive social and psychological outcomes in Blacks. Toward the latter part of the book, we turn our attention to the application of cultural values in a positive, strengths-based approach to counseling and psychotherapy with Black Americans and people of African descent. We argue that it is essential that mental health professionals, in fact, all people and professionals who work with Black people, grasp these critical aspects of Black culture. It is imperative that these cultural practices and beliefs, rather than social and cultural deficits, be comprehended to effectively deliver competent care and mental health treatment for Black Americans.

References

Alang, S. (2019). Mental health care among blacks in America: Confronting racism and constructing solutions. *Health Services Research, 54*, 346–355.

Ali, B., Rockett, I., Miller, T., & Leonardo, J. (2022). Racial/ethnic differences in preceding circumstances of suicide and potential suicide misclassification among US adolescents. *Journal of Racial and Ethnic Health Disparities, 9*(1), 296–304.

American Psychiatric Association (2017). *Mental health disparities: Diverse populations*. Washington, DC: American Psychiatric Association.

American Psychological Association (2021). *Apology to people of color for APA's role in promoting, perpetuating, and failing to challenge racism, racial discrimination, and human hierarchy in U.S.* Washington, DC: American Psychological Association.

Anglin, D., Ereshefsky, S., Klaunig, M., Bridgewater, M., Niendam, T., Ellman, L., DeVylder, J., Thayer, G., Bolden, K., Musket, C., Grattan, R., Lincoln, S., Schiffman, J., Lipner, E., Bachman, P., Corcoran, C. Mota, N. & van der Ven, E. (2021). From womb to neighborhood: A racial analysis of social determinants of psychosis in the United States. *American Journal of Psychiatry, 178*(7), 599–610.

Assari, S., Gibbons, F. X. & Simons, R. (2018). Depression among Black youth: Interaction of class and place. *Brain Sciences, 8*, 108–124.

Assari, S., Lankarani, M., & Caldwell, C. (2017). Discrimination increases suicidal ideation in Black adolescents regardless of ethnicity and gender. *Behavioral Sciences, 7*(4), 75–84.

Barnes D.M., Keyes K.M., Bates L.M., (2013). Racial differences in depression in the United States: how do subgroup analyses inform a paradox? *Social Psychiatry and Psychiatric Epidemiology, 48*(12), 1941–9. doi: 10.1007/s00127-013-0718-7.

Barnes, A. (2013). Race and schizophrenia diagnosis in four types of hospitals. *Journal of Black Studies, 44*(6), 665–681.

Barnes, D., & Bates, L. (2017). Do racial patterns in psychological distress shed light on the Black-White depression paradox? A systematic review. *Social Psychiatry and Psychiatric Epidemiology, 52,* 913–928.

Barnes, D., Keyes, K. & Bates, L. (2013). Racial differences in depression in the United States: how do subgroup analyses inform a paradox? *Social Psychiatry and Psychiatric Epidemiology, 48,* 1941–1949.

Becares, L., Nazroo, J., & Jackson, J. (2014). Ethnic density and depressive symptoms among African Americans: Threshold and differential effects across social and demographic subgroups. *American Journal of Public Health, 104*(12), 2334–2341.

Bridge, J. A., Horowitz, L. M., & Fontanella, C. A. (2018). Age-related racial disparity in suicide rates among US youths from 2001 through 2015. *JAMA Pediatrics, 172*(7), 697–699.

Britt-Spells, A. M., Slebodnik, M., Sands, L. P., & Rollock, D. (2018). Effects of perceived discrimination on depressive symptoms among Black men residing in the United States a meta-analysis. *American Journal of Men's Health, 12*(1), 52–63.

Carter, R. T. (1995). *The influence of race and racial identity in psychotherapy: Toward a racially inclusive model.* New York, NY: John Wiley & Sons.

Carter, R. T., & Pieterse, A. (2020). *Measuring the effects of racism: Guidelines for the assessment and treatment of race-based traumatic stress injury.* New York, NY: Columbia University Press.

Centers for Disease Control and Prevention. (2023). *Youth Risk Behavior Survey data summary & trends report 2011–2021.* Retrieved from www.cdc.gov/yrbs

Congressional Black Caucus. (2020). *Ring the alarm: The crisis of Black youth suicide in America.* Washington, DC.: Emergency Taskforce on Black Youth Suicide and Mental Health.

Cook, B. L., Zuvekas, S. H., Carson, N., Wayne, G. F., Vesper, A., & McGuire, T. G. (2014). Assessing racial/ethnic disparities in treatment across episodes of mental health care. *Health Services Research, 49*(1), 206–229.

Council on Criminal Justice (December, 2023). *Trends in homicide: What you need to know.* Retrieved from https://counciloncj.org/homicide-trends-report/

Cummings Center for the History of Psychology (2021). *Examining psychology's contributions to the belief in racial hierarchy and perpetuation of inequality for People of Color in the United States.* Cummings Center for the History of Psychology (proposed for vote to receive in Council of Representatives meeting scheduled for October 2021).

Davenport, S., Darby, B., Gray, T. J., & Spear, C. (December, 2023). *Access across America: State-by-state insights into the accessibility of care for mental health and substance use disorders.* Retrieved from https://www.milliman.com/en/insight/access-across-america-state-insights-accessibility-mental-health-substance-use

DeVylder J.E., Jun H.J., Fedina L., Coleman D., Anglin D., Cogburn C., Link B., & Barth R.P. (2018) Association of exposure to police violence with prevalence of mental health symptoms among Urban residents in the United States. *JAMA Netw Open.* 1(7): 30646377; PMCID: PMC6324385.

Dohrenwend, B. P., Turner, J. B., Turse, N. A., Lewis-Fernandez, R., & Yager, T. J. (2008). War-related post-traumatic stress disorder in Black, Hispanic, and majority White Vietnam veterans: The roles of exposure and vulnerability. *Journal of Traumatic Stress, 21*(2), 133–141.

Eack, S., Bahorik, A., Newhill, C., Neighbors, H., & Davis, L. (2012). Interviewer-perceived honestly as a mediator of racial disparities in the diagnosis of schizophrenia. *Psychiatric Services, 63*(9), 875–880.

Elisha, I., & Collins, R. (2022). Resilience: Within-group variations in the impact of racial discrimination on Black youth's mental health. *Behavioral and Brain Sciences, 9*(1), 11–17.

Erving, C., Thomas, C., & Frazier, C. (2019). Is the Black-White mental health paradox consistent across gender and psychiatric disorders? *American Journal of Epidemiology, 188*(2), 314–322.

Faber S.C., Khanna R. A., Michaels T.I., & Williams M.T. (2023). The weaponization of medicine: Early psychosis in the Black community and the need for racially informed mental healthcare. *Frontiers in Psychiatry, 14*, 1098292. doi: 10.3389/fpsyt.2023.1098292. PMID: 36846217; PMCID: PMC9947477.

Ford, E. (2015). First-episode psychosis in the criminal justice system: Identifying a critical intercept for early intervention. *Harvard Review of Psychiatry, 23*(3), 167–175.

Gara, M., Minsky, S., Silverstein, S., Miskimen, T., & Strakowski, S. (2019). A naturalistic study of racial disparities in diagnoses at an outpatient behavioral health clinic. *Psychiatric Services, 70*, 130–134.

Gara, M., Vega, W., Arndt, S., Escamilla, M., Fleck, D., Lawson, W., Lesser I., Neighbors H.W., Wilson D.R., Arnold L.M., & Strakowski S.M., (2012). Influence of patient race and ethnicity on clinical assessment in patients with affective disorders. *Archives of General Psychiatry, 69*(6), 593–600.

Geary, D. (September 14, 2015). The Moynihan Report: An annotated edition. *The Atlantic*. Retrieved on 8 April 2023 from

Gibbs, T., Okuda, M., Oquendo, M., Lawson, W., Wang, S., Thomas, Y., & Blanco, C. (2013). Mental health of African Americans and Caribbean blacks in the United States: Results from the National Epidemiological Survey on alcohol and related conditions. *American Journal of Public Health, 103*, 330–338.

Goodwill, J. R. (2024). Reasons for suicide in Black young adults: A latent class analysis. *Journal of Racial and Ethnic Health Disparities, 11*, 425–440.

Gray-Little, B., & Hafdahl, A. (2000). Factors influencing racial comparisons of self-esteem: A quantitative review. *Psychological Bulletin, 126*(1), 26–54.

Grossi, E. (2021). Truth in numbers? Emancipation, race, and federal census statistics in debates over black mental health in the United States, 1840–1900. *Endeavor, 45*(1–2), 10076.

Guerra, M. (2022). Black mental health: Black Americans' behavioral health needs outpace access to care. *RTI Health Advance*. Retrieved from https://healthcare.rti.org/insights/black-mental-health-and-behavioral-health-disparities

Guthrie, R. V. (1998). *Even the rat was white: A historical view of psychology.* Boston, MA: Allyn and Bacon.

Hill, L., Ndugga, N., & Artiga, S. (2023). Key data on health and health care by race and ethnicity. *KFF*. Retrieved from https://www.kff.org/racial-equity-and-health-policy/report/key-data-on-health-and-health-care-by-race-and-ethnicity/

Himle, J., Baser, R., Taylor, R., Campbell, R., & Jackson, J. (2009). Anxiety disorders among African Americans, blacks of Caribbean descent, and non-Hispanic whites in the United States. *Journal of Anxiety Disorders*, *23*, 578–590.

Horowitz, A. (2002). *Creating mental illness*. Chicago, IL: University of Chicago Press.

Hughes, M., Kielcolt, K. J. & Keith, V. (2022). Racial identity and the racial paradox in mental health. In M. Elliot (Ed.) *Research handbook on society and mental health* (pp.115–135). Northampton, MA: Edward Elgar Publishing.

Kardiner, A., & Ovesey, L. (1951). *The Mark of Oppression*. New York, NY: Norton.

Keyes, C. L. M. (2009). The Black-White paradox in health: Flourishing in the face of social inequality and discrimination. *Journal of Personality*, *77*(6), 1677–1705.

Li, K., Richards, E., & Goes, F. (2023). Racial differences in the major clinical symptom domains of bipolar disorder. *International Journal of Bipolar Disorders*, *11*(1), 17–24.

Lopez, L., Kirzinger, A., Sparks, G. & Brodie, M. (2022). KFF/CNN mental health in America survey. *KFF*. Retrieved from https://www.kff.org/mental-health/report/kff-cnn-mental-health-in-america-survey/

Louie, P., Upeneiks, L., Erving, C., & Tobin, C. (2022). Do racial differences in coping resources explain the Black-White paradox in mental health? A test of multiple mechanisms. *Journal of Health and Social Behavior*, *63*(1), 55–70.

Lu, W., Lindsey, M. A., Irsheid, S., & Nebbitt, V. E. (2017). Psyhcometric properties of the CES-D among Black adolescents in public housing. *Journal of the Society for Social Work and Research*, *8*(4), 2334–2315.

Lu, W., Silverstein, S., Mueser, K., Minsky, S., Bullock, D., Buchbinder, S., Chen, Q., Eubanks R., Guillaume-Salvant. (2023). Undocumented PTSD among African American clients with serious mental illness in a statewide mental health system. *Psychological Trauma: Theory, Research, Practice, and Policy*, *15*(5), 781–790.

Madubata, I., Spivey, L. A., Alvarez, G. M., Neblett, E. W., & Prinstein, M. (2022). Forms of racial/ethnic discrimination and suicidal ideation: A prospective examination of African American and Latinx youth. *Jorunal of Child & Adolescent Psychology*, *51*(1), 23–31.

Marcotte, D. E., & Hansen, B. (2023). *The re-emerging suicide crisis in the U.S.: Patterns, causes and solutions*. Working Paper 31242. Cambridge, MA: National Bureau of Economic Research.

McLaughlin, K. A., Alvarez, K., Fillbrunn, M., Green, J. G., Jackson, J. S., Kessler, R. C., Sadikova, E., Sampson, N. A., Vilsaint, C. L., Williams, D. R., & Alegría, M. (2019). Racial/ethnic variation in trauma-related psychopathology in the United States: A population-based study. *Psychological Medicine*, *49*(13), 2215–2226.

Mental Health America (n.d.). *Black and African American communities and mental health*. Retrieved from https://www.mhanational.org/issues/black-and-african-american-communities-and-mental-health

Metzl, J. (2009). *The protest psychosis*. Boston, MA: Beacon Press.

Meza, J. I., Patel, K. & Bath, E. (2022). Black youth suicide crisis: Prevalence rates, review of risk and protective factors, and current evidence-based practices. *Focus*, *20*, 197–203.

Misra, S., Etkins, O., Yang, L., & Williams, D. (2022). Structural racism and inequities in incidence, course of illness, and treatment of psychotic disorders among Black Americans. *American Journal of Public Health*, *112*(4), 624–632.

Oh, H., Waldman, K., Koyanagi, A., Anderson, R., & DeVylder. (2020). Major discriminatory events and suicidal thoughts and behaviors amongst Black Americans: Findings from the national survey of American life. *Journal of Affective Disorders*, *263*, 47–53.

Olbert, C. M., Nagendra, A., & Buck, B. (2018). Meta-analysis of Black vs. White racial disparity in schizophrenia diagnosis in the United States: Do structured assessments attenuate racial disparities. *Jorunal of Abnormal Psychology, 127*(1), 104–115.

Opara, I., Assan, M.A., Pierre, K., Gunn, J.F., Metzger, I., Hamilton, J., & Arugu, E. (2020). Suicide among Black children: An integrated model of the Interpersonal Psychological Theory of Suicide and Intersectionality Theory for researchers and clinicians. *Journal of Black Studies, 51*(6), 611–631.

Pamplin, J. R., & Bates, L. M. (2021). Evaluating hypothesized explanations for the Black-white depression paradox: A critical review of the extant evidence. *Social Science & Medicine, 281*, 114085.

Panchal, N. (February 6, 2024). Recent trends in mental health and substance abuse concerns among adolescents. *KFF*. Retrieved on March 23, 2024 from https://www.kff.org/mental-health/issue-brief/recent-trends-in-mental-health-and-substance-use-concerns-among-adolescents/

Panchal, N., Saunders, H., & Ndugga, N. (2022). Five key findings on mental health and substance use disorders by race/ethnicity. *KFF*. Retrieved from https://www.kff.org/racial-equity-and-health-policy/issue-brief/five-key-findings-on-mental-health-and-substance-use-disorders-by-race-ethnicity/

Peters, Z. J., Santo, L., Davis, D., & DeFrances, C. J. (2023). Emergency department visits related to mental health disorders among adults, by race and Hispanic ethnicity: United States, 2018–2020. *National Health Statistics Reports*; no 181. Hyattsville, MD: National Center for Health Statistics.

Pieterse, A. L., Carter R.T., Evans S. E., & Waters R., (2010) An examination of the relationship between racial/ethnic discrimination, and trauma-related symptoms in a college student population, Journal of Counseling Psychology, 57(3), 255–263.

Price, J. H., & Kubchandani, J. (2019). The changing characteristics of African American adolescent suicides, 2001–2017. *Journal of Community Health, 44*, 756–763.

Roberts, A. L., Gilman, S. E., Breslau, J., Breslau, N., & Koenen, K. C. (2011). Race/ethnic differences in exposure to traumatic events, development of post-traumatic stress disorder, and treatment-seeking for post-traumatic stress disorder in the United States. *Psychological Medicine, 41*(1), 71–83.

Robinson, W. L., Whipple, C. R., Keenan, K., Flack, C. E. & Wingate, L. (2022). Suicide in African American adolescents: Understanding risk by studying resilience. *Annual Review of Clinical Psychology, 18*, 359–385.

Rockett, W., Stack, De Leo, Frost, D., Walker, & Kapusta, N. (2010). Race/ethnicity and potential suicide misclassification: Window on minority suicide paradox? *BMC Psychiatry, 10*, 35–41.

Romanelli, M., Sheftall, A. H., Irsheid, S. B., Lindsey, M. A., & Grogan, T. M. (2022). Factors associated with distinct patterns of suicidal thoughts, suicide plans, and suicide attempts among US adolescents. *Prevention Science, 23*(1), 73–84.

Schwartz, R. C. & Blankenship, D. M. (2014). Racial disparities in psychotic disorder diagnosis: A review of empirical literature. *World Journal of Psychiatry, 4*(4), 133–140.

Sheftall, A. H., Vakill, F., Ruch, D. A., Boyd, R. C., Lindsey, M. A. & Bridge, J. A. (2022). Black youth suicide: Investigation of current trends and precipitating circumstances. *Journal of the American Academy of Child & Adoclescent Psychiatry, 61*(5), 662–675.

Shim, R., Koplan, C., Langheim, F., Manseau, M., Powers, R. & Compton, M. (2014). The social determinants of mental health: An overview and call to action. *Psychiatric Annals, 44*(1), 22–26.

Sibrava, N. J., Bjornsson, A. S., Pérez Benítez, A. C. I., Moitra, E., Weisberg, R. B., & Keller, M. B. (2019). Posttraumatic stress disorder in African American and Latinx adults: Clinical course and the role of racial and ethnic discrimination. *American Psychologist, 74*(1), 101–116.

Stone, D. M., Mack, K. A., & Qualters, J. (2023). Notes from the field: Recent changes in suicide rates, by race and ethnicity and age group – United States, 2021. *Morbidity & Mortality Weekly Report, 72*(6), 160–162.

Substance Abuse and Mental Health Services Administration. (2015). *Racial/ethnic differences in mental health service use among adults.* HHS Publication No. SMA-15-4906. Rockville, MD: Substance Abuse and Mental Health Services Administration.

Substance Abuse and Mental Health Services Administration. (2023). *Key substance use and mental health indicators in the United States: Results from the 2022 National Survey on Drug Use and Health* (HHS Publication No. PEP23-07-01-006, NSDUH Series H-58). Center for Behavioral Health Statistics and Quality, Substance Abuse, and Mental Health Services Administration. https://www.samhsa.gov/data/report/2022-nsduh-annual-national-report

Talley, D., Warner, S. L., Perry, D., Brissette, E., Consiglio, F. L., Capri, R., Violano, P. & Coker, K. L. (2021). Understanding situational factors and conditions contributing to suicide among Black youth and young adults. *Aggression and Violent Behavior, 58*, 101614.

Twenge, J. M. & Crocker, J. (2002). Race and self-esteeem: Meta-analyses comparing Whites, Blacks, Hispanics, Asians, and American Indians and comment on Gray-Little and Hafdahl (2000). *Psychological Bulletin, 128*(3), 371–408.

Tyrell, F., Neville, H., Causadias, J., Cokley, K., & Adams-Wiggins, K. (2023). Reclaiming the ntributions of Black scholars in psychology. *American Psychologist, 78*(4), 367–375.

Upeneiks, L., Louie, P., & Hill, T. D. (2023). The role of religious/spiritual struggles in the Black-White mental health paradox. *Society and Mental Health, 13*(2), 151–168.

Villarroel, M. A., Blackwell, D. L., & Jen, A. (2019). *Tables of summary health statistics for U.S. adults: 2018 national health interview survey. National Center for Health Statistics.* Retrieved from https://www.cdc.gov/nchs/nhis/SHS/tables.htm.

Warren, C. (2016) Black interiority, freedom, and the impossibility of living. *Nineteenth-Century Contexts, 38*(2), 107–121.

Willoughby, C. (2018). Running away from drapetomania: Samuel A. Cartwright, medicine, and race in the Antebellum South. *Journal of Southern History, 84*(3), 579–561.

Chapter 3

Black American Culture and the Debate about What It Is or Is Not

It was, and still is, the belief of most Americans that Black people, once captured and enslaved, lost any connection to their culture(s) of origin and relied on Whites as models for proper behavior and moral lives. In essence, since Africans came from a primitive place and lived as uncivilized people prior to their encounter with Europeans, Whites offered them ways to live; and it was through Whites' kindness, generosity, and example that Negros learned how to live and raise a family, and the value of hard work and moral behavior; or so goes the prevailing view. The short of it is that it was assumed that Black people in America had no culture of their own.

Herskovits (1990) outlines several scholars' perspectives on whether Black people had retained any of their African cultural ways and practices. He documents at least five arguments on this topic and presents the words of various scholars who held such views. In essence, the arguments were that: (a) Black people are by nature childlike and adaptable to their situations, they accepted their lot without protest or resistance unlike Native Americans who elected to die rather than be slaves; (b) the Africans who were captured and enslaved, more often than not, were less able, since the stronger avoided capture; (c) the diversity in language, customs, and traditions of the varied Africans captured and their distribution in the New World made it impossible for any common knowledge, behaviors, or understandings, to be held or shared; (d) in the unlikely instance that some who shared their heritage were together, in this instance, the low level of civilization and the savage ways of the African people meant that White cultural ways would prevail, and the Africans exposed to such superior culture, behavior, and language would willingly give up their traditional ways in the face of such superior people; and therefore, (e) Black people have, nor could have had, a past.

Herskovits provides examples of these points of view. For instance, E. Franklin Frazier stated, "Probably never before in history has a people been so nearly completely stripped of its social heritage as the Negros who were brought to America" (cited in Herskovits, 1990, p. 4). It was not possible, Frazier argues,

DOI: 10.4324/9781003083221-4

for African descendants to hold on to memories of the past or stories about Africa or their ancestors. Another scholar notes that

> in the course of capture, importation, and enslavement they lost every vestige of the African culture... the suppression of religious exercises. The supernatural beliefs and practices completely disappeared. The native forms of family life and codes and customs... were destroyed by the circumstances of slave life...
>
> (cited in Herskovits, 1990, p. 4)

Embree believed that the Negro was cut-off from his/her African home. He stated,

> The old African tribal society was completely destroyed... The only folkways that had elements in common for all the slaves were those they found about them in America... They began to speak English, to take up the Christian religion, to fall into labor patterns demanded by American needs and customs, to fit themselves as best they could into the mores of the New World.
>
> (cited in Herskovits, 1990, p. 5)

Scholars believed that whatever Africans knew was lost once they were brought to America. Stampp (1956) wrote,

> In Africa the Negroes had been accustomed to strictly regulated family life and a rigidly enforced moral code. But in America the disintegration of their social organization removed the traditional sanctions which had encouraged them to respect old custom. Here they found the whites organized into families having great social and economic importance but regulated by different laws (...) Actually, the differences [between Black and white family life] resulted from the fact that slavery inevitable made much of the white caste's family pattern meaningless and unintelligible – and in some ways impossible – for the average bondsmen. Here as at so many other points, the slaves had lost their native culture without being able to find a workable substitute and therefore lived in a kind of cultural chaos.
>
> (p. 340)

Webber (1978) writes about the slave experience and points out how many of the positions taken by historians, researchers, and scholars were not supported by an analysis of the writings and stories of Whites and Blacks about their experiences in the 1800s. He states, while naming the various scholars:

> Blacks under slavery were not the bearers of an inferior culture slowly enlightened and civilized by a superior culture (Ulrich Philips). Nor were

slaves torn from their African culture and placed in a slave system where their only choice was to mimic white culture (Stanley Elkins) or to slowly assimilate into white culture following the lead of favored house servants and slave artisans (E. Franklin Frazier, Robert Fogel, and Stanley Engerman). Slaves did not live in a state of cultural chaos "in a twilight zone between two ways of life (…) unable to obtain from either many of the attributes which distinguished man from beast" (Kenneth Stampp). The relationship between plantation blacks and whites was not so completely and reciprocally paternalistic that slaves were unable to "express the simplest human feeling without reference" to their masters (Eugene Genovese).

(p. xxi)

In fact, to the contrary of the positions taken by many of these scholars,

By the time of the Civil War black persons in America had actively fashioned a new culture from both the cultural foundation of their African past and the crucible of their experiences under slavery in the South. Slave culture has at its heart a set of cultural themes, forms of artistic expression, a religion, a family pattern, and a community which set blacks apart from whites and enabled them to form and control a world of their own values and definitions. The architects of this culture were these black men and women from whose common experiences sprang the songs and stories of American slavery, who nurtured the rites and beliefs of their community and religious life and who instilled in their children and other slaves the cultural themes of the community.

(Webber, 1978, pp. xxi–xxii)

Contrary to what some would have us believe, Blacks had a culture and sense of community that helped and aided in maintaining their dignity. In essence, as people discussed how to understand Black people's social and cultural status, three models emerged that have been and continue to be used to explain Black Americans' status and purported lack of culture: (a) Blacks were inherently biologically and socially inferior; (b) Blacks were culturally deprived; (c) and then it was argued that Blacks were culturally different. When a particular perspective is ascendant, it is used to explain situations and circumstances people find themselves in and it dominates other viewpoints and perspectives. The concepts and beliefs associated with a particular point of view are used for problem-solving and to create and establish policies, procedures, programs, and interventions directed at social, clinical, and mental health needs (Carter, 1995). The three points of view about Black culture that have been, and continue to be, used to explain the status of Africans and their decedents will be presented. Each of the three will be described and discussed in terms of how each particular point of view influenced what was known about the status of Black people.

It is important to remember that while each theory is primarily associated with a particular period in the nation's history, none of the three is confined by that period. Therefore, the models overlap, they have been employed simultaneously, and the assumptions derived from each are embedded, to varying degrees, in current social, political, health, and educational beliefs, institutions, policies, and practices.

Historical and Social Context

Through race, culture took on importance in human relations in the Americas and Caribbean Islands from the time Europeans landed on the shores of the New World and encountered Indigenous people. The explorers who were mostly White Europeans considered themselves superior in relation to the Indigenous people they met, and from the outset, they subjugated these people to their wishes, cultural practices, and beliefs.

Between 1619 and 1640, a small number of Africans were introduced into Virginia as "servants. Some, and perhaps most, of these early arrivals were freed after a limited term of service" (Fredrickson, 1988, p. 193). Horton and Horton (2005) observed that the

> Africans brought to Jamestown in the early seventeenth century were bound laborers, not all were treated as slaves (…) During the early colonial period, American concepts about race, slavery, and standards for race relations were still being formulated and were not yet as fixed as they would become in the eighteenth century.
>
> (p. 29)

Nevertheless, societal racism, the belief, and conviction that Africans and People of Color (Latinx, Native Americans, Asians) in general were inferior because of their race and should be treated accordingly, held sway in the early 17th century (1600s) (Horton & Horton, 2005). Sometime later, an explicit racial ideological justification based on the natural inferiority of Blacks was promulgated and used to maintain slavery in the 19th (1800s) century. That Africans (or Blacks) were inferior to Whites was written in the Bible and therefore was all the evidence needed for the subjugation of Africans, during the years when the British colonies were established and grew to be states of the Union. According to Kendi (2016), the Bible said that Black people "were the children of Ham, the son of Noah, and they were singled out to be black as the result of Noah's curse, which produced Ham's colour and the slavery God inflicted upon his descendants" (p. 21).

The issues of race and cultural differences are endemic and ingrained in all aspects of North American life, first as religious belief, then as custom, then as law, and then as tradition. As such, race has been fluid and constantly changing, yet deeply troubling, and nevertheless a central feature in the United States' social, political, and economic life. It was not possible for the field of mental health practice and theory to evolve without addressing race as well in efforts to deliver mental health services and treatment to Americans.

Members of American society believe that Whites are superior, and their culture is normative. As far as Black people were concerned, they had no culture, which cemented the notion of their inferiority and justified their low caste status. As Webber notes,

> Whites saw blacks as people without a culture, without... educational instruments of their own. Whites saw blacks as savages to be civilized, as children at best and animals at worst. As such, slaves were assumed to be without strong values or beliefs and certainly without a coherent culture or social organization of their own. For this reason, white teaching reflected an unstated attitude of filling up empty brains, of scratching white understandings upon the tabula rasa of limited black intelligence. That the content of white teaching directly contradicted understandings, attitudes, values and feelings which slaves had learned from birth in an educational process created and controlled by slaves themselves was a notion too incredible and too dangerous to entertain. To suggest that slaves were capable of molding their own culture, of fashioning and maintaining their own educational instruments would be to undermine the most fundamental arguments with which whites rationalized their enslavement of other human beings.
>
> (Webber 1978, pp. 249–250)

So, Whites did not entertain the idea that Blacks could have their own culture or attitudes that were not derived from White teaching. Instead, they constructed the notion that Blacks were like children, dependent upon them for care and guidance. At the same time, it should be noted that it would not be possible for a plantation to be profitable if the people who worked on it were not competent and able to perform myriad tasks, many requiring considerable skill and expertise. Nevertheless, uncivilized was the core notion about Black people. It seemed to help to think that their low status was natural and ordained by scripture.

Black people had to assimilate into White culture and society to obtain any measure of social participation. Fredrickson (1988) observes:

> On the whole [Americans have] treated blacks as if they were inherently inferior, and for at least a century of its history this pattern of rigid racial stratification was buttressed and strengthened by a widely accepted racist ideology. Although few would deny that explicit or ideological racism--the formal doctrine of inherent biological inferiority--became popular at a relatively late date in American history, recent historians have tended to see implicit... racism as having sprung up very early, partly because of certain pre-existing

European attitudes towards blacks which gave a special character to the natural antipathy of English settlers toward any people who were obviously strange and different.

(pp. 190–191)

According to Gould (1981), people did not question ideas or behaviors sur- rounding the notions of the race-based inferiority of Black people. He states,

... we must first recognize the cultural milieau of a society whose leaders and intellectuals did not doubt the propriety of racial ranking--with Indians below Whites and Blacks below everybody else... Under this universal umberella, arguments did not contrast equality with inequality. One group--we might call them "hard-liners" – held that Blacks were inferior and thus their biologi- cal status justified enslavement and colonization. Another group – the "soft- liners," if you will--agreed that Blacks were inferior, but held that a people's right to freedom did not depend upon their level of intelligence. Soft-liners held various attitudes about the nature of Black disadvantage. Some argued that proper education and standards of life could "raise" Blacks to a White level; others advocated permanent Black ineptitude.

(pp. 31–32)

The theory of Blacks' inferiority is based on beliefs of biological and genetic limitations that made Black people deficient in comparison to Whites. There- fore, any differences in behavior, culture, and mental status between Whites and Blacks, including the ones structured into society that limited Blacks' move- ment, educational access, and work options, could be attributed to the inher- ent inferiority of Blacks (Carter, 1995). Many noted scientific leaders from the country's most esteemed institutions have accepted and promoted the inferiority perspective.

The idea and belief that Africans were inferior to Europeans was a notion taken for granted during the country's colonial era since these people lacked cul- ture and proper Christian practices. Even so, the religious premise served their purposes well and was used effectively before it became necessary to develop a theory of biological and genetic inferiority in the 19th century (1800s). As was pointed out, before the 1800s, the notion and conviction that Africans were infe- rior was socially accepted custom and operated without question (Fredrickson, 1988). As Marger (1991) notes,

Although societal racism--the treatment of Blacks as if they were inher- ently inferior for reasons of race [and lack of culture]--dates from the late seventeenth (1600's) and early eighteenth (1700's) centuries, a rationalized racist ideology did not develop until the nineteenth (1800's) century.

(pp. 201)

In the 1800s, scientists and scholars set out to establish scientifically the specific characteristics of racial differences using biological and genetic information to show racial differences. Guthrie (1976) describes the early work of anthropologists who tried to classify races according to skin-color measures, hair texture, and lip thickness. It was during the 1800s that psychology emerged as a distinct science that studied the mind. And psychology used the well-established sciences of biology and physics, while joining applied anthropology (a branch of anthropology pre-occupied with classifying human races and groups) and ethnology (the specific discipline concerned with racial studies). Thus, the new science of psychology focused primarily on laboratory and experimental research and methods. In this way, psychology distinguished itself from anthropology as the field that studied human behavior using scientific methods. Guthrie (1976) points out,

> A number of racial classifications were made, all which placed the black [person] at the bottom of the human family hierarchy. The relative question of racial categorization reached such ridiculous proportions in the country that the U.S. senate commissioned Daniel and Elnora Folkmar to prepare for the Immigration Commission, a Dictionary of races or Peoples… The Black person in the dictionary of races was described as "belonging to the lowest division of mankind".
>
> (p. 32)

The classification system reflected the government's of identifying racial groups and promoting doctrine of Biological Determinism. The biological determinist doctrine, according to Gould (1981) "holds that shared behavioural norms, and the social and economic differences between human groups – primarily races, classes, and sexes – arise from inherited, inborn distinctions and that society, in this sense, is an accurate reflection of biology" (p. 20).

There were two ways to illustrate the tenants of biological determinism. One was to measure a single characteristic thought to reflect cognitive ability, that is, intelligence. The measurement of intelligence dominated the intellectual discourse about human worth since it was held up to be both scientific and objective. Yet, the proponents of measures of intelligence relied, on craniometry (the study of human skulls) during the 19th century and intelligence testing developed by psychologists during the 20th century. Both measures were used to demonstrate the inferiority of Blacks.

One of the leading contributors to craniometry was Samuel Morton. He believed that races could be ranked by the size of their skulls, revealing the capacity of the brain. He published three volumes: one in 1839 focused on Americans; a second in 1844 focused on Egyptian skulls; and a third in 1849 focused on his complete skull collection. Morton's work was highly acclaimed and hailed as "good" and credible science. His findings were "reprinted repeatedly during the nineteenth century as irrefutable 'hard' data on the mental worth of human races... whites on top, Indians in the middle, and blacks on the bottom" (Gould, 1981, pp. 53–54). In examining Morton's data, Gould (1981) reports several errors in calculations and omissions which make his findings questionable. Nevertheless, the belief in racial inferiority had taken hold. Other scientists held similar beliefs as Morton while engaged in their pursuits. For example, consider the work of Stanley Hall, the first president of the American Psychological Association, who stated in his book *Adolescence* (1904) that Black Americans were members of a race that was not civilized, and Louis Terman, a Stanford University professor and psychologist, who brought the Binet intelligence test to America, and proclaimed that People of Color could not be educated and that they could not be productive citizens due to their low levels of intelligence (Thomas & Sillen, 1972). Decades later, the same perspective is offered in new research, using different measures of intelligence, but with the same result. Arthur Jensen (1968) found that Blacks as a group, in comparison to Whites, were less intelligent. But one critic noted that social scientists were "detached from the reality of a history of racism in the United States and tend to view People of Color as inferior, troublesome, and a blemish to the notion of national excellence" (Cross, Long, & Ziafka, 1978, p. 263).

From a mental health vantage point, the inferior perspective led many to see Black people as not mentally sophisticated enough to suffer from mental disorders.

> There was also the common opinion that the "uncivilized races" (for example, Indians and Africans/Blacks) had much less or almost no mental illness. Psychological theorists asserted that the constitution of the civilized was initially more sensitive, more liable to creativity and, unfortunately, to insanity. The lower races, the uncivilized, were less emotionally sensitive and were thereby protected from the strains of progress. Therefore, the American Indian, the Black slave, and various other apparently sluggard groups gave evidence of their retardation through an almost embarrassing lack of insanity, the presence of which thus became considered as a sign of progress.
>
> (Willie, Kramer, & Brown, 1973, pp. 29–30)

Psychologists, psychiatrists, and other scientists embraced the doctrine of biological determinism. Belief in biological determinism led to the idea of biological limitations that naturally resulted in pathological personalities and limited social and psychological functioning in Blacks. It seems people wanted to have it both ways: the lack of culture meant less mental illness, yet as Blacks advocated for and gained more civil rights, then it turns out they exhibited greater psychological distress. According to one noted medical professional, psychologically normal Negroes were faithful and happy-go-lucky; the mentally afflicted ones raised disturbances (Carter, 1995). The idea here being that people who lacked culture or complex thought could not exhibit disruptions in their thoughts and behaviors.

In the first issue of the *Psychoanalytic Review* (1913), there were articles about the mental health of Black people. The editor of the issue observed,

> The existence side by side of the white and colored races in the U.S. offers a unique opportunity not only to study the psychology of a race at a relatively low cultural level, but to study their mutual effects on one another...
>
> (Evarts, 1913, p. 388)

So, Blacks were uncivilized people who had low levels of mental distress because they were too simple minded to have such concerns, and at the same time they were rebellious and troubled. The source for Blacks' problems had to do with their lack of family structure and cohesion. The family system was not the same as that of White families and thus it was judged to be a family system that was damaged and harmed its members.

Failed Family and Cultural Structures

For most societies, the family is the primary mechanism to transmit cultural learning and to help its members learn their respective roles and functions. Yet, for the Black family, the family structure was altered or was transient and, as such, was viewed as dysfunctional and chaotic, a state attributed to the Negro and their natural inability to cope without the guidance of their White masters. Stampp (1956) notes,

> Indeed, the typical slave family was matriarchal in form, for the mother's role was far more important than the father's. In so far as the family did have significance it involved responsibilities which traditionally belonged to women, such as cleaning house, preparing food, making clothes and raising children. The husband was at most his wife's assistant...
>
> (p. 344)

Therefore, regardless of how the Africans arrived in the country, and irrespective of their situations and circumstances, which they had little say about, they longed to be like Whites, and they actively worked to reject their past beliefs and values. Their families, such as they were, seemed to be characterized by chaos and instability. What was clear was their lack of a clear culture of their own, as many scholars would have us believe (Stampp, 1956). Yet, the arguments shifted from inferiority to cultural disadvantage, mostly based on their social status and the limits that came with their status. These limits meant that Blacks could not participate in the benefits of mainstream White cultural practices. Men could not be providers and heads of households; adults lacked education and knowledge of the society and its institutions; children were born to unwed mothers, who seldom held jobs and were dependent on society. Men were often criminals and unemployed, and so on. These myriad factors amounted to cultural disadvantage or deprivation.

Cultural Deprivation

Because of the social activism of the 1950s and 1960s there was a shift from the inferiority perspective about Blacks, that held sway for two centuries, to the cultural deprivation view. The focus on biological and genetic explanations for racial group differences changed, and scholars and policy makers took up the idea that social-class disparities and the caste structure of the United States contributed to racial group differences. Black people comprised a large segment of the lower social classes and thus the issues and problems associated with poverty became the focus for explaining racial group disparities. Ornstein notes that,

> Educators have become increasingly concerned with the need to study the problems of the poor, in order to remedy their plight. The term "disadvantaged" and its derivative terms "deprived" and "underprivileged" began to appear with reference to the children and youth of lower-class and minority groups.
>
> (1982, pp. 197)

The cultural deprivation theories used the social and biological meaning of race to create a criterion whereby non-White racial group members are compared to a White normative standard to demonstrate the various ways in which they were deprived or were different from the norm (Conant, 1961; Harrington, 1963; Riessman, 1962). In fact, this new emphasis seemed like a shift in perspective from that of inborn inferiority from God or nature since it was centered on social conditions. Yet the shift, while real, seems subtle a best. In both points of view, White culture and social structure are the norms to be attained.

The cultural deprivation view attributes the differences between White and Black people to cultural disadvantage, which effects not only social position but also variation in behavior and personality. Therefore, advocates for this perspective assert than inequality in economic, social, and cultural experiences are the basis for any psychosocial differences between the "races." While structural barriers are noted, they are given less emphasis or importance.

The emphasis on the characteristics of social disadvantage led to investigations, which continue to this day, that document the presumed abnormal effects of poverty and racial discrimination. Consequently, most typically report on such issues as juvenile delinquency, mental illness, emotional disturbance, lack of education, crime, poverty, and so forth. The focus on the outcomes surrounding a group's socio-political, economic, and psychosocial life presents a distorted picture of Black people that has become ubiquitous in the social and behavioral sciences and has persisted over time. As Black scholars have noted, the literature on Black people and families, for example, displays a "selected focus on the negative aspects" (Thomas & Sillen, 1972, pp. 46).

For instance, one government report, The Moynihan Report (1966; 2018), received considerable attention when it proclaimed that the Negro family existed in a tangle of pathology, which was characterized by a female headed family that blocks the growth of the Negro group. The report was issued, it was said, to improve the situation of Black families. Moynihan outlined various events and efforts that brought about what he called the Negro Revolution that was led by Black action and non-violent protests, federal legislation, administrative actions, and court rulings, and that promoted civil rights long-denied Black people. Yet, even acknowledging these facts, Moynihan states that "at the heart of the deterioration of the fabric of Negro society is the deterioration of the Negro family" (The Moynihan Report, 1966; 2018, p. 5).

The evidence he presented of this crisis, as it was called, was the high rate of divorce, births out of wedlock, female headed households, and welfare dependency, among other factors. The roots of the problems encountered by Negros were, according to Moynihan's report, slavery, Jim Crow, migration to Northern cities from the South, low pay, and lack of employment and education, which together created many of the problems described. Yet here we have a situation that worries Moynihan; while giving credit to the Negro, he also presents a dire situation that he calls a tangle of pathology. First, "that the Negro has survived at all is extraordinary... the Negro community has not only survived, but... entered national affairs... the highest testament to... the creative vitality of the Negro people" (p. 29). He notes further that the Negro community paid a high price for survival and centuries of racial oppression, in that they have been forced into a female-headed family structure and this has blocked the traditional role for Black men in the family. He notes that about half of Negro families were middle-class and adhered to the traditional family structure. But because they lived in proximity to the lower-class Negros, they were not free of the troubles the poorer ones had. He states,

> Half of the Negro community falls into the middle class. However, the remaining half is in desperate and deteriorating circumstance. Moreover, because [of] housing segregation it is immensely difficult for the stable half to escape from the cultural influences of the unstable one...
>
> (The Moynihan Report, 2018, p. 29)

So, even Black middle-class children are exposed to the "tangle of pathology" and the "disturbed group." The culture that best describes Black people according to Moynihan is one of poverty that deviates from mainstream White America.

Since, in American society, males are the leaders of society, families, and guardians of the culture, it is an aberration for women to head Negro families. In essence, Negros were failing because of their weak and pathological family struc-ture. While there is some recognition of the social forces that were and are aligned against Negros, yet the weak and dysfunctional family system is presented as the failings of Negros themselves. The system of slavery contributed to the destruc-tion of the Negro's will and ability to be free from dysfunction and pathology. It is also stated in this analysis that the Negro male is indicted for his failure to lead his community and family. There is little male guidance for children or for women, since many men cannot be adequate providers and bread winners. In this situation, the Negro family suffers and fails to contribute to society or their own well-being.

It is fair to argue that a life of poverty, discrimination, and exclusion from many social institutions (e.g., schools) has an adverse effect. Yet it is wrong to assume that all Black people have been permanently psychologically destroyed or crippled by the damaging influences of racism in our society or that they have no cultural moorings. It is important to identify the social obstacles that obstruct and hamper a group or an individual's potential. Yet this does not mean that the obstacles "crippled him/her." Thus, the studies on "cultural disadvantage" serve a useful purpose by calling attention to the obstacles that Black families face. But these studies often assumed that Black people have been and are inevitably and permanently damaged by the conditions associated with racial discrimina-tion such as, mental stress, poverty, lack of education, and poor health.

For example, Kardiner and Ovesey's influential book *The Mark of Oppression* (1951), which defines Black peoples' "basic personality" in terms of the stigma of racial oppression in America, was based on the psychoanalysis of 25 patients. Kardiner and Ovesey believed that racial oppression produced an unerasable mark which damaged the Black person's psyche. Furthermore, the authors con-tended that Blacks had no culture of their own and relied on White society for meaning and guidance in all things. These scholars argued that every personality trait of Black people, without exception, could be traced to their "difficult living conditions," resulting in "a wretched internal life" (Kardiner & Ovesey, 1951, p. 3). They contended that the oppression that Black people endure also denies Black people the possibility of developing a positive self-esteem:

> The Negro has no possible basis for a healthy self-esteem and every incentive for self-hatred. The basic Negro personality is a caricature of the correspond-ing White personality, because the Negro must adapt to the same culture and must accept the same social goals, but without the ability to achieve them.
>
> (Kardiner & Ovesey, 1951, p. 317)

These conclusions and generalizations were based on people who were dis-turbed. They state,

> Our contrast control is the American White man; we require no other con-trol. Both he and the Negro live under similar cultural conditions with the

exception of a few easily identifiable variables existing for the Negro only. This means we can plot the personality differences of the Negro in terms of these variables against the known personality of the White.

(Kardiner & Ovesey, 1951, p. 11)

Kardiner and Ovesey ignored healthy Blacks or assumed no psychologically healthy Blacks existed. According to these authors, oppression had crippled every Black person, each of whom failed in social relations with other Blacks because every Negro they encountered projected self-contempt.

Kardiner and Ovesey's work was roundly criticized for not acknowledging the variety of individual responses to oppression and stress. Kenneth Clark (1965) noted that while people forced to live under circumstances and conditions that communicate to them a complete lack of respect or dignity will certainly come to doubt their self-worth, this impact on self-esteem is not necessarily uniform across all members of the group. He argued that while some may experience reduced self-esteem, others will develop "appropriate anger at the injustices they suffer and focus their energies on the struggle against oppression" (pp. 63–64). He continued that others might have different responses in different situations, some unhealthy and some healthy.

Given the social-political-historical and contemporary salience of race in our society, it seems reasonable to conclude that it is not possible to be socialized into this society without being presented with myriad opportunities to internalize beliefs and attitudes about one's racial group. In the sciences and popular culture, the message is that anything other than White society and family structure is unacceptable as the "American way." Black Americans and Native Americans, as well as members of other racial groups, have for centuries been the repository for negative projections, distortions, and destructive myths about their race, and through race, their cultures (Williams & Mohammed, 2013).

Such myths and beliefs have been internalized by most Americans; consequently, these messages and the boundaries due to race are maintained to this day. No person or professional group – including mental health professionals – are immune to the infectious influence of racism. Few mental health training programs adequately equip their developing professionals with the knowledge, attitudes, and skills that would allow them to work across the racial boundaries that exist in our society. Consequently, much of what is known about Blacks is overwhelmingly negative. We know that talk about race stimulates intense emotions and tremendous confusion. We contend that this is by design; if it is difficult to talk about a thing, then it is not possible to know about it or to come to understand how it works.

Some have argued (e.g., Sue, Sue, Neville, & Smith, 2019) that Black culture is not deprived or absent but different from that of White culture. More important, Black culture evolved from the same conditions of oppression that brought about the ideas that Black people had no culture. The truth is, Black culture was always visible, it is/was just devalued and denigrated. For instance, let's consider the female-headed household. When social circumstances changed, and divorce and female-headed households became more frequent and common among White families, the reference to families of this type shifted to an acceptable reference, of single parent households, and these familes were/are not seen as damaged or pathological.

Cultural Difference

During the last several decades, policymakers and social scientists have argued that cultural difference is not synonymous with deprivation. The cultural difference viewpoint holds that psychological and behavioral differences between Whites and People of Color are best explained in terms of the various influences related to racial and cultural background. Difference advocates reject the notion that race and culture for People of Color is lacking. At the outset of the movement to recognize that Black people had distinct cultural practices and values, culture was synonymous with racial groups. The argument was that members of distinct racial groups had retained and developed their own unique cultural patterns, in part, due to their isolation and segregation from mainstream society. Social scientists established the cultural difference ideas by focusing their efforts on describing the cultures of various historically disenfranchised American racial groups and studying the various psychological and social variables associated with their specific experiences. It needs to be noted that as time passed, the term "culture" was broadened and is now called "diversity," which includes *any* difference that is currently considered cultural, although many of these memberships are best understood as reference groups rather than a distinct cultural group, since they are all members of American or related cultural groups (e.g., age, social class, gender, sexual orientation, religion, and ableness). In terms of mental health practice, the impact of the cultural difference perspective has been that mental health training and practice settings have developed interventions and instructional guidelines that include some aspects of the racial-cultural experience of Americans of Color.

There has been increased and intensified interest in cross racial-cultural issues in many spheres of American life, as evidenced by many books and research activities in this area. The number of texts, books, and journal articles has increased. Authors, scholars, and researchers have offered, and continue to offer, guidelines, suggestions, research findings, and clinical observations about the status, circumstances, and needs of racial-cultural group members (i.e., Native Americans, Latinx, Asian Americans, African Americans or Blacks, and immigrants and refugees; Carter, 2016). Much of the diversity literature has involved awareness-building, increasing participants' knowledge regarding racial groups' cultures, and building awareness to enhance cross-racial effectiveness (Sue, Sue, Neville, & Smith, 2019). So, there is now some recognition that Blacks have a culture that differs from Whites, yet in some respects, the belief that racial disparities dictate the behavioral patterns of Blacks remains.

Cultural Values and Mental Health

Many scholars have suggested that in psychotherapy relationships, conflicts may arise due to the differing racial-cultural values of the participants. Stewart and Bennet (1991) argue that culture consists of patterns of thinking and behavior that can be very difficult for people to develop awareness of because they are so deeply internalized. One's "reality" is based on deeply held cultural assumptions and values that define "the goodness and desirability of certain actions or attitudes," thereby "prescrib[ing] which actions and ways of being are better than others" (p. 14). Cultural values are thought to influence several aspects of the psychotherapy process. Writers have argued that therapists and mental health professionals must understand their patient's culture, if they are different or have varied reference group memberships, to provide effective services. More specifically, Carter and Pieterse (2020) describe several aspects of the psychotherapy relationship that are influenced by the participants' respective race and cultures. These include: the therapist's and patient's racial/cultural backgrounds; the assumptions that each in the therapy dyad make about the nature of illness, helping, relationships, and the source of their problems; and how the environment where therapy takes place is influenced by social norms and the dominant racial-cultural group's beliefs and practices. As can be seen, many elements of the therapeutic relationship are subject to racial-cultural socialization factors and professional training. A person's expectations, perceptions, feelings, thoughts, behaviors, and the way he or she organizes information represent his/her racial/cultural learning, in which the family and the social-political environment are the primary sources of such learning.

Katz (1985) and Carter (2005) describe White Americans' common racial/cultural values and beliefs, and they suggest that White culture is the integration of ideas, values, and existential propositions from White European ethnic groups in the United States. Thus, White culture is characterized by adherence to principles and practices governed by notions of rugged individualism such that the individual's needs come before that of the group or family; self-expression is focused on action or doing defined by an individual's external achievements; decision-making is determined by the majority when Whites are in power--otherwise, a top-down structure is used usually when Whites are at the top; language-based communication relies on written and "standard" English forms and devalues oral traditions and languages that are not standard English; the temporal focus is on what is to come or the future and in this way time is treated as a commodity; the religious system is based on Christian ideals, and social customs (e.g., holidays) are founded on celebrations of Christian religions, White Euro-American history, and male leaders; family systems are male-centered and tend to be nuclear including immediate members of the family; and aesthetics are European-based and emphasize music and art from European society.

Katz (1985) contends that White American cultural values are the basis of theories of human development and personality that guide mental health practice:

> The similarities between White culture and the cultural values that form the foundations of traditional counseling [psychotherapy] theory and practice exist and are interchangeable. Because counseling theory and practice developed out of the experience of White therapists and researchers working almost exclusively with White client systems, it comes as no surprise that the profession reflects White cultural values. The continued use of this theory base predicated on one world view, one set of assumptions concerning human behavior, and one set of values concerning mental health limits our abilities to be effective cross-culturally.
>
> (Katz, 1985, p. 619)

Therefore, what happens in instances when people in therapy are from and employ different racial-cultural practices, and what if their thinking and emotions vary as well?

Black American Cultural Values

Some scholars believe that, because of their low social status, members of non-dominant racial groups develop negative attitudes and beliefs toward themselves and their racial group. Jones (2003) and other scholars argue that this is not so; he contends that oppressed people can have positive regard for themselves and their group. And he presents an African-based cultural worldview associated with positive psychological well-being for Black Americans.

For Jones, a peoples' worldview is comprised of both psychological and cultural elements (i.e., having existential propositions that guide behavior and attitudes). With both elements, one's worldview is reflected in their ways of thinking, in emotional expression, and behavioral actions that are shared by a people and communicated through symbols, ideas, and values which serve as guides for action. Jones states that present-day Black American culture is connected to their African origins. The way Black culture evolved is best described by two processes: one reactionary (i.e., the practices and values that developed in reaction to their lives in America), and the other evolutionary (i.e., the practices and values that existed prior to being captives).

Black people had to cope and adapt (react) to their circumstances as oppressed captives and had to do so over time (evolve new ways to act). They had to learn how to handle the loss of their freedom and how to deal with being dehumanized. It was the evolutionary mechanism that held the core African cultural ethos. That is, these aspects of their being enabled "the recovering [of] certain forms of physical and psychological freedom" (Jones, 2003, p. 223), and set the basis for regaining humanity in a hostile setting. Blacks' struggle for freedom and opportunity is motivated by the desire for self-protection (survival) and self-enhancement (growth). Africans and their descendants used their cultural socialization and psychological perspective prior to their arrival in the New World to adapt. For Jones, these cultural patterns are/were comprised of Time, Rhythm, Improvisation, Orality, and Spirituality or TRIOS, among others (Jones, 2003).

Time in African culture is present and past-oriented. Rhythm characterizes most activities and places them in an internal and external context that allows for the activity to have shape, energy and psychological meaning. Thus, rhythm connects the person to his or her environment. Improvisation is like rhythm in that it is both a personal and social form of expression and connects the person and environment. It allows the person to control and structure self-expression while interacting with others. He or she can find or create ways of expressing self that emerge in the moment, and yet are still unique and personal. Oral practices capture the power of spoken words, stories, and songs which communicate the group's beliefs. It is this aspect of the culture that connects the present with the past and is the means through which the significance of life's events is communicated. Spirituality, a central element of African culture, is the conviction that there are forces that exist beyond humans that affect the things that happen daily. Thus, multiple forces are at play that determine or explain events and it is not possible to know such forces since many are beyond what humans can comprehend,

> Africans believed that the spirits of their ancestors had great power over their lives, in this as in every aspect of African life, the kinship group was important... a similar high regard was held for the spirits that dwelt on the family land, in the trees, and rocks.
>
> (Franklin & Moss, 2000, p., 25)

They observe further that

> survival of African culture is obvious. When it comes to measuring or evaluating the persistence of African culture in the New World and especially in the United States the problem becomes much more difficult. It can be seen in the language. . . In literature the persistence of African culture can be seen in the folk tales that have been recorded by American writers. In religion, some beliefs, practices, and musical forms can be traced to the African background. In work, in play, in social organizations and in various aesthetic manifestation there are some evidences of African culture.
>
> (Franklin & Moss, 2000, p. 32)

Jones (2003) states,

> The ecological challenges of slavery engaged the patterns of TRIOS in adapting-coping sequences. In this oppressive environment, the opportunities

for expression, social organization, and control demanded each of the TRIOS elements. Creole or pidgin languages emerged to enable oral communication among people who may have spoken somewhat different languages or dialects... Improvisation was a means of creating linguistic meaning that were privileged among the native speakers, and thus, shielded the speaker from adverse consequences when speech was heard by a person hostile to his well-being. Expression of the human spirit was made possible through music, song, and dance [rhythm]. Social organization was necessarily improvised as were strategies for control of self-protective collective action. The cultural patterns became practical means of coping, adapting, and surviving. Thus, humanity was preserved through employing known and deep cultural principles and practices.

(p. 228)

More importantly, the nature of being dehumanized brought forth strong and powerful actions on the part of Black people, as Berlin, Favreau, and Miller (1998) observed:

But slavery's brutality inhered less in the brutish and sadistic outbursts than in the routine, systematic, violence of slaveowners found necessary to reduce men and women to things (. . .) *Violence called forth powerful resistance. Slavery's heroes and heroines should no more be forgotten than the adversity they confronted... it is equally important to appreciate the silent, everyday heroics of the men and women who stoically took the slaveholders worst and quietly educated their children to take back piecemeal what the "masters" had appropriated... In short, men and women recognized their inability to overthrow slavery, taught their children to survive until their moment arrived.*

(emphasis added, pp. xxii–xxiii)

In addition to TRIOS, over the centuries Black people exercised significant psychological resolve and taught and practiced several other cultural values, such as beliefs in the value of community, racial socialization, racism-related coping, and racial identity status development (i.e., psychological orientation to one's race). Slave narratives show how life in the slave quarter community occurred and what was important, as documented by Webber (1978),

Though the chains with which whites controlled black bodies were very real, try as they might, whites could not control black minds. These [Black minds] were molded from birth in an educational process created and managed by the [Black] quarter community. By passing their unique set of cultural themes from generation to generation, the members of the quarter community were able to resist most white teaching, set themselves apart from white society, and mold their own cultural norms and group identity. While legally slaves, the black men, women, and children of the quarter community successfully protected their psychological freedom and celebrated their human dignity.

(p. 262)

Webber documents and describes several cultural themes endemic to the slave quarter community. These communities varied in size and type but were ubiquitous in American society. It is also where Black culture was nourished and prospered. Webber (1978) states,

> By the time of the Civil War black persons in America had actively fashioned a new culture from both the culture foundation of their African past and the crucible of their experiences under slavery in the South. Slave culture has at its heart a set of cultural themes, forms of artistic expression, a religion, a family pattern, and a community structure which set blacks apart from whites and enabled them to form and control a world of their own values and definitions. The architects of this culture were the field hand masses and their house and town allies. It was these black men and women from whose common experiences sprang the songs and stories of American slavery, who nurtured the rites and beliefs of their community and religious life and who instilled in their children, and other slaves the cultural themes of their community.

(pp. xii–xiii)

The themes established in the 19th century remained active into the 21st century as scholars noted. Black American cultural values are characterized by beliefs in a group-focused form of sharing, spirituality, present time orientation, and harmony-with-nature (Carter & Helms, 1987). Hill (1972) suggests that while slavery and racial oppression attempted to destroy the existence of Black families, the family survived because of their strong kinship bonds, flexibility of family roles, and high value placed on religion, education, and work. Black families, according to Hines and Boyd-Franklin (1982) and Boyd-Franklin (2006), are organized around extended kinship networks which may include blood and non-related persons. Family roles and responsibilities, jobs, and functions are often interchanged among family members as was the case in the past, and strangely enough were deemed by outsiders to be signs of pathology. This sharing of roles and functions occurs across generation and gender roles. Blacks also participate in social equalizer roles and activities in the community or churches. These types of activities are used by Blacks to reinforce their self-worth. The cultural values of Blacks and their families may lead them to mental health professionals who might not share or know Blacks' worldview.

Black Culture and Treatment Issues

The Black client may enter therapy with several defenses associated with race. She may have anxieties about the therapist, regardless of the race of the therapist. Sanders Thompson, Bazile, and Akbar (2004) noted that Blacks view therapists (White or Person of Color) as reflecting the perspectives of mainstream American society. Thus, the Black client may be less forthcoming, less verbal, and less likely to self-disclose. They may perceive their therapists as being distant and unable to relate to their experiences. More importantly, many Black clients may simply desire a therapy relationship in which they can self-disclose without educating. The Black client also may be beset with anxieties associated with his or her Blackness and status in American society. Consequently, the client may tend to be less active and involved and may react negatively to some interventions attempted by the therapist. In such instances, one would expect that either the client would terminate therapy early or leave with little symptom relief.

It has been argued by some authors that because of their shared experience of oppression and discrimination and their shared racial background, Black mental health professionals are better suited to treat Black clients. However, this may not be so. A criticism of mental health training programs is that they do not train mental health professionals to be racially-culturally competent. Black therapists are usually trained to work with White clients. So, racial-cultural differences are seldom included in the techniques and theory of human development offered in mental health training programs. Therefore, Black and therapists of Color are subject to the same pitfalls as are White therapists when working with Black clients.

Conclusion

During their training, clinicians are often taught about the pitfalls attendant with lack of racial-cultural knowledge, such as failure to examine one's own racial background and the foundations of one's professional training. However, many psychotherapists and mental health professionals are still poorly equipped to handle race and Black culture in psychotherapy. In fact, some clinical scholars have explained the cultural values, patterns, and behavioral distinctions described above as important aspects of therapy impasses. As Abel, Metraux, and Roel (1987) point out, the treatment situation characterizes the importance or salience of cultural patterns:

> It is important to note that cultural patterns do not themselves create transference and countertransference--the conditions of treatment do that. Rather, any issue from the patient's past (for example being misunderstood as a child) can be exacerbated by cultural factors (for example, having a therapist from a different culture who does not understand the influence of a particular cultural factor on a patient's life). Cultural factors, then, are persistent issues

in psychotherapy. Language, religion, time orientation... become ways the patient's conflicts surface or disguise themselves to help or hinder the therapeutic work.

(pp. 154–155)

Thus, cultural factors produce misunderstandings by the therapist and can hamper the therapy relationship. Therapists who operate from a worldview with relatively fixed expectations and role behaviors might expect self-disclosure from patients and may presume that the patient is autonomous from their family. They may expect that the past, present, and future will be appropriately distinguished such that the client will strive for a life in which the future is different from the present. The client is supposed to see the therapist as a powerful, knowledgeable expert. The therapist sees his or herself also as responsible, able to judge what is real for his or her patient, capable of objectivity or neutrality, and using a non-judgmental stance. The expectation is that the therapist will not bring his or her own personal values into treatment and can therefore aid the client to uncover important aspects about past and present in the service of the client's future. Yet, when cultural values conflict, as reflected in racial dynamics, therapists and patients encounter innumerable problems. It seems that under these circumstances, race and culture introduce difficulties that must be overcome or resolved before effective therapeutic work can occur.

The therapy literature suggests that race and culture impact therapy as the racial attitudes of both the therapist and the client affect therapy. What we know from the literature is how the race of clients creates problems in treatment. What is unclear from the literature is what characteristics of patients and therapists predict or determine specific types of influences. How does one determine if a client is operating from a particular cultural worldview?

To date, despite the vast literature on the topic of race or culture in therapy, little consistent and reliable information is available to mental health professionals. Barriers exist that prevent a clear set of theoretically derived guidelines for comprehending Black cultural practices that influence psychotherapy and treatment interventions. Some barriers that hinder understanding of the influence of race; are intellectual, some emotional, and some socio-political. When social scientists and mental health professionals attempt to explain race-related social and psychological boundaries, divisions, and conflicts, they typically engage in an intellectual shell game in which they substitute economics, education, values, and/or communication styles for race. The tendency to substitute something else for race reflects the strength of the emotional, social, political, and psychosocial resistance most Americans have been taught when it comes to examining and understanding racial-cultural issues in our society. Generally, racial-cultural differences and perspectives, when discussed, are often described in emotional terms. According to White American cultural traditions, this renders the topic inaccessible to enlightened discourse since emotionalism is considered irrational and therefore not subject to rational discourse. Hence, intellectual boundaries have been created to limit meaningful discourse and hamper understanding about race and the cultural beliefs of Black people.

Another obstacle particular to psychology and mental health is the absence of theory and race's marginal status in human development and personality theory. The lack of theory-based models keeps the discourse about race speculative and emotional and prevents insight. Another obstacle is the tendency to use racial-cultural group categories or membership as the primary unit of analysis. This practice implicitly promotes a belief that racial issues are the exclusive province of Black people, while most Whites deny or are unaware of the racial-cultural context in which they live. Therefore, when conflicts or cultural differences arise, racial issues are generally construed as marginal or as a concern for the non-dominant group member. For some, racial issues and conflicts would not exist if People of Color did not raise them. The assumption seems to be that White Americans do not as individuals need to consider racial issues as important to them. Yet, if race is one-sided, how do we understand the influence of race and culture in our work as helping professionals?

The psychological significance of race and culture for everyone varies as a function of his or her interpretation of the socialization and psychosocial developmental processes. The psychological significance of race and one's culture affects how one thinks, feels, acts, and consequently sees the world and others who are in the same and different racial groups. Because race has personal meaning for everyone, it follows that it would matter in interpersonal and helping relationships.

Race and cultural issues in American society and specifically in the mental health profession are complex and multi-leveled. The complexity associated with racial-cultural issues stems from United States history and how these issues have been integrated into the social fabric of our society. Mental health professionals and other helpers continue to perpetuate the sociocultural milieu surrounding culture and race. One reason for perpetuating racial-cultural barriers is the tendency of most people to approach these issues as absent history and without any theoretical basis.

References

Abel, T. M., Metraux, R., & Roll, S. (1987). *Psychotherapy and culture* (rev. ed.). Albuquerque: University of New Mexico Press.

Berlin, I., Favreau, M., & Miller, S. F. (1998). *Remembering slavery*. New York, NY: The New Press.

Boyd-Franklin, N. (2006). *Black families in therapy: Understanding the African American experience*. New York: Guildford.

Carter, R. T. (1995). *The influence of race and racial identity in the psychotherapy process: Toward a racially inclusive model*. New York, NY: Wiley.

Carter, R. T. (2005). A cultural-historical model for understanding racial-cultural competence and confronting dynamic cultural conflicts: An introduction. In R. T. Carter (Ed.),

Handbook of racial-cultural psychology and counseling: Training and practice (Vol. 2) (pp. ix–xxvi). Hoboken, NJ: Wiley.

Carter, R.T., (2016). The road less traveled: Research on race, In J.M., Casas, Suzuki L.A., Alexandria, C.M., & Jackson, M.A., (Eds. 4th Edition), (pp. 71–80) *The Handbook of* Multicultural Counseling. Thousand Oaks, CA: Sage.

Carter, R. T., & Helms, J. E. (1987). The relationship of Black value-orientations to racial identity attitudes. *Measurement and Evaluation in Counseling and Development, 19*, 185–195.

Carter, R. T., & Pieterse, A. (2020). *Measuring the effects of racism: Guidelines for the assessment and treatment of race-based traumatic stress injury.* New York, NY: Columbia University Press.

Clark, K. B. (1965). *Dark ghetto.* New York, NY: Harper & Row.

Conant, J. B. (1961). *Slums and suburbs.* New York: McGraw-Hill.

Cross, D. E., Long, M. A., & Ziafka, A. (1978). Minority cultures and education in the United States. *Education and Urban Society, 10*, 263–276.

Evarts, A. B. (1913). Dementia precox in the colored race. *Psychoanalytic Review, 1*, 388–403.

Franklin, H. J., & Moss, A. A. (2000). *From slavery to freedom: A history of African Americans* (8th Ed.). Boston, MA: McGraw Hill.

Fredrickson, G. M. (1988). *The arrogance of race. Historical perspectives on slavery, racism and social inequity.* Middleton, CT: Wesleyan University Press.

Gould, S. J. (1981). *The mismeasure of man.* New York: Norton.

Guthrie, R. V. (1976). *Even the rat was white: A historical view of psychology.* New York: Bantam.

Harrington, M. (1963). *The other America.* Baltimore: Penguin.

Herskovits, M. J. (1990). *The myth of the Negro past.* Beacon Press.

Hill, R. B. (1972). *The strengths of black families.* New York: Emerson Hall.

Hines, P. M., & Boyd-Franklin, N. (1982). Black families. In M. McGoldrick, J. K. Pearce, & J. Giordano (Eds.), *Ethnicity and family therapy.* New York, NY: Guilford Press.

Horton, J. O., & Horton, L. E. (2005). *Slavery and the making of America.* New York, NY: Oxford University Press.

Jensen A. R. (1968). Social class, race, and genetics: Implications for education. *American Educational Research Journal, 5*(1), 1–42.

Jones, J. M. (2003). TRIOS: A psychologcial theory of the African legacy in American culture. *Journal of Social Issues, 39*(1), 217–242.

Kardiner, A., & Ovesey, L. (1951). *The mark of oppression.* New York, NY: Norton.

Katz, J. H. (1985). The sociopolitical nature of counseling. *The Counseling Psychologist, 13*(4), 615–624.

Kendi, I. X. (2016). *Stamped from the beginning.* New York, NY: Nation Books.

Marger, M. (1991). *Race and ethnic relations: American and global perspectives* (2nd Ed.). Belmont, CA: Wadsworth/Thomson Learning.

Moynihan, D. (1966; 2018). The Moynihan Report: The Negro family – the case for national action. *Office of Policy Planning and Research of U.S. Department of Labor.* New York: Cosimo Classics.

Ornstein, A. (1982). The education of the disadvantaged: A 20-year review. *Educational Researcher, 24*, 197–211.

Riessman, F. (1962). *The culturally deprived child.* New York: Harper & Row.

Sanders Thompson, V. L., Bazile, A., & Akbar M. (2004). African Americans' perceptions of psychotherapy and psychotherapists. *Professional Psychology: Research and Practice, 35*(1), 19–26. doi: 10.1037/0735-7028.35.1.19.

Stampp, K. M. (1956). *The peculiar institution.* New York, NY: Vintage Books.

Stewart, E.C. & Bennett, M.J., (1991). *American Cultural Patterns: A cross-cultural perspective.* Nicholas Brealey Publishing.

Sue, D. W., Sue, D., Neville, H., & Smith, L. (Eds.). (2019) *Counseling the culturally diverse: Theory and practice* (8th Ed.). Hoboken, NJ: Wiley.

Thomas, A., & Sillen, S. (1972). *Racism and psychiatry.* New York: Carol Publishing.

Webber, T. L. (1978). *Deep like the rivers: Education in the slave quarter community, 1831–1865.* New York, NY: W.W. Norton.

Williams, D. R., & Mohammed S. A. (2013). Racism and health I: Pathways and scientific evidence. *American Behavioral Scientist, 57*(8), 1152–1173. doi: 10.1177/0002764213487340.

Willie, C. V., Kramer, B. M., & Brown, B. S. (1973). *Racism and mental health.* Pittsburgh: University of Pittsburgh Press.

Chapter 4

Digging Deeper into Black Americans' African Cultural Legacy

Reference Group Identity and Socialization

In this chapter, we will focus on identity development and cultural awareness. We will also discuss Africans' cultural values before European contact, Black Americans' beliefs and values, and how they evolved racial identity, as well as the cultural mechanisms that were employed by Blacks to navigate the society in which they were born. People grow up in families and communities, thus we will examine the role that socialization plays in the development of racial awareness and racial identity development. But first, we visit the African past because we argue that Black people have a culture that is unique to them, despite claims that they do not. So, we trace Black Americans' cultural practices to their African roots. We also present how it is possible for these ancient cultural ways to be present among Black Americans today.

Culture in Africa

To learn about Black African ancestors' legacy, we discuss in brief, some aspects of African society that set the foundation for the cultural practices and beliefs of people of African descent. While a fuller description of African history is beyond the scope of the book, we endeavor to offer an overview to frame the presence of cultural themes and core aspects of an African-centered world view.

Many scholars across disciplines and lay people, irrespective of race, held that Africans and their descendants had no distinct culture of their own. Africa was depicted as a "primitive society in an arrested state of development," and people of African descent as "congenitally backward people" who were physically, morally, and politically inferior, and "destined... to occupy a condition of servile dependency" (Berlin, 2010, p. 3). Europeans are said to have had a negative perception of Africans based on early contact with Africa in the 15th century (1400s), and assumptions Europeans made about the meaning of differences in physical appearance and cultural practices between them and Africans. In the language and customs of Europeans, Blackness was equated with being uncivilized, and dark skin color was associated with evil. In these early contacts, the rich and long history of civilization, learning, and wealth that existed in Africa

DOI: 10.4324/9781003083221-5

during and before these encounters was ignored (Bennett, 1988; Horton & Horton, 2005). Africans were not savages; they lived different lifestyles than Europeans, and they observed distinct and complex cultural practices, as did all people around the world (Horton & Horton, 2005).

The history of people on the African continent extends back more than 5,000 years. Five hundred years after the decline of Egypt, three large and powerful empires existed in the Western Sudan or the west coastal region of the continent. These empires reveal the fact that Africans lived in complex social systems and generated considerable wealth; they built homes, villages, and cities. And they created systems and organizations to administer their governments and ruling bodies.

Located between the Sahara to the North and the forest of the Guinea Coast to the South, theses empires were known as Ghana (not the current country), Mali, and Songhay. These empire states reached the peak of their power during the Middle Ages in Europe (during the 5th–17th centuries). And fell into decline around the time that Europeans visited the west coast of the continent, around the 15th and 16th centuries.

Harms (2018) points out that the various settlements, villages, and towns in the regions in question were numerous yet independent in their governance. The African people created distinct kinship-based political organizations in which a village chief was selected to govern. Such towns and villages often expanded to encompass many villages, which combined to form a kingdom, with its leader known as its King. Kingdoms, like villages, could also grow and expand to the size of an empire. However, when expansion occurred there was no effort to remove the former leaders. Chiefs and kings remained and became vassals to the leader of the empire if one was established (Harms, 2018). In this way, it is possible that an Empire could be formed when a greater power overtook a weaker kingdom(s) or chiefdom(s), and the weaker rulers would pay tribute to the stronger ruler of the Empire and agree to its status as a vassal or lesser state. In this instance, the former state remained intact with its ruler and political structure. What changed was the addition of a new administrative structure. As Empires weakened, vassal entities could break away and re-establish their local rulers. Thus, there was always some form of stability.

It is difficult to reconstruct the events that preceded the rise of these Empires in Africa since not many records exist, and as Harms (2018) tells us, much of what is known is drawn from oral histories and traditions which have advantages and disadvantages. The oral histories, an honored African tradition, can be added to what few written documents exist. In fact, Asante (2019) used the writings of several ancient scholars such as Ibu Battuta and Leo Africanus and others for information about this period in history.

What is important about these Empires is the wealth and prosperity they created, and that many were centers of world-wide education and commerce and were repositories of books and manuscripts. The seats of the three Empires were large cities with populations in the hundreds of thousands, renowned for their forward leaning advancements and influence. These three Empires were dominant for over a millennium. Their wealth was built from trade in gold, ivory, and other commodities, often with Europeans, through the Sahara Desert. Ghana ruled the region from the 5th century until the 13th century, and Mali emerged as the next great empire, located between the Senegal and Niger Rivers. Three hundred fifty miles to the southeast of Ghana, the Mali Empire was in an area with good water and grasslands, with proximity to the Bure gold mines. Mali was controlled by the Mande people, who through conquest were able to enlarge their empire. The Mali Empire was distinct since the Mande people used a social system that was divided by categories and groupings, such as nobles, commoners, slaves, and guilds (i.e., blacksmiths, woodcarvers, bards). Membership was based on birth and linage, and intermarriage was forbidden among the various guilds and groups. Its cities and states were recognized far and wide. Some like Timbuktu (a city of some 100,000) were known as centers for education and advanced learning.

After Mali's rise as the center of power in the region in the 13th century, it declined in the 15th century, and was replaced by the Songhay Empire, which declined in the 17th century (1600s).

> the reign of the great West African States came to an end. The decline is attributed to clashes between Islam and Christianity, and the terrain in which the states were built was open, and last some attributed it to the "corrupting influence of the slave trade... The popular myth depicts the conquering European carrying the blessing of civilization to the naked "savages" who sat under trees, filled their teeth and waited for fruit to drop into their hands. The truth is less flattering to the European ego. On the west coast of Africa, from whence came most of the ancestors of American Blacks, there were complex institutions ranging from extended family groupings of village states and territorial empires. Most of these units had all the appurtenances of the modern state, armies, courts and internal revenue departments.
>
> (Bennett, 1988, p. 22)

Common African Cultural Themes

What we learn from the overview of the early centuries of African people is that there are some points of commonality among them in the face of considerable diversity of language, place, climates, social organizations, and history (Franklin & Moss 2000). One common theme at the core of African societies was the family unit and kinship ties. Many societies were formed around kinship, and inheritance was often determined by women (matrilineal). Some men had multiple wives (polygamy) if the man could afford them. In the social order, the community cared for all its members, including the old, sick, and disabled. Learning and knowledge was conveyed through oral traditions and practices.

Scholars and historians have focused their attention on West African societies because it is from this region of the continent that most Africans brought to the New World colonies were located. There are several aspects of African life that characterize the many ethnic groups and peoples. Africans established governing entities around the family that in some instances grew to reflect state kingdoms, or Empires. States also evolved that were not kin-related but had leaders or small councils that provided the needed decision-making its people required (Thornton, 2012).

Africans were spiritual. For them, the spirits were real and located in many places and things, thus it was wise to honor and live in harmony with nature, and Africans believed in

> a supreme God who created the earth... There were lesser gods... (as well as) cults of fate and ancestor worship. Undergirding all was the basic concept of "life forces." The life force of the Creator was thought to be present in all things, animate and inanimate. This force... continued to exist even after the death of the individual... in a pure and perfect state which could influence the lives of living things.
>
> (Bennett, 1988, pp. 24–25)

In terms of religious practices, it is said that Africans had complex systems of beliefs and practices. Some followed Islam, others were Christian, and still others followed traditional African religious beliefs in which the spirits of one's ancestors "had great power over their lives," and the spirits that dwelled in inanimate objects such as one's family land, rocks, and trees, were held in high regard (Franklin & Moss, 2000, p. 25).

Economic life was, for the most part, agricultural where land was worked by its first occupants and was considered beyond them to belong to the entire community, not individuals. According to Franklin and Moss (2000), Africa was, "therefore never a series of isolated, self-sufficient communities, but an area that had far-flung interest based on agriculture, industry, and commerce" (p. 20). Their industry and commerce meant that they traveled and traded with others near and far. In some regions, trade was a centuries old endeavor.

Like their political life, social life in Africa was centered around the group, family, or clan. Males usually were the heads of clans and families, but relationships were determined by mothers not by fathers. This difference made women important figures in African society, "because they were, through marriage, the keys to appropriating land and through their labor and that of the children they bore, the means to cultivating land" (Franklin & Moss 2000, p. 20). Like any social group, Africans had a pecking order in which the "nobles" held top positions, followed by workers, and then there were those who enjoyed no rights or preferences and were referred to as war captives, or servants. But the people at the lower rungs of the African social order had privileges and were accorded respect because they were important and necessary participants in the society and their contributions were valued. They could move freely and climb up the social ladder.

There are cultural practices that survived over the course of many generations, and some traveled to the New World. Franklin and Moss (2000) argued that there is evidence that African culture survived in language, literature, folk tales, religion, beliefs and practices, musical forms, social organizations, and aesthetics. African people who were captives and their descendants managed to hold on to various aspects of their original cultures. And due to their interactions with White Europeans, these cultural practices were transformed and altered so they could adapt to their situations of bondage and racial oppression.

During Slavery

In whatever situation, one is born, one must evolve an identity, a self-concept that contains information about who you are and how you matter in the world where you live. Usually, this identity formation is influenced by interactions between the environment and circumstances in which one is raised, and one's psychological and physical being.

The enslavement and racial oppression of Black people in the North American colonies and the United States, from 1619 to 1964, some 350 or so years, has left a long-standing system of racial oppression in the United States (Feagin, 2006; Williams & Mohammed, 2009). The racial subjugation of Black people meant that they did not participate in the larger social system, and therefore it was believed that anything they knew or did were byproducts of their interactions with Whites. Stevenson (1998) points out that prior to the 1960s, the way that Black families functioned was characterized as negative and dysfunctional, yet at the same time scholars and researchers have documented differences in Blacks' cultural behavior and ways of being.

We will discuss several aspects of Black cultural life that reveal a different course than maladjustment or White influence. The cultural practices that Blacks used during their enslavement and racial oppression have been identified as their strong kinship bonds (not just family by blood), a vital work ethic, flexible family roles (not using rigid male and female role definitions), the importance of achievement (pushing family to do better), and spiritual practices as well as other practices (Belgrave & Allison, 2019).

Psychologically, there is and was a determination on the part of Africans and their descendants to value and honor their traditions and ways of living regardless of place and situation. Africans had a wide range of languages, social practices, religions, beliefs, and psychological perspectives prior to being captives. Once they began to function as a group with common goals and objectives, they used their core values and psychological orientations and resolutions as fuel to believe they would overcome their new situation as slaves and restricted free people. More importantly, they taught the new generations the thoughts and behaviors that reflected their hope for a better life.

It is also true that the decades of harsh oppression resulted in significant damage to members of the group. Many individuals were and have been pressed into submission, and some harmed themselves and other members of the group. Nevertheless, many others have held on and taught valuable lessons or left legacies that have guided those that followed (Thornton, 2012). Black people were successful at handling racial oppression because they held on to the beliefs and values, altered by their circumstances, that reflected and honored their ancestors. In addition to what was mentioned before (i.e., strong kinship bonds, a vital work ethic, flexible family roles, and the value of achievement), some aspects of Black culture are expressed in their temporal focus on the past/present; their use of rhythm (i.e., this was infused in movement and work practices, as well as in personal expressions); oral traditions; spirituality; and communal cultural practices, expressed as racial group identity that placed a high value on an individual's actions as inextricably related to the well-being of the group.

Across the sweep of centuries of racial oppression and indignity in the face of ever growing and elaborate efforts to deny them, free and enslaved Africans, and their decedents, found ways to establish and pass along the needed beliefs and psychological mechanisms necessary to maintain and create communities, families, and institutions, even in the face of shifting locations and the harsh and degrading ways they were treated. Therefore, while Africans were captives, many did not surrender nor did they lose their minds, culture, or their values. Africans and their decedents were forced to be isolated in their communities, and yet this is where they passed on lessons to their offspring about the value of their community, the strength of their spirit, the wisdom of their ancestors, and about how to deal with racial oppression. There were a range of differences employed as to how best to cope, or even if survival was warranted. But Africans and their descendants did persevere as a people, and they managed to reclaim and have control over portions of their lives, little by little:

> In the 1800's the center of slave life was the family which was enmeshed in a dense network of kin relationships… It was typical that they would marry and maintain long-term relationships. A web of distinctive customs and beliefs sustained those lifelong relationships.
>
> (Berlin, Favreau, & Miller, 1998, p. xxxviii)

> Scarcely less important than the family was the slaves' religion… the dense network of kinship that knit together the slave communities of the 17th (1600's) and 18th (1700's) centuries,… the slaves' religious beliefs and practices nevertheless stood apart.
>
> (Berlin et al., 1998, pp. xxxix–xii)

Black enslaved people passed on how to cope with racial oppression and how to believe in one's own people (racial identity). The transmission of the essential messages and ways of living were critical to the group's well-being and were sources of cultural, psychological, and emotional strength that contributed to the people's psychological health.

Black Life After Emancipation

During the Jim Crow era (1877–1964), Blacks were subjected daily to domestic terror at the hands of Whites with little or no protection. Their freedom was extremely limited, as was their personal safety. They were in effect still treated as slaves without the explicit legal designation. They were brutalized and killed at random, usually by lynching. They were second-class citizens, forced to bow to the wishes of Whites, no matter the situation or circumstances. Blacks had to give way to Whites if they encountered them on the street. They had to address White people as Sir and Madam, while being referred to as Aunt or Uncle, or worse by the N-word. They could be arrested for most any pretense and sold to corporations or farms as laborers for little or no pay, since they were paying off made up fines or debts and were in essence criminals (Blackmon, 2008). The era of Black racial oppression began in 1877 when political considerations led to the withdrawal of federal troops from the South, thus abandoning Blacks and the promises of freedom that was proclaimed in federal law. In time, the status of Blacks was sealed and closed, many thought, for all time. The 20th century opened with the clear pledge that Blacks, the majority of whom resided in Southern states, would be held to the lower rungs of society. Their status was codified in state and soon federal laws (Woodward, 1974). Packard (2002) describes it this way,

> From the end of reconstruction until the Supreme Court's *Plessy v. Ferguson* decision in 1896, Jim Crow spread like a pestilence. The virus settled in community after community, in county after county, state after state, until its cells had taken over the entire body of the South [and country]. From a hazy and undocumented existence as simply "custom" until it was armored in the full force of statutory law, Jim Crow became what it meant to be Southern.
>
> (p. 65)

In *Remembering Jim Crow*, Chafe, Gavins, and Korstad (2001) point out that their more than 1,200 interviews with Blacks who lived through this era in history revealed several important facts. Black people in the South and North managed to find ways to sustain collective and community will that was used to fight back, endure, and define their lives on their terms (Stevenson, 2014). Members of the Black community created ways and means to aid one another and established organizations and institutions that contributed to their well-being.

It was also true that "families nurture(d) each other and especially their children" (Chafe et al., 2001, p. xxx). Parents taught their children what to expect and what to do, while teaching racial and personal pride and self-worth. Their work lives were double-edged swords providing essential means and the prospect of further and deeper levels of humiliation. Chafe et al. observed that "the workplace was a perennially contested ground, potentially a source of pride and accomplishment, but just as often, a site of threat, danger, and unpredictable cruelty" (p. xxxi).

Blacks turned to their own institutions for hope and investment. They supported their segregated schools and teachers and aligned with Black churches as core organizations that sustained the people and held them together. The church and its leaders also sustained the struggle for a better life and equal rights and bolstered personal and racial pride. In short, in the face of unimageable hostility, Blacks mounted considerable resistance to Jim Crow, by way of their cultural practices through community, family, religion, and personal and cultural pride.

It was not until 1965 that equal opportunity employment laws were enacted, and 1967 that the legal ban on interracial marriage was lifted (Loving v. Virginia; Carter & Scheuermann, 2020). Nevertheless, race-based oppression in the United States continues to exist. Black people continue to be the targets of racism in many forms, including institutional racism in education and employment that reproduces and reinforces social and economic oppression; systemic inequity in the criminal legal system ranging from police bias and brutality to mass incarceration; and the perpetuation of stereotypes and negative depictions of Black people in the media (Carter & Scheuermann, 2020; Vera & Gordon, 2003). The cumulative impact of the structures and systems of racial oppression, which were established and practiced for 400 years prior to the passage of Civil Rights legislation, continues to affect every aspect of the lives of Black people and communities to this day.

Since the 1965 laws were passed, we have witnessed racist scientific practices across several disciplines seeking to prove White racial superiority. For example, Jensen's (1969) and Herrnstein and Murray's (1994) reports, which were both challenged and debunked by social scientists (e.g., Alland, 2002; Jacoby & Glauberman, 1995), suggested heredity was the major contributing factor explaining differences in IQ scores between Blacks and Whites. However, how Blacks held on to their culture and survived is less often discussed. What strengths did they draw upon to maintain their relative psychological resolve and focus in the face of long-standing racial oppression and violence? Each generation taught the next about race, how to cope, the value of community and family, and what was important in life.

Blacks Passed on Cultural Beliefs and Ways

Blacks today exhibit cultural preferences that include oral traditions, as reflected in their use of the spoken word and song as a critical means of communication passed to them through their heritage and socialization messages. Since for many centuries reading and writing was unlawful, forbidden, and punished, oral expression was and continues to be a means of cultural transmission and socialization. It is this aspect of the Black culture that connects the present with the past and is the mechanism through which meaning in life is communicated. There is also spirituality. A central element of African and Black American culture, it is the conviction that there are forces that exist beyond humans that affect the things that happen daily. Thus, multiple forces are at play that determine or explain events. Adherence to Black American cultural practices is varied among Black people. Some embrace Black culture and others do not; and many are not certain of the value of the practices.

There are several ways that differing ways of responding to racial oppression can be described. One is in psychological and cultural terms. Some theorists argue that a Black person's psychological orientation to his or her racial group membership, or racial identity, determines his or her cultural preferences. As such, if one devalues their racial group membership and values that of Whites, then that person would be invested in the cultural practices of the dominant racial group and would reject and devalue the cultural worldview of Black people. In this way racial identity is related to one's cultural worldview.

Racial Identity: Psychological Orientation to Racial Group Membership

Racial identity theorists argue that one's race or skin color alone does not determine the type of psychological resolution one adapts with respect to one's racial group membership (Helms, 1990). The variability in racial identity is reflected in a range of behaviors and thoughts. To illustrate, some individuals believe race does not matter, others are confused about the importance of race, while some think and act in ways to suggest that race is all that matters and, therefore, they fight to end or maintain racial inequality. Lastly, others regard race as a complex aspect of their personality and behave accordingly. The variation in how people understand the meaning of their race can influence a person's identity development, interpersonal interactions, socialization messages, and social relationships. As such, an understanding of racial identity and how it works to influence race-related information processing, and how to apply that understanding, is highly meaningful in mental health service and treatment interventions.

Children are born and grow physically, emotionally, psychologically, and socially among their families, communities, and larger social system. The family and community are directly involved in the growth and care of the child, and they foster its development. In the United States and colonies, children were raised for the most part in racially homogeneous settings. That is, American society was/is racially divided or stratified, such that racially different people rarely live together, but did/do interact quite a bit. Moreover, physical growth and development of a child is very much influenced by the nature of the environment one is exposed to and the resources that parents and families have available, which was/is itself a function of their social and economic status. The environment also influences the growing child's psychological and emotional experiences and his/her interactions with parents and family members. Developmental theorists have mapped the process of human development across the years. What we know now is that self-awareness begins early in life, but abstract and complex thinking takes time to develop, and it is not until adolescence that people are able to develop more complex thinking abilities and emotional awareness. It is at this stage of development that people also begin to have a firmer sense of social and personal identity.

The human development process occurs in a racial-cultural context that has not been explicit in most theories of human development or personality, but exists, nevertheless. The physical-social environment and worldview of a racial group is guided by distinct propositions and assumptions about the nature of humankind and the world in which we live. Carter (1995) states,

> Because race is an aspect of American culture, it is reasonable to conclude that, in early intellectual and social development, a child will internalize the respective psychosocial meanings assigned to his or her racial group. For instance, racial groups vary in terms of family structure and values attached to particular activities (e.g., cognitive vs interpersonal skills) and to forms of language... These variations are also influenced by social customs and stereotypes regarding members of each racial/ethnic group.
>
> (p. 78)

One's development also involves the emergence of one's personality or the expression of the uniqueness of their personhood. There are many theories of how human's personalities come into being. There is agreement among theorists that nature and nurture interact to shape and influence the development of the personality, and that the process occurs over the course of a lifetime (Carter, 1995). Since the child begins life dependent on others, they must learn moral and social behavior through the process of socialization. At the time, Carter noted that more was known about how socialization influences gender identity or gender-related behavior than racial identity or race-related behavior. He argues that just as gender is learned, so are race-appropriate roles and behaviors. He states,

> Social and personality development is intertwined with prevailing assumptions about race that are learned through imitation, internalization, and reinforced by a need to conform to cultural norms and be accepted by society at large. As an individual matures, he or she develops a personality that is informed by social and moral attitudes, behaviors and feelings.
>
> (Carter 1995, p. 80)

Thus, personality, aided by the process of socialization, guides interpersonal and social interactions, the person expresses what comes from their genes and their environment, and most of what a child learns comes from his family and community. In the case of race, children exhibit racial awareness by the age of three or four. The four-year-old can distinguish her race from that of others and can assign meaning and values to the racial groups in question. Research has found that White children viewed Blacks and other racial groups in negative terms, while Blacks saw other racial group members in more positive ways (Carter 1995; 2005; 2025).

It is safe to say that, given the legacy of race in our social system, it shapes psychosocial and racial identity development. While people in the United States have and are subject to similar racial norms and attitudes, people vary in how they receive and respond to racial information. Thus, members of a racial group are seldom culturally uniform. Models that address the psychological differences with respect to race within racial groups are known as racial identity theories. When theories of racial identity emerged in the psychological literature, how racial identity was shaped by families was not clear as these processes do not appear to be a focus of the early racial identity frameworks. There are some who contend that socialization and racial identity are related. We will explore that connection, but we first present a snapshot of the racial context that we believe influenced and influences people's understanding and beliefs about race as well as the ways they handle racial information in the context of mental health.

Racial Identity Models: Understanding the Foundations of Black Cultural Strengths

Several racial identity models have been proposed since the early 1970s (see Carter, 2005a; Helms, 1990; Sellers, Smith, Shelton, Rowley, & Chavous, 1998 and Cross, 1991). These models address the racial identity of People of Color and Whites. We focus here on racial identity models that pertain to Blacks. In our effort to understand how Black Americans have managed to stay alive and viable as a people throughout time, it is important to describe how racial identity was conceptualized and applied. We contend that an individual's racial identity influences other Black cultural worldviews and practices such as racial socialization and related cultural values.

While many scholars wrote explicitly about racial identity in the years after the Civil Rights movement, we believe that the psychological variation that became more evident at that time has always existed from the time Africans set foot in the New World and on North American soil. The different psychological stances were more apparent during the Civil Rights movement (1950–1970) because they were publicly visible as individual psychological expressions of, race-based identity. That is, the larger group of people who were known as "Colored" or "Negro" transformed themselves into a group that proclaimed themselves to be "Black" – a once deeply offensive term. People of African descent took what was once an insult that often would lead to fights and anger and made it a term of pride and honor. Seeing these psychosocial and cultural issues unfold in public view, as part of the social and Civil Rights movement for racial equality, helped scholars to document something that existed but was less visible before the Civil Rights era. In the same way, current activists for dismantling systemic and structural racism have embraced the notion that Black Lives Matter and are advocating for changes in law enforcement. Their cause has been taken up by Black people, as well as people from other racial groups, and has spread across the country and the world. Many aspects of Black life have come to light.

We know that Africans of various ethnic backgrounds were held as slaves and became colored, Negros, and Blacks in America and in other parts of the New World. Furthermore, their ways of thinking about themselves as a people and as racial beings varied, and they found ways to cope and adapt to the racial violence and terrorism directed at them. Blacks also found ways to teach and socialize their children to navigate the racial world they inhabited. Yet many of the practices referred to occur on the level of the individual and thus, the person's psychological and emotional states are important to grasp. Individuals comprise groups and form, as members of groups, cultural beliefs and practices expressed through beliefs, behaviors, and psychological mechanisms. One's environment and circumstances contribute to the nature of the group's cultural worldview and particular activities that guide their well-being and shape their developmental context.

The social transformation that occurred during the Civil Rights and Black Power movements of the 1950s–1970s is described by psychologists in terms of individual psychological changes and identity development and was/is called racial identity. *Racial identity* refers to the notion that all people, regardless of their race, ascribe different psychological meanings to, and have different levels of cultural investment in their racial group membership. It is this meaning, and the associated cultural value preferences, that determine how an individual makes sense of the world and themselves as racial beings (Helms, 1990). Racial identity comprises a person's thoughts (cognitions), feelings (affective states), behaviors, and cultural worldview (Carter, 1995; Helms, 1990; Thompson & Carter, 2013). It is for this reason that racial identity is important in understanding interactions in therapy since it goes beyond a mere recognition of one's skin-color and physical features and includes both psychological and emotional states as well as one's cultural worldview.

Over time, multiple perspectives regarding racial identity have been advanced by researchers and scholars. It was first thought to be stages of development that were linear, and scholars held that racial identity was primarily a group-orientation, divorced from one's personality. Some only presented racial identity as a non-dominant group experience (i.e., something only Blacks or non-Whites experienced), while others contended that all racial groups share in the racial identity developmental process (Carter, 1995; 2025). The broader notions about racial identity also held that it was, in fact, an aspect of personality and was a part of the ego that processed race-related information about self and other racial groups. In this way, racial identity ego statuses were not linear and could co-exist, with one or more being dominant, depending upon how effective it was at the task of handling race-related information. When a particular racial identity ego status could not handle the current racial content, then the person could draw upon other statuses to process the information, and as such these could become stronger and used more often. These trends and differing perspectives are apparent in the overview of the history of thinking about racial identity that follows. More than anything, racial identity was about an aspect of the psychology of race and racial group membership which was significantly more complex than social demographic race denoted by skin-color and physical features.

Scholars proposed types and some introduced linear stages of Black identity. One of the earliest models is called Nigrescence and it described the developmental course of becoming Black. For some scholars, Black racial identity referred to how one thought about and judged oneself and one's social or reference group, as well as ones' opposing racial group (i.e., White people). Scholars (cf, Helms, 1990) suggested that racial identity was related to one's personality. It was suggested that for healthy development to occur, Black people needed to reject identification with White culture and White standards, and that being White-identified was unhealthy even if it was a perspective that was rewarded in dominant mainstream society. The position that being White-identified was not healthy was a direct departure from the notion of assimilation that prevailed in American society. In the beginning for the most part theorists, working independently of one another, put forth similar Black racial identity models in which one moved from one racial identity level to another. In essence, this progression meant moving from a White-identified to a Black-oriented racial and cultural identification.

Thomas' (1971) and Cross' (1971) models were used in psychology more than others and were subjected to the most empirical inquiry and investigation (Parham & Helms, 1981). Cross' (1971) Black identity theory had five stages. The last stage received little attention and was overlooked as time passed, so we present the four that have been used. The stages were *Pre-encounter, Encounter, Immersion-Emersion, and Internalization. Pre-Encounter* involved the idealization of White American worldviews. Thus, Black people in this stage of racial identity perceive themselves as human-beings, not a Black person. *Encounter* occurred as a jolting experience or encounter with racism that led to questions about their old Negro worldview and to testing their new perceptions about being Black. *Immersion-Emersion* is the stage where transformation occurs and the effort to dismantle the old identity happens, and it becomes necessary to with-draw into a Black world either physically or psychologically. Several thoughts and behaviors emerge during this phase:

> The person's level of Blackness is high, but the degree of internalization of the new identity is minimal. This period of emergent identity or "just dis-covered Blackness" is manifested in the construction of the correct ideol-ogy and/or world view, glorification of African heritage, either/or thinking, blacker-than-thou attitudes, unrealistic expectations concerning the efficacy of Black Power, and the tendency to denigrate White people and White cul-ture, while simultaneously deifying Black people and Black culture...
>
> (Cross, 1980, p. 85)

Immersion is followed by an Emersion, characterized by a leveling off of intense emotions and thoughts, and one is able to be more critical in his/her analysis of race and cultural differences. It is possible to see both the pluses and minuses of Black society, and psychological and emotional control returns marking the end of the stage and the beginning of *Internalization*. In *Internalization*, conflicts between worldviews of the Negro and the Black aspects of one's identity are resolved and thus, one can use one's race and culture as their main reference group.

Parham and Helms (1981) created the Black Racial Identity Attitudes Scale (BRIAS) to predict Black people's preferences for counselors' race. They intro-duced psychological variation of Blacks into the area of mental health and com-pared racial identity attitudes with racial self-designation (social demographic race designation). The study found that Black Pre-encounter attitudes were related to a preference for White counselors, while Encounter and Immersion-Emersion attitudes were related to a preference for Black counselors and oppo-sition to having a White counselor, while Internalization did not reveal any preferences for counselor race. Thus, the study established the merit of the theory that within-group psychological differences existed among Black Americans.

The application of racial identity theory to the process and outcomes of therapy was also tested. In this research White racial identity was also used. The theory proposed that relationship types were formed in therapy pairs by the combination of racial identity attitudes of the participants. Helms' (1984; 1990) interaction model and Carter's (1995) racially inclusive model of therapy used racial identity attitudes measures to describe how such attitudes influence therapy process and outcome. Four different types of potential pairings were described in therapist-client dyads or groups or social interactions: *Parallel* (i.e., same level of racial identity), *Crossed* (opposite levels), *Progressive* (helper is more advanced), and *Regressive* (client is more advanced), regardless of their respective socio-demographic racial group (Helms, 1984). The pairings create the dynamics both for the process (i.e., the manner and nature of the exchanges between therapy participants) and outcomes of the clinical encounter or social interaction since it is not the therapy participants' social demographic race, as such, that characterize relationship types, but how their psychologically based racial identity status attitudes combine and interact. Moreover, Carter (1995) suggested that varied cognitive processes, affective states, actions, and reactions to the therapy relationship characterize the different types of relationships, and he presented evidence of how the therapy process was in fact so affected.

Helms (1990) stated that racial identity was an aspect of personality and part of one's racial self-concept. The view of racial identity as a component of self is based in the notion that it is also related to one's cultural values and racial group preferences. Carter and Helms (1987) reported,

> Racial identity attitudes predicted three of the five Afro-centric value alternatives (Harmony with Nature, Doing Activity, and Collateral Social Relations and none of the Euro-centric based on Euro-American philosophy) alternatives. Immersion-Emersion and Internalization attitudes significantly predicted belief in Collateral Social Relations... (meaning the will of the group over the wishes of individuals). In addition,... Internalization attitudes were also predictive of a belief in Harmony with Nature and Doing Activity orientations... empirical support for Boykin's (1982) and Nobles (1980) contentions that vestiges of African philosophy beliefs have been retained by Afro-American culture and are expressed by the self-actualizing Afro-American...
>
> (p. 193)

Further, development in understanding of racial identity was offered by Helms and Piper (1994) who suggested that, rather than thinking of racial identity as stages, as had been presented by other theorists, it would be more accurate to conceive of racial identity resolutions as existing in a circumplex or ego space, depicted as a circle, where one status may occupy more space than another and thus would be more dominant. Their notions shifted thinking about racial identity from the linear approach to seeing statuses wherein a person possessed all racial identity statuses at the same time, but to varying degrees of influence. The status that was used more than others tended to be more dominant, and thus occupied more space in the psyche. If information was not processed effectively by the dominant status, then one might begin to rely on other statuses and these statuses would grow to have more influence. The revised thinking also meant that measurement procedures also needed to be revised, and instruments had to be used differently to capture the complexity of racial identity status attitudes (Carter & Johnson, 2019). The process of racial identity is sequential, wherein "increasingly more sophisticated differentiation of the ego evolves from earlier or less mature statuses" (Helms, 1996, p. 155), and there are variations in how racial identity is expressed which can be measured. To be clear, ego status refers to how race-related information is handled via one's thoughts and emotions. Helms (1996) argued that how a person's racial identity matures or differentiates is determined by their racial socialization and personal growth. As we have noted, there are other models of racial identity such as the Multidimensional model.

Multidimensional Theory of Racial Identity

In the late 1990s, Sellers and colleagues (Sellers et al., 1998) introduced both the multidimensional theory of racial identity and the Multidimensional Inventory of Black Identity (MIBI). In their model, Sellers and colleagues define racial identity as "the significance and qualitative meaning that individuals attribute to their membership within the Black racial group within their self-concept" (p. 23). The model is grounded in three notions: (1) one's identity is influenced by situations and is a stable aspect of one's self, though change is possible and intense situations foster change; (2) people have multiple aspects to their identities which are ordered, but the model is focused on race (social class, gender, etc.); (3) MIBI is more concerned with the state of a person's racial identity rather than its development, so there is less interest in locating a stage of racial identity. The MIBI has several dimensions, which are: (a) *racial salience*, the importance of one's race as part of their self-concept; (b) *centrality*, how the person defines him or herself in terms of race; (c) *regard*, the positive and negative emotions about being Black, with private and public (how others view Blacks as a group) areas of focus; (d) *ideology*, one's personal perspective about how racial group members should behave. There are four possible ideologies: (1) *nationalist*, wherein one believes that Blacks should be in charge of their world and environments; (2) the *oppressed minority*, wherein Blacks seek to work with other minority groups to address social inequities; (3) *assimilationist*, wherein Blacks seek to be accepted into mainstream society, and though they may be aware of their Blackness and racism, they work for social change within existing systems; and (4) *humanist*, which focuses on the betterment of all humans.

Five decades of theoretical and empirical work on racial identity has produced a large body of theory and research (e.g., Carter, 1995; 1996; Cross, 1991; Flowers, Levesque, & Fischer, 2012; Helms, 1990; Oparanozie, Sales, DiClemente, & Braxton, 2012; Sellers & Shelton, 2003; Thompson & Carter, 2013; Vandiver, Fhagen-Smith, Cokley, Cross, & Worrell, 2001). Positive racial identity has been associated with higher levels of self-esteem, a greater sense of mastery, greater psychological well-being, fewer anxiety and depression symptoms, and improved health outcomes, and has been found to serve a protective function against suicide and to buffer the psychological impact of racial discrimination (Blassingame et al., 2023; Hughes, Kiecolt, Keith, & Demo, 2015; McClain et al., 2016; Pierre & Mahalik, 2005; Twenge & Crocker, 2002;

Zapolski, Beutlich, Fisher, & Barnes-Najor, 2019). The research and scholarship on racial identity development has helped shape and influence how the discipline of psychology conceptualizes, investigates, and treats the impact of racial group membership and ethnicity on people's lives and has helped build a better understanding of cultural preferences among Blacks.

Historians, sociologists, and educators have written about the unwavering importance of the Black family (Gutman & Berlin, 1987; Martin & Martin, 1985). The racial identity of the elders (grandparents, parents, uncles, and aunts) has historically been an important mechanism by which information and stories (oral tradition) are passed down from generation to generation. The absence of a developed Black racial identity in some individuals may foreclose the important transmission of important lessons and messages about one's race to Black children, thus creating a deficit in their ability to reach a developed and positive Black racial identity. A positive racial identity is first and foremost, a necessity in maintaining Black cultural strength through generations. Once one has developed a positive racial identity, s/he can pass on Black cultural values and beliefs to younger Blacks. It is also possible that as the individual matures, s/he can come to grasp the meaning of their racial group membership, despite what was taught by parents and some members of the community. The process by which racial practices are encouraged and by which racial orientations are fostered is racial socialization.

Racial Socialization and Racial Identity

Stevenson (1994) states that the "phenomena of family socialization processes that contribute to the healthy racial identity development of African American men, women, and children have been and continue to be of clinical and research interest" (p. 445). Like all parents, Black people need to help their young mature and aid them in learning what is needed in our social system. At the same time, they need to arm their children to handle the racial hostility and violence that characterizes their lives. Racial oppression has existed for more than 400 years and while its form and function has changed over time, the fact of its existence has not. A stark example is in the frequency with which Black men are killed by police officers. According to scholars between 2013 and 2019, some 4,000 people have died by police use of lethal force, and of those, Black people were twice as likely to be killed than any other racial group (Fagan & Campbell, 2020).

Thus, Black people have multiple tasks to perform in socializing their children and in caring for their families. Stevenson notes that members from various disciplines have contributed to understanding how the family helps build racial identity but points out the focus of racial identity research and theory has been on college age populations, with some attention given to young children, and less attention given to adolescences (Phinney & Rotheram, 1987). He observes further that the idea that Black families have the added task of softening the impact of racism and of promoting and fostering cultural pride is a critical activity. He reports that researchers documented that socialization and racial identity were linked in that racial group identity was formed in part by parental socialization. When parents taught their children to prepare for racism, such individuals were more likely to exhibit stronger feelings of closeness to other Blacks. Stevenson (1995) defines racial socialization as the "process of communicating messages and behaviors to children to bolster their sense of identity given the possibility and reality that their life experiences may include racially hostile encounters" (p. 51). He argues that it is important to consider racial socialization as comprising cultural interactions that exceed reactions to racial oppression and include creative adaptations as well. He states that racial socialization should be more than responses to racial hostility.

> It is proposed that reactive and creative racial socialization messages and behaviors are relevant for different contexts and that the flexible application of both messages by youth should result in greater interpersonal competence and coping. This is, instead of viewing racial socialization as preparing the child only for oppressive experiences (e.g., protective African American culture), it is proposed that these processes also include teaching children how to be proud of their culture because its substance is historic, African derived, culturally empowering, and not dependent on oppressive experiences. A second perspective… about… a socialized identity is the view of self as extended and interactional as opposed to individualistic… we can improve our understanding of Black adolescent identity development by knowing what the individual thinks of self in context through the activities, experiences and interactions that happen outside himself or herself and through experiences that represent the group. This definition is akin to the concept of reference group orientation.
>
> (Stevenson, 1995, pp. 51–52)

Racial socialization offers a way to examine the Black cultural orientation to social relations. It is defined as teachings about race relations and protection against racism, as well as the process of learning about how to function as a member of the Black cultural group. Overall, racial socialization is aimed at instructing Blacks about their individual and social realities and how to navigate the world with this knowledge. Racial socialization is communicated through the direct and indirect messages an individual receives *or* the beliefs a person holds because they receive race-related messages. Elmore and Gaylord-Harden (2013) emphasize the importance of racial socialization as the process of rearing children toward a positive racial identity and often involves preparing children for racial encounters. Peters (1985) noted that Black parents have the additional task of "raising physically and emotionally healthy children who are Black in a society in which being Black has negative connotations" (p. 161). Lesane-Brown (2006) considers racial socialization to be reflected in both verbal and non-verbal messages sent to youth with the purpose of instilling in them values, attitudes, and beliefs that guide how the youth understands the meaning and importance of their race and social status due to race, as well as their interactions with people of the same and different racial groups. For Black Americans in general over time, racial socialization has been one mechanism through which generations pass down instructions about not only the rules and meaning of being a member of the Black racial group but also how to exist and flourish as a Black person in U.S. society.

Racial socialization exists within a system beyond the nuclear family and can involve the interaction of social issues, direct and indirect messages, the influence of parents, as well as others besides parents, and the impact of the views and behaviors of their targets. Current racial socialization literature aims to understand and address the full complexity of this process and the many factors such as time, who delivers the messages, and the composition of an individual's environment (Barr & Neville, 2014). To examine the cultural transmission in more detail and how it may have worked across the years, we will discuss this cultural practice in more detail in the next chapter. We will examine what the messages were and how they were passed on to promote a positive Black identity.

References

Alland, A. (2002). *Race in mind*. New York, NY: Palgrave Macmillan.

Asante, M. K. (2019). *The history of Africa: The quest for eternal harmony* (3rd Ed.). New York, NY: Routledge.

Barr, S. C., & Neville, H. A. (2014). Racial socialization, color-blind racial ideology, and mental health among Black college students an examination of an ecological model. *Journal of Black Psychology, 40*(2), 138–165.

Belgrave, F. Z., & Allison, (2019). *African American psychology: From Africa to America (4th Ed.)*. Los Angles, CA.: Sage

Bennett, L. (1988). *Before the Mayflower: A history of Black America*. Chicago, IL: Johnson Publishing.

Berlin, I. (2010). *The making of African America: The four great migrations*. New York: Viking.

Berlin, I., Favreau, M., & Miller, S. F. (1998). *Remembering slavery*. New York, NY: The New Press.

Blackmon, D. A. (2008). *Slavery by another name*. New York: Random House.

Blassingame, W.-S., N. N., Au, J., Mekawi, Y., Lewis, C. B., Ferdinand, N. L., Wilson, T. E., Dunn, S. E., & Kaslow, N. J. (2023). Racial identity profiles and indicators of well-being in suicidal African American women. *Journal of African American Studies 27*(4), 1–18. doi: 10.1007/s12111-023-09638-1.

Boykin, A. W. (1983). The academic performance of Afro-American children. In J. T. Spence (Ed.), Achievement and achievement motives: Psychological and sociological approaches (pp. 321-371). San Francisco: W. H. Freeman.

Carter, R. T. (1991). Cultural values: A review of empirical research and implications for counseling. *Journal of Counseling and Development, 70,* 164–173.

Carter, R. T. (1995). *The influence of race and racial identity in psychotherapy.* New York: John Wiley & Sons.

Carter, R. T. (1996). Exploring the complexity of racial identity attitude measures. In G. R. Sodowsky & J. Impara (Eds.), *Multicultural assessment in counseling and clinical psychology* (pp. 193–224). Lincoln, NE: Buros Institute of Mental Measurement.

Carter, R. T. (Ed.) (2005). *Handbook of racial-cultural psychology and counseling,* Vol. 1, *Theory and research.* Hoboken, NJ: Wiley.

Carter, R. T. (2025). *Recognizing the psychological and cultural strengths of Black Americans: Historical, social, and psychological perspectives.* New York, NY: Routledge.

Carter, R. T., & Helms, J. E. (1987). The relationship of Black value-orientations to racial identity attitudes. *Measurement and Evaluation in Counseling and Development, 19,* 185–195.

Carter, R. T., & Helms, J. E. (1992). The counseling process defined by relationship types: A test of Helms' interactional model. *Journal of Multicultural Counseling and Development, 20*(4), 181–201.

Carter, R. T., & Johnson, V. (2019). Racial identity statuses: Applications to practice. *Practice Innovations, 4*(1), 42–58.

Carter, R. T., & Pieterse, A. (2020). *Measuring the effects of racism: Guidelines for the assessment and treatment of race-based traumatic stress injury.* New York, NY: Columbia University Press.

Carter, R. T., & Scheuermann, T. D. (2020). *Confronting racism: Integrating mental health strategies with legal reform.* New York, NY: Routledge.

Chafe, W. H., Gavins, R., & Korstad, R. (2001). *Remembering Jim Crow.* New York, NY: The New Press.

Cross, W. E. Jr (1971). The Negro-to-Black conversion experience: Toward a psychology of Black liberation. *Black World, 20*(9), 13–27.

Cross, W. E. Jr (1980). Models of psychological Nigrescence: A literature review. In R. L. Jones (Ed.), *Black psychology* (2nd ed.) (pp. 81–98). New York, NY: Harper & Row Publishers.

Cross, W. E., Jr (1991). *Shades of Black.* Philadelphia, PA: Temple University Press.

Cross, W. E., Parham, T. A., & Helms, J. A. (1998). Nigrescence revisited: Theory and research. In R. L. Jones (Ed.), *African American identity development* (pp. 3–73). Berkeley CA: Cobb & Henry Publishers.

Elmore, C. A., & Gaylord-Harden, N. K. (2013). The influence of supportive parenting and racial socialization messages on African American youth behavioral outcomes. *Journal of Child and Family Studies, 22*(1), 63–75.

Fagan, J. A., &. Campbell, A. D. (2020). Race and reasonableness in police killings. *Boston University Law Review,* 100, 951–1010; Columbia Public Law Review Research Paper No.14–655 (2020). https://scholarship.law.columbia.edu/faculty_scholarship/2656

Feagin, J. R. (2006). *Systemic racism.* New York, NY: Routledge.

Flowers, K. C., Levesque, M. C., & Fischer, S. (2012) The elationship between maladaptive eating behaviors and racial identity among African American women in college. *Journal of Black Psychology 38*(3), 290–312.

Franklin, H. J., & Moss, A. A. (2000). *From slavery to freedom: A history of African Americans* (8th ed.). Boston, MA: McGraw Hill.

Gutman, H. G., & Berlin, I. (1987). *Power and culture: Essays on the American working class.* New York, NY: Pantheon Books.

Harms, R. (2018). *Africa in Global History with sources.* New York, NY: W.W. Norton and Company.

Helms, J. E. (1984). Toward a theoretical explanation of the effects of race on counseling: A Black and White model. *The Counseling Psychologist, 12*(3–4), 153–165. doi: 10.1177/0011000084124013

Helms, J. E. (1990). *Black and white racial identity: Theory, research and practice.* New York, NY: Greenwood Press.

Helms, J. E. (1996). Toward a methodology for measuring and assessing racial as distinguished from ethnic identity. In G. Roysircar Sodowsky & J. Impara (Eds.), *Multicultural assessment in counseling and clinical psychology.* Lincoln, NE: Buros Institute of Mental Measurement University of Nebraska-Lincoln.

Helms, J. E., & Piper, R. E. (1994). Implications of racial identity theory for vocational psychology. *Journal of Vocational Behavior, 44*(2), 124–138. doi: 10.1006/jvbe.1994.1009.

Herrnstein, R. J., & Murray, C. A. (1994). *The bell curve: Intelligence and class structure in American life.* New York: Free Press.

Horton, J. O., & Horton, L. E. (2005). *Slavery and the making of America.* New York, NY: Oxford University Press.

Jacoby, R., & Glauberman, N. (1995). *The bell curve debate.* New York, NY: Three Rivers Press.

Jensen, A. R. (1969). How much can we boost IQ and scholastic achievement? *Harvard Educational Review, 39*(1), 1–123. doi: 10.17763/haer.39.1.l3u15956627424k7.

Lesane-Brown, C. L. (2006). A review of race socialization within Black families. *Developmental Review, 26*(4), 400–426.

Martin, J. M., & Martin, E. P. (1985). *The helping tradition in the Black family and community.* Silver Spring, MD: National Association of Social Workers, Inc.

McClain, B., S. T., Jones, B., Awosogba, O., Jackson, S., & Cokley, K. (2016). An examination of the impact of racial and ethnic identity, impostor feelings, and minority status stress on the mental health of Black college students. *Journal of Multicultural Counseling and Development, 44*(2), 101–117.

Nobles, W. E. (1980). African philosophy: Foundations for Black psychology. In R. L. Jones (Ed.), *Black Psychology* (2nd ed.) (pp. 23–36). New York: Harper & Row.

Oparanozie, A., Sales, J. M., DiClemente, R. J., & Braxton, N. D. (2012). Racial identity and risky sexual behaviors among Black heterosexual men. *Journal of Black Psychology, 38*(1), 32–51.

Packard J.M., (2002). *American nightmare: The History of Jim Crow.* New York, St. Martin's Press.

Parham, T. A., & Helms, J. E. (1981). The influence of Blacks students; racial identity attitudes on preference for counselor's race. *Journal of Counseling Psychology, 28*, 250–257.

Peters, M. F. (1985). Racial socialization of young Black children. In H. P. McAdoo (Ed.), *Black children: Social, educational, and parental environments* (pp. 159–173). Thousand Oaks, CA: Sage Publications, Inc.

Phinney, J. S., & Rotheram, M. J. (1987) *Children's ethnic socialization: Pluralism and development.* Newbury, CA: Sage.

Pierre, M. R., & Mahalik, J. R. (2005). Examining African self-consciousness and Black racial identity as predictors of Black men's psychological well-being. *Cultural Diversity & Ethnic Minority Psychology, 11*(1), 28–40.

Sellers, R. M., & Shelton, J. N. (2003). The role of racial identity in perceived racial discrimination. *Journal of Personality and Social Psychology, 84*(5), 1079–1092. doi: 10.1037/0022-3514.84.5.1079

Sellers, R. M., Smith, M. A., Shelton, J. N., Rowley, S. A., & Chavous, T. M. (1998). Multidimensional model of racial identity: A reconceptualization of African American racial identity. *Personality and Social Psychology Review, 2*(1), 18–39.

Stevenson, H. C. (1994). Validation of the scale of racial socialization for African American adolescents: Steps toward multidimensionality. *Journal of Black Psychology, 20*(4), 445–468.

Stevenson, H. C. (1995). Relationship of adolescent perceptions of racial socialization to racial identity. *Journal of Black Psychology, 21*(1), 49–70.

Stevenson, H. C. (1998). Theoretical considerations in measuring racial identity and socialization: Extending the self-further. In R. Jones (Ed.), *African American identity development: Theory, research, and intervention* (pp. 227–263). Hampton, VA: Cobb & Henry.

Stevenson, B. (2014). Just mercy: A story of justice and redemption. New York, NY: Spiegel & Grau.

Thomas, C. (1971). *Boys no more.* Beverly Hill, CA: Glencoe Press.

Thompson, C. E., & Carter, R. T. (Eds.) (2013). *Racial identity development theory applications to individual, group and organizations.* Hillsdale, NJ: Lawrence Erlbaum.

Thornton, J. K. (2012). *A cultural history of the Atlantic world, 1250–1820.* New York, NY: Cambridge University Press.

Twenge, J. M., & Crocker, J. (2002). Race and self-esteem: Meta-analyses comparing Whites, Blacks, Hispanics, Asians, and American Indians and comment on Gray-Little and Hafdahl (2000). *Psychological Bulletin, 128*(3), 371–408.

Vandiver, B. J., Fhagen-Smith, P. E., Cokley, K. O., Cross, W. E., Jr., & Worrell, F. C. (2001). Cross's Nigrescence model: From theory to scale to theory. *Journal of Multicultural Counseling and Development, 29,* 174–200.

Vera, H. & Gordon, A., (2003). *Screen saviors: Hollywoods Fiction of Whiteness.* New York: Rowman & Littlefield.

Williams, D. R., &. Mohammed, S. A. (2009). Discrimination and Racial Disparities in Health: Evidence and Needed Research. *Journal of Behavioral Medicine, 32,* 20–47. doi: 10.1007/s10865-008-9185-0.

Woodward, C. V. (1974). *The strange career of Jim Crow.* New York, NY: Oxford University Press.

Zapolski, T. C. B., Beutlich, M. R., Fisher, S., & Barnes-Najor, J. (2019). Collective ethnic-racial identity and health outcomes among African American youth: Examination of promotive and protective effects. *Cultural Diversity & Ethnic Minority Psychology, 25*(3), 388–396.

Chapter 5

Black American Cultural Legacy

Parents and Community Teaching About Race

We discussed racial socialization in the last chapter and noted some of its definitions and that it involved the transmission of messages about how to cope with a range of experiences that children will encounter as they grow up, including racial events. In this chapter, we will continue the discussion of racial socialization, present more detail about it, and look into the past to see how and in what ways Black Americans passed on their values to their offspring during the times when they were forbidden to read or write by law and custom.

We start with visiting the past to consider what intergenerational messages were conveyed and how, and what were the core communications and mechanisms used to teach the young how to manage their lives and that of their children. We know that socialization was an effective strategy to pass on messages to new generations on how to navigate the often-harsh realities of living as a Black person in American society. Furthermore, we also know that most racial socialization messages were designed to foster positive Black racial identity and to strengthen the bonds among members of the community, raise their spirits, and instill cultural pride. We know that children were taught to value oral traditions, as reflected in the use of stories and songs to teach and communicate. Black people were taught to be able to recognize and move to the rhythms of nature as in song and dance and other physical activities; to work; to value family; to take part in religious ceremonies; and to hold the community in high esteem. Lastly, the individual was taught the value of improvisation as a mechanism to express her/his unique personality in the context of the community. However, as racial identity theorists have contended, being a psychosocially healthy Black person in America involves not only a positive image of oneself as a Black person but also a positive social orientation toward the larger racial group. As mentioned, kinship is a central feature of Black Americans' culture dating back to African ancestry (Stack, 1974). That is, socializing Blacks toward the Black racial culture ideally includes messages about the collaborative and communalistic orientation that characterize Black communities.

After our look back, we return to the present and discuss how racial socialization is related to other Black cultural practices and review the research evidence

DOI: 10.4324/9781003083221-6

about the various messages sent and received by children, parents, families, relatives, peers, and others. But first we visit the past.

Lesson in Time: Historical Foundation of Racial Socialization

Although Africans and their descendants lived, to some extent, in isolation for two and one-half centuries, they were nevertheless, watched and monitored, constantly. In their private moments and openly, they passed on lessons to their offspring to teach them about the value of community, the strength of their spirit, the wisdom of their ancestors, and about how to deal with the racial oppression they faced. There was variation among them regarding their beliefs and practices. There were a range of differences employed as to how best to cope and survive, or even if survival was warranted. But Africans and their descendants did endure as a people, and they also reclaimed portions of their lives: Berlin, Favreau, and Miller (1998) state:

> Playing on the slaveholders' dependence on the slaves' natural increase, slaves struggled for control of the reproductive process. They asserted the right to choose their partner and control the birthing process. Slaves women, or elderly "grannies," served as midwives; only rarely, and in dire emergencies, did slaveholders and their agents usher slave infants into the world (...) During the nineteenth century, the hallmark of the slave's domestic life was a nuclear family enmeshed in a dense network of kin relationships.
>
> (pp. xxxvii–xxxviii)

It was typical that slaves would marry and maintain long-term relationships [contrary to popular beliefs]. A web of distinctive customs and beliefs sustained those lifelong relationships and separated the family life of Black American slaves from that of others (Berlin et al., 1998). The transmission of the essential messages and ways of living are and were critical to Black Americans' continued existence and are/were sources of cultural strength that contributed to Black people's psychological health. As one looks back to learn about Africans and their descendants, there is less written about their lives from their perspective and more about what was done to them. But there is evidence in the sources that are available to document some of the cultural practices and psychological mechanisms and patterns that are and were used in the service of their continued existence. Narratives from free Blacks and former slaves, as documented by Webber (1978), reveal their lives and their communities and tell about the ways that Whites did not control Blacks' thoughts and actions. These narratives demonstrate that Blacks taught their children their cultural ways, and that they acted daily in ways that "protected their psychological freedom and celebrated their human dignity" (p. 262).

Webber documents and describes several cultural themes endemic to the slave quarter community, the area of the home plantation where slaves lived and experienced their worlds. These communities, or slave quarters, varied in size and type but were ubiquitous in American society. It is also where Black culture was nourished and prospered. Webber presented several cultural themes (that are also described by Jones, 2003) that characterized Black communities, free and slave. A central theme among them was "communality" defined as a group spirit and identification, or reference group orientation, held together by a commitment to solidarity, and moral and behavioral rules that members of the community followed in order to have the trust of other community members. People could not betray confidences or share the community's secrets. Trust was not based on skin-color but on deeds. It was the code and practice of the community to share, protect, and care for each other as family as best as they could. There was pride in the ability of Black people to handle adversity with intellect and wisdom. The core of the community was family, often extended, but not always defined by blood. Webber (1978) described the family in this way,

> This... family pattern included not only what is referred to as the "extended family," but also other persons not necessarily related by blood or marriage. Such individuals might include step-parents, peer group members, community leaders, religious meeting brethren, nursery teachers, doctors, conjurors special friends, and any other individual who, for reasons other than kinship by blood, felt a familial responsibility to help nurture, protect, and educate any given black child.
>
> (Webber, 1978, p. 157)

Transmitting, from one generation to the next, the values, psychological principles, and cultural beliefs that Black people held dear and cherished involved using many mechanisms. The religious congregation was one. They would often meet in secret, away from the slave quarters. The community, family, and peers were also mechanisms used to convey critical cultural messages and to teach the rules used to endure. Songs and stories were told as part of the oral traditions and, given the prohibitions against learning to read and write, were the concrete tools for learning. Even though forbidden, a small number of Blacks learned to read and write, and they taught others in secret. Regarding the songs and stories, Webber (1978) notes,

> Both the narratives and numerous complications of slave songs and stories lend weight to the conclusion that, though they differed from region to region, the songs and stories of the quarter community expressed similar values, beliefs and attitudes throughout the ante-bellum South. In addition to giving voice to the themes of the quarter community, songs and stories were also

an essential medium by which those themes were evoked, supported, and transmitted from generation to generation.

(p. 207)

More important was the reality that while Blacks were being held and treated as property and lacked resources, they nevertheless were able to maintain psychological focus and to develop and transmit their unique cultural values and beliefs. They fended off the teachings of Whites, dismissed much of what they were being asked to believe, and rejected how they were told they should behave. Enslaved Blacks did have a culture and beliefs and were intelligent and inventive. Survival came at a high cost, since many died or were harmed in ways that are unthinkable or horrific. Some surrendered, and still others fought back with their lives (Bouie, 2019). Yet, in the end, Webber describes how Blacks resisted the teachings of Whites, who regarded them as empty vessels. They silently forged their own educational process and taught their own what was needed for their safety.

The Jim Crow Era

The idea that Blacks had no culture, values, or processes of their own is a theme Whites explicitly and intentionally promoted throughout slavery until at least the Civil Rights movement, and that in many ways is still taught in the 21st century, albeit often in less explicit ways. Although slavery was officially abolished in 1865, the reality is that slaves were slow to be emancipated and the true end of racial domination was/is gradual, dragging well into the 21st century (Feagin, 2006).

What followed the Civil War was a time of Reconstruction in the South (1863–1877) and the establishment of Jim Crow laws, which meant separate and unequal status for Blacks (1877–1964; Feagin, 2006; Silverstein, 2019). The notion that Blacks were inferior held firm after they were freed. For Whites who depended upon their labor, Black people were thought of as children in need of guidance and rules (although, children could not be the backbone of a nation). So, they were the targets of exploitation in many forms (e.g., forced prison labor and share cropping). As always, Blacks resisted, even in the face of domestic terrorism and lynching. Throughout the Great Migration, they moved out of the South and settled in America's cities, only to be isolated into ghettos and inner-city neighborhoods. The narratives began to shift and change about them and their abilities or lack thereof in part because Blacks and like-minded Whites advocated for their Civil Rights. Historians, writing in the 1970s and 1980s about past eras, noted that many ideas about Blacks needed to be revised or restated, and scholars in 2019 made similar points. For instance, in introducing the 1619 project which appeared in the *New York Times* magazine, Silverstein (2019) notes that 1619 is a notable date in history, even though most would mark July 4th 1776 as the birth date of the nation. He contends,

What if, however, we were to tell you that this fact, which is taught in our schools and unanimously celebrated every fourth of July, is wrong, and that the country's true birth date, the moment that its defining contradictions first came into the world, was in late August of 1619? ... that was when a ship arrived at Point Comfort in the British colony of Virginia, bearing a cargo of 20 to 30 enslaved Africans. Their arrival inaugurated a barbaric system of chattel slavery that would last for the next 250 years. This is sometimes referred to as the country's original sin, but it is more than that: It is the country's very origin. Out of slavery – and the anti-black racism it required – grew nearly everything that has truly made America exceptional: Its economic might, its industrial power, its electoral system, diet and popular music, the inequities of its public health and education, its astonishing penchant for violence, its income inequality, the example it sets for the world of freedom and equality, its slang, its legal system and endemic racial fears and hatreds that continue to plague us to this day.

(Silverstein, 2019, pp. 4–5)

Therefore, from this vantage point, much of what makes America unique was intrinsically related to the presence of Black people, and their contributions are numerous, even if unrecognized. During the Jim Crow era, Blacks were subjected on a daily basis to domestic terror at the hands of Whites with little or no protection, yet they still managed to find ways to sustain collective will and they fought back, endured, and defined their lives (B. Stevenson, 2014). Chafe, Gavins, and Korstad (2001) state that the Black people who were interviewed and talked about their experiences during Jim Crow told

compelling [stories] of accommodation and resistance, love and fear, pride and humiliation that constituted the everyday working lives of black Americans who lived through the era (...) the era [was characterized by the] ... dailiness of the terror blacks experienced at the hands of capricious whites... From lynching to being denied the right to be called "Mr." or "Mrs." ... black citizens, ... individually and collectively, found ways to endure, fight back, and occasionally define their own destinies... another "lesson", therefore, is the capacity of the black community to come to each other's aid and invent means of sustaining the collective will to survive... There was also the enduring capacity of families to nurture each other, and especially children. In the face of a system so dangerous and capricious that there was no rules one could count on for protection. One informant(s) recalled how his father taught him to watch out for whites... he told us what to expect, how to act, how to stay away from them... so we... know what we were supposed to do...

(p. xxx)

In the circumstances of Jim Crow, that lasted into the mid-1960s, parents still taught things like personal pride and the importance of sustaining efforts to achieve even in the face of hostility and powerlessness. They taught that it was a virtue to be good and honest and to believe in yourself (Chafe et al., 2001).

The Civil Rights Era

Although equal opportunity employment laws were enacted in 1965 (Carter & Scheuermann, 2020; Romano, 2003). Even now, race-based oppression in the United States continues to exist. Black people continue to be the targets of racism ranging from social and economic oppression, police bias, mass incarceration, and the negative depictions of Black people in television, film and other media controlled mostly by Whites (Carter & Scheuermann, 2020; Vera & Gordon 2003). In fact, Alexander (2012) argues, what replaced legal segregation was mass incarceration veiled by colorblind policies and practices. Alexander explains how resistance to Civil Rights was presented under the guise of law and order. Arguments for the need for law and order came about during eras of social unrest, much of which was associated with the struggle to obtain equal rights and social justice for Blacks and other minorities. Alexander observes that what happened in regard to race was that the structure of American society actually did not change, what did change was the language that was used to produce the same goal (i.e., racial oppression).

People advocated for colorblindness, saying that we should not consider race, and thus race should not be used in the law (Carter & Scheuermann, 2020). At the same time, there was an urgent need to respond to the rise in criminal activity. So, the criminal justice system was used instead "to label people of color 'criminals' and then engage in all the practices we supposedly left behind" (Alexander, 2012, p. 2), since today it is legal to discriminate if someone is a felon. Alexander notes that once designated as criminals, Black people face the same types and degree of discrimination as felons as was true for Black people before the Civil Rights era:

> Once you're a felon, the old forms of discrimination employment, housing discrimination, denial of the right to vote, denial of education opportunities, denial of food stamps, and other public benefits, and exclusion from jury service are suddenly legal... We have not ended racial caste in America; we have merely redesigned it.
>
> (Alexander, 2012, p. 2)

Yet, the role of racial socialization cannot be underestimated, nor its link to racial identity and other cultural practices, as these beliefs and behaviors contribute to Black people's status and will to push ahead. We now turn to a more detailed discussion of racial socialization and how it works.

Socialization and Race: An Aspect of Black Culture

Socialization is a way to examine the Black cultural orientation to social relations and family. As was noted in the previous chapter, Black people raised their children as human and as racial beings. The context in which human development occurs matters and affects what skills, knowledge, and awareness are needed to effectively and successfully contribute to one's life and well-being, and to manage to live and care for one's family and loved ones. Human development is an interactional process that occurs between the person and his/her environment, and from birth, it is on-going and reciprocal. Thus, much in the process of development depends on the characteristics of the factors that interact in dynamic ways with the person in the course of development. The factors that are critical to our discussion are racial group membership, racial socialization, and identity development, as well as the sociocultural, economic, and familial settings in which human development takes place.

Racial groups have been separated into distinct and racially homogenous communities, schools, and often workplaces. For the most part, Black people have been relegated to neighborhoods with concentrated poverty, substandard housing, and under-resourced schools, leading to employment in lower status and menial jobs. Thompson and Carter (2013) argue that segregation in housing and work influences socialization and identity formation by way of establishing institutional and cultural practices that

> reinforce and sustain racial myths and foster the idea [that] … *sociorace* is equated with dramatic and distinct difference beyond skin color and physical appearance. Skin color and physical appearance also become associated with moral, intellectual, and behavioral characteristics. The mass media contributes to the socialization process by reinforcing the lessons and rules that are taught in our immediate environment.
>
> (p. 7)

How race is defined combines both biological markers and the social meaning assigned to particular racial groups in society. The notion of race, based on the racial group one is assumed to be part of, determines for many expectations for social roles, achievement, values, moral codes, and norms for both in-group and out-group members. In most social situations race is assigned to the non-dominant group. Such a social system operates efficiently in situations where the biological markers, such as skin color and physical features, identify members of the respective racial groups.

Racism is a system established on the basis of identifiable racial categories and therefore, complex systems operate beyond the will of the individual. It is possible for organizations and institutions to have structures and processes that establish and promote different outcomes based on racial group membership, and this occurs on its own without any conscious racial bias on the part of individuals. The race-based outcomes advantage the favored group and disadvantage the marginal group or members of the marginal group who are deemed less worthy. An example is the separate racial worlds created during the Jim Crow era. Thompson and Carter (2013) note,

> Institutional and cultural racism appear to have begun taking shape centuries before the *Plessy v. Ferguson* decision. According to social historians, institutional and cultural racism began when Europeans created social systems of subordination and when they began to exploit people who were culturally different from them. In North America, ideas of the racial supremacy of Whites began when Europeans had their first contact with Native Americans in the 15th century. In most cases, this involves the physical and violent taking of land, attempts to destroy Native American culture, and the displacement of indigenous people.
>
> (pp. 5–6)

It is in the context of racism in North America that Black parents and families raise their children, yet the reality is that many Black parents may not wish to address race during the process of socialization. Stevenson et al., (1996) point out that there is considerable variation in attitudes about whether to teach about race and if so, how. Stevenson and colleagues report that, in earlier studies of race-related messages from Black parents (e.g., Spencer 1983), 50% of them thought teaching about race was important. Bowman and Howard (1985) found that less than 40% of adolescents received messages about race and that 54% did not. Thornton, Chatters, Taylor, and Allen (1990) reported from the National Survey of Black Americans that 64% of parents did teach about race while raising their children, while 36% did not. These researchers point out that some Black parents did not want their children to be aware of racism. Some believed that to teach about race would discourage their children before their lives began. Others thought such teaching would make their children bitter and angry, while some considered the matter of racism to be too big an issue for children to grasp, and still others thought racism was not a big problem. These differences reinforce the reality that Black Americans are not a monolith, and likely reflect the different experiences and racial identities of the parents in these studies.

While researchers recognized the variation among parents, they also sought to document the perspectives of children, adolescents, and other members of the extended family systems that operated in Black communities. It was thought early on that identity development was influenced by race and that for a healthy Black identity a person had to address the matter of race, thus the link between racial identity, personal identity, and socialization in a racial context, which we discussed in the previous chapter.

H. Stevenson (1998) argues that social science scholars and researchers described Black families from a deficit perspective and that this viewpoint was destructive and misguided. He points out how scholars have presented evidence to the contrary demonstrating that Blacks were culturally different, not deficient. He states that there are "five key areas in which... to think about the strengths resident within African American family life. Those areas identified include *strong kinship bonds, strong work orientation, adaptability of family roles, strong achievement orientation,* and *strong religious orientation"* (emphasis added, p. 230).

Black people learned that they needed to draw on their cultural values to counter the racially hostile society in which they lived and to protect community and individual identity development (Stevenson, 1998). Boykin and Toms (1985) presented a framework for understanding the socialization challenges for Black families called the "triple quandary" that reflected the areas to which families had to react. They included teaching children according to: (a) mainstream social norms and values; or (b) helping children learn how to face the facts of oppression and being a minority person in America; and (c) teaching children a Black cultural worldview that is distinct from mainstream society. Understanding how Black parents and families prepare their children to live and grow as psychologically healthy people in a racially hostile society is important to understand. H. Stevenson (1995) states that socialization about race is more than responding to racial hostility,

> These processes also include teaching children how to be proud of their culture because its substance is historic, African derived, culturally empowering, and not dependent on oppressive experiences. A second perspective... about... a socialized identity is the view of self as extended and interactional as opposed to individualistic... This definition is akin to the concept of reference group orientation.
>
> (pp. 51–52)

Racial socialization is defined as teaching about race relations and protection against racism, as well as the process of learning about how to function as a member of the Black cultural group and as an American. It is aimed at instructing Blacks about their individual and social realities and how to navigate the world with this knowledge. Racial socialization includes both the direct and indirect messages that an individual receives, and which are communicated during the socialization process, as well as the beliefs a person holds as a result of receiving these race-related messages. However, racial socialization also refers to the process of rearing children toward a positive racial identity and often involves preparing children for racial encounters. Racial socialization theorists contend that the messages taught by parents and community members have a protective benefit to both parents and child. For Blacks in general over time, racial socialization has been one mechanism through which generations pass down instructions not only about the rules and meaning of being a member of the Black racial group but also about how to exist and flourish as a person in U.S. society.

A critical issue for Stevenson (1995) was how to measure racial socialization. He argued that, with regard to the concept and its application or the measurement of both of racial identity and racial socialization,

> The primary worldview orientation espoused is a dialogical, diunital, "both-and" epistemology that assumes opposites are synthesized. This view has implications for how identity and socialization are conceptualized and how measurement is developed. The two salient ethos differences of an African-centered experiential community mirror this epistemology and are called "survival of the tribe" and "oneness of being." These two guiding principles are contrasted with the Euro-American principles of "survival of the fittest" and "control over nature...
>
> (p. 245)

Blacks strive to be in harmony with their world and nature and to act to benefit the community while acting as an individual. For Stevenson (1995), research on racial socialization should include the assessment of both socialization and racial identity. Moreover, he argues that the stress of racism is offset by parents who communicate to their children that much of what they encounter in a racially hostile society is not of their making and that they should not think or assume any responsibility. He states further that racial socialization is a key factor in racial identity development, and both are sources of support from families that contribute to a holistic sense of oneself as a racial being. The various participants in the socialization process are family, peers, community members, and the social system, all of which influence the expression of racial identity. Further, he argues that "racial socialization is a major process in the survival of African American youth if it protects the youth from certain racial hostilities experienced within different ecologies" (Stevenson, 1998, p. 245). Thus, to measure racial socialization, it is necessary to do so from various vantage points: from what parents say they teach; from what children say they learned or were taught; from what other family members communicate; and from what the messages are and how they are communicated (i.e., directly or indirectly). Therefore, instruments need to capture the many facets of the racial identity and racial socialization process. We turn our attention now to the research literature and review selectively what scholars and researchers have found regarding racial socialization. First, we examine research on how racial socialization functions in the therapy domain.

H. Stevenson and Renard (1993) state that therapists and mental health professionals need racial-cultural competence strategies in delivering psychological treatments to Black individuals and families, and that their strategies require an understanding of the underlying societal dynamics that influence Black people's lives. As was noted earlier in this chapter, Hill (1972) and other scholars (Jones, 2003) have documented several strengths of Black families and people. Stevenson and Renard contend that the socialization process, which employs various forms of direct teaching and demonstrations, as well as indirect behavioral lessons, is the place to learn about and understand how Blacks transmit the values of their culture.

These authors also describe Boykin and Toms' (1985) values of Black American life as: (a) *spirituality*; (b) *harmony*; (c) *the call-and-response communication style*; (d) *rhythmic-movement* and *music, or verve*; as well as (e) *improvising*; (f) *affect or emotional expression*, (i.e., how feelings, thoughts, and actions are intermingled); (g) *communalism*; (h) *expressive individualism* (i.e., a unique style as creative expression); and (i) *orality* (i.e., the traditions of spoken communication) and the use of stories and social time, (i.e., human events are important). These join the previous list of values. There are barriers to understanding how best to apply cultural strengths in treatment. Next, we review what we have learned from the racial socialization literature.

Racial Socialization Research Evidence

Stevenson (1993; 1994) reports on the development of a parent's version and adolescent's version of a scale to measure racial socialization called the Scale of Racial Socialization (SORS, A and P). The SORS-A Scale consists of 44 items utilizing a Likert-type response format in which items capture several domains of racial socialization. In the 1993 study, 120 adolescents were given the scale and two dimensions were revealed: spiritual appreciation, which involved messages about religious and cultural expression, and societal apprehension, which includes messages that warn the child about the possibility of negative social encounters. In his 1994 study with the SORS-A, 229 participants were included and items that captured the following domains were included: perception of education, which included items regarding messages about racism in schools; awareness of racism in society, which included items about how racism functions in society; appreciation of spirituality and religion, which included items about belief in God and related activities; promotion of Black heritage and culture, which included items that ask if parents teach about black history and culture; appreciation of extended family, which included items that inquire about the role of relatives in the family; and acceptance of child rearing, which includes items about the importance of child-rearing. The SORS-A was administered with a skin color question and another about whether the family taught about racism. The SORS-A was factor analyzed and the resulting factors were correlated with one another and with the other items in the study. In essence, five factors emerged, yet four were considered viable and one was dropped from further analyses. The factors were: (1) spiritual and religious coping; (2) extended family caring; (3) cultural pride messages; (4) racism awareness; and (5) life achievement, which was dropped. In further analyses, it was found that spiritual coping, extended family, and cultural pride grouped together to reflect a proactive dimension, and protective actions were reflected in the Racism Awareness factor in that those who scored high on this factor did not harbor racist attitudes toward Blacks or Whites. Based on the outcomes of the research, it seems that adolescents' perspectives provided important information about the value of the content and the types of messages received from parents and other family.

In a follow-up study, H. Stevenson (1995) examined racial identity and racial socialization also in adolescents. His objective was to learn about what Black teenagers believed about race and gender identity from interpersonal and intrapersonal perspectives. He notes that researchers had not studied racial identity in youth and that less was known about family, peer, and community contexts as influences on racial identity development. He explored racial identity development in young adolescence because identity develops during these years. He used the Black Racial Identity Attitude Scale and factor analyzed it to see if the various stages would emerge with adolescents, and then correlated them with the racial socialization domains. He found that three Black racial identity subscales could be identified (Encounter did not emerge) and that Pre-Encounter was inversely related to two SORS-A Scales: racial awareness and spiritual coping. Internalization attitudes were related to three of the SORS-A factors, but not racial awareness. Stevenson was instrumental in the assessment of racial socialization, yet other researchers also introduced instruments and Stevenson updated and revised his measures. In a review of the racial socialization literature, Lesane-Brown (2006) documented the presence of some eight instruments.

Thomas and Speight (1999) explored racial socialization messages used by Black American parents and their racial identity attitudes; specific messages according to the gender of children; and the relationship between racial socialization and racial identity attitudes. One hundred four African American parents participated in the study. Racial socialization was seen as important to the vast majority of parents (96%) and they reported a wide variety of socialization messages. These were in the categories referred to as: the presence of racism; the need to be aware of race; the importance of being ready for challenges; how best to function effectively; cultural enrichment; and self-development. The messages were about achievement, racial pride, overcoming racism, Black heritage, religion, self-pride, the reality of racism, the importance of respecting others and being fair, as well as the need to support other Blacks and not to trust Whites. Analysis suggests that parents with Internalization attitudes are more likely to view racial socialization as important, while people with Pre-Encounter attitudes did not communicate about race to their children. The study found that Encounter and Immersion-Emersion attitudes of parents were not related to racial socialization messages. Furthermore, boys and girls received different messages; boys tended to be taught about racial barriers and to be fair, while girls received messages about racial pride.

In a related study, Stevenson et al., (1996) examined the relationship between kinship social support and racial socialization for adolescents. They examined the frequency of racial messages reported by the young people, demographic variation, and degree of kinship support. They found considerable variation in youth's reports of receiving messages about race from parents or family. Overall, 49% said they received such messages sometimes or often, with no gender or other differences. More messages were communicated by more highly educated and middle- and upper-socioeconomic groups. Higher levels of kinship support were related to greater frequency of cultural pride messages. Lastly, kinship support was not related to teaching racial awareness.

We have learned that racial socialization can be measured for parents and youth, and that it is related to the racial identity development of both parents and adolescents but varies by gender and racial identity attitude. While some parents intend to teach about race, many others do not, and some youth do not receive the racial socialization messages sent by family members. But those that do seem to benefit. Furthermore, we discovered that there are several areas and types of messages that are sent by parents, family members, and others; some that are race-related and others that are not. For example, some messages encourage children to be the best person they can be, irrespective of their racial situation.

Lesane-Brown, Brown, Caldwell, and Sellers (2005) found that the majority (77.8-85.3%) of adolescents and college students in their sample received racial socialization messages from multiple sources including parents, family, friends, and other adults. This finding is consistent with the way in which Black culture's child-rearing responsibilities are extended beyond blood-relatives to members of the community (Collins, 2005). The source of these messages may be an important factor in understanding the impact of racial socialization on the psychological functioning of Blacks. Most research has focused solely on the impact of parent to child racial socialization messages while neglecting how messages from church members, neighbors, and older adult relatives may differentially impact the racial socialization process. In addition, the frequency of the messages need to be considered (Lesane-Brown, 2006).

The rate or frequency at which the different types of messages are received may also affect the relationship between racial socialization messages and potential outcomes or lessons learned. While the content of messages has been shown to be important in psychosocial functioning, the frequency of the types of messages can also be considered a vital part of the socialization process. For instance, the psychological distress one may experience may be greater if more messages focus on building awareness to discriminatory practices than on developing cultural heritage and pride (Hughes, Rodriquez, & Smith, 2006; Lesane-Brown, 2006). Moreover, the frequency of the different areas of content of racial socialization messages has been shown to differentiate between sources. For instance, in one study, Black college students reported receiving the message that "Whites think they are better" more often from parents than friends (Lesane-Brown et al., 2005). Knowing when racial socialization messages were first and last received may also be helpful in fully understanding the racial socialization process for Blacks. The temporality and duration of this process may differ from individual to individual and additionally impact psychosocial functioning. By looking at the onset and recency of racial socialization messages, it may be possible to determine when and how often the racial socialization process occurred for an individual.

Lesane-Brown and colleagues (2005) examined which messages were most useful to recipients given an individual's point in life. More concretely, the researchers found that college students were more likely to identify messages about how their hard work can help them achieve anything as most helpful, while adolescents found that messages communicating that race does not matter were the most helpful. This difference in the utility of these types of messages from adolescent to college student may be a product of political and historical changes in race relations, where the individual is in their academic trajectory, and/or the racial make-up of the neighborhoods or schools where the study subjects spent most of their time, or all three.

As mentioned, Black people are not passive recipients of racial socialization messages. Based on a number of individual differences, they may accept, reject, or ignore certain types of messages. Some racial socialization messages are the types that someone would pass on to their children. In effect such messages reveal which lessons were well-received and thus likely to be passed on. Examination of this area of an individual's racial socialization not only highlights the importance of ascertaining which messages they accepted but also attends to the intergenerational nature of the racial socialization process for Blacks in America.

The process of racial socialization takes place both verbally and non-verbally. More attention is given to verbal messages, yet other socializing behaviors are non-verbal and are communicated through actions or interactions about race. For example, consider being taken to Black museums and monuments and attending Black churches as ways to communicate about race and life messages (Lesane-Brown et al., 2005). This non-verbal component of the socialization process may differentially impact mental health outcomes than do verbal messages.

Despite variations in the definition and conceptualization of racial socialization, much work has been done to not only create a nuanced and comprehensive understanding of this process but also unveil the effects of many aspects of racial socialization on Black Americans. While utilizing a multitude of measurement tools, researchers have found generally that racial socialization is an important aspect of Black life and that different types of messages come with differential psychosocial outcomes. These outcomes span different domains of life including education, occupation, and psychological functioning (Hughes et al., 2006; Lesane-Brown, 2006).

Racial socialization has been documented as a strong correlate in the psychosocial health of Black Americans. In general, it has been associated with higher levels of anger management, academic and future orientation, academic performance, quality of interpersonal relationships, motivation and engagement, and ability to cope with discrimination, as well as lower levels of externalizing problems, stress, substance use, and problem behaviors (Elmore & Gaylord-Harden, 2013; Grills, Cooke, Douglas, Subica, Villanueva, & Hudson, 2016; Hughes et al., 2006; Neblett et al., 2008; Neblett, Terzian, & Harriott, 2010; Wang, Henry, Smith, Huguley, & Guo, 2020; Wang, Smith, Miller-Cotto, & Huguley, 2020b). Berkel and colleagues (2009) found that the more racial socialization the parent(s) or caregiver(s) used, the higher the children's self-pride. However, a closer examination shows the content of specific messages seem to have variable impact on psychosocial health, some appearing more helpful than others. Black pride messages have been associated with fostering psychosocial health. Cultural pride reinforcement messages have been associated with lower levels of anxiety and increased peer self-esteem (Bannon, McKay, Chacko, Rodriguez, & Cavaleri, 2009). Not surprisingly, Davis and Stevenson (2006) found that cultural pride reinforcement was inversely related to lethargy and low self-esteem. In addition, racial pride messages have been related to resilience in the face of discrimination, increased self-esteem, less unprovoked anger, and higher academic achievement (Barnes, 1980; Branch & Newcombe, 1986; Branscombe, Schmitt, & Harvey, 1999; Rumbaut, 1994; Spencer, 1983; Stevenson, Reed, Bodison, & Bishop, 1997; Smith, Walker, Fields, Brookins, & Seay, 1999). Bennett (2006) found a positive relationship between racial socialization and achieved ethnic identity.

Racial socialization messages have been found to have a protective effect, reducing symptoms of anger and depression for adolescents exposed to personal racial discrimination (Saleem & Lambert, 2016), and buffering the relationship between discrimination and substance use (Neblett et al., 2010). Researchers have examined whether messages that increase awareness about the inevitability of racial discrimination, along with messages aimed at preparing targets for these incidences, are associated with psychosocial health in Blacks. Some researchers have suggested that preparation for bias messages may serve to counteract negative expectations or stereotypes about minority student academic abilities (Mendoza-Denton, Downy, Purdie, Davis, & Pietrzak, 2002; Steele & Aronson, 1998). Conversely, some studies have documented negative effects of messages about racial bias on youth, documenting associations of decreased self-esteem and increased depression with these types of messages (Barnes, 1980; Branch & Newcombe, 1986; Branscombe et al., 1999; Rumbaut, 1994; Spencer, 1983). Further, Biafora et al. (1993) found that cultural mistrust was positively associated with deviant behavior. While it seems messages that are anticipatory in nature help to prepare and offset the negative impact of racial discrimination and negative racial stereotypes, messages simply teaching about racial bias and to not trust other cultural groups may leave youth both informed but unarmed for negative racial encounters. In fact, two studies show Black youth who expected discrimination or who had been taught racial mistrust exhibited more depression, deviant behavior, and greater conflict with parents (Rumbaut, 1994; Biafora et al., 1993). Other research showed that coupling messages about preparation for bias and cultural pride yielded lower levels of initiation of fights and fighting overall (Stevenson, Herrero-Taylor, Cameron, & Davis, 2002). While preparing Blacks for discrimination can be beneficial, it seems too much of these messages, and particularly when not paired with other racial socialization messages, can yield negative outcomes. To this point, Davis and Stevenson (2006) found that messages communicating awareness of discrimination led to a decrease in irritability; however, an increase in instrumental helplessness. Saleem and Lambert (2016) found that, while high racial socialization messages were protective against interpersonal racism, neither cultural pride messages nor racial barrier messages had a protective effect against anger and depression for adolescents facing institutional racism.

Relatedly, messages about the benefit of Blacks involving themselves in mainstream institutions led to more instances of low energy, pessimism, guilt, low self-esteem, irritability, sad mood, and overall depression. These socialization messages may impair functioning because often this goal and the reality for Blacks are incongruent. Distress may result as the goal of fitting into mainstream environments and the reality of discriminatory behavior clash.

The findings are related to Black racial identity development, wherein individuals who exhibit a positive Black self-image seem to show less psychological distress and more well-being. An inverse relationship between racial socialization and Pre-encounter racial identity attitudes was found (Stevenson, 1995). As discussed previously, it is possible that messages about the harsh reality of a racially oppressive society without additional messages aimed at how to cope, may leave targets feeling hopeless and unprepared in the face of such incidents. As discussed, while the content of racial socialization messages matter, not all messages are explicitly stated. Some come in the form of implicit messages. Caughy, O'Campo, Randolph, and Nickerson (2002) demonstrated the impact of non-verbal racial socialization practices. The number of Afrocentric items in the household was associated with greater factual knowledge and better problem-solving skills in Black children. While taking on a more implicit form, these non-verbal messages may be highly correlated and an extension of verbal messages of Black cultural pride. Burt, Simon, and Gibbons (2012) found cultural socialization messages were not helpful in mitigating the effects of racial discrimination on criminal behavior. Elmore and Gaylord-Harden (2013) found no significant effect of racial pride or racial bias messages on internalizing behaviors, such as withdrawing and somatic complaints, and externalizing behaviors, such as delinquent or aggressive behavior, in African American children.

Overall the process of racial socialization seems to be an effective strategy to pass on how to navigate the often harsh realities of living as a Black person in American society. Further, most racial socialization messages foster positive racial identity for Blacks. However, as racial identity theorists have contended, being a psychosocially healthy Black person in America involves not only a positive image of self as a Black person but also a positive social orientation toward the larger racial group. That is, socializing Blacks toward Black culture ideally includes some messages about the collaborative and communalistic orientation of Blacks. The cultural value of kinship can be traced to West African practices and is not solely the result of U.S. social dynamics. Stewart and Bennett (1991) report American cultural social relationships generally are devoid of obligation with an aversion to any social indebtedness. They point out how this cultural pattern does not seem to hold up in subcultures of the United States such as that of Blacks in the United States, who are seen to adopt an affiliative orientation to social relationships (Stewart & Bennett, 1991).

Beginning as an African cultural value, this prioritizing of the needs of the community over the needs of the individual may have survived because of the extreme economic oppression Blacks have faced. A need to share resources and responsibilities is extended from the immediate family to other members of the community at large. Not only does this include sharing resources and goods, but also the shared responsibility of child rearing, teaching, etc. Researchers have attempted to understand this social interdependence in Black culture in a number of ways including the examination of collectivism and individualism. One reason offered for this culture of affiliation is that the sense of identity and belongingness that is bred in this type of cultural orientation lends itself to more social and political leverage (Stewart & Bennett, 1991).

References

Alexander, M. (2012). *The New Jim Crow: Mass incarceration in the age of colorblindness*. New York, NY: The New Press.

Bannon, Jr, W. M., McKay, M. M., Chacko, A., Rodriguez, J. A., & Cavaleri, Jr, M. (2009). Cultural pride reinforcement as a dimension of racial socialization protective of urban African American child anxiety. *Families in Society: The Journal of Contemporary Social Services, 90*(1), 79–86.

Barnes, E. J. (1980). The Black community as the source of positive self-concept for Black children: A theoretical perspective. *Black Psychology, 2*(1), 106–130.

Bennett, M. D. (2006). Culture and context: A study of neighborhood effects on racial socialization and ethnic identity content in a sample of African American adolescents. *Journal of Black Psychology, 32*(4), 479–500.

Berkel, C., Murry, V. M., Hurt, T. R., Chen, Y. F., Brody, G. H., Simons, R. L., Cutrona, C., & Gibbons, F. X. (2009). It takes a village: Protecting rural African American youth in the context of racism. *Journal of Youth and Adolescence, 38*(2), 175–188.

Berlin, I., Favreau, M., & Miller, S. F. (1998). *Remembering slavery*. New York, NY: The New Press.

Biafora, F. A., Warheit, G. J., Zimmerman, R. S., Gil, A. G., Apospori, E., Taylor, D., & Vega, W. A. (1993). Racial mistrust and deviant behaviors among ethnically diverse Black adolescent boys1. *Journal of Applied Social Psychology, 23*(11), 891–910.

Bouie, J. (August 20th, 2019). Undemocratic democracy. *1619 Project. The New York Times*, 50–55.

Bowman, P., & Howard, C. (1985). Race related socialization, motivation and academic achievement: A study of Black youths in three generation families. *Journal of American Academy of Child Psychiatry, 24*, 134–142.

Boykin, A. W., & Toms, F. D. (1985). Black child socialization: A conceptual framework. In H. McAdoo (Ed.), *Black children: Social, educational, and parental environments* (pp. 33–51). Thousand Oaks, CA: Sage Publications, Inc.

Branch, C. W., & Newcombe, N. (1986). Racial attitude development among young Black children as a function of parental attitudes: A longitudinal and cross-sectional study. *Child Development, 1*, 712–721.

Branscombe, N. R., Schmitt, M. T., & Harvey, R. D. (1999). Perceiving pervasive discrimination among African Americans: Implications for group identification and well-being. *Journal of Personality and Social Psychology, 77*(1), 135.

Burt, C. H., Simons, R. L., & Gibbons, F. X. (2012). Racial discrimination, ethnic-racial socialization, and crime: A micro-sociological model of risk and resilience. *American Sociological Review, 77*(4), 648–677.

Carter, R. T. & Scheuermann, T.D. (2020). *Confronting racism: Integrating mental health strategies with legal reform.* New York, NY: Routledge.

Caughy, M. O. B., O'Campo, P. J., Randolph, S. M., & Nickerson, K. (2002). The influence of racial socialization practices on the cognitive and behavioral competence of African American preschoolers. *Child Development, 73*(5), 1611–1625.

Chafe, W. H., Gavins, R., & Korstad, R. (2001). *Remembering Jim Crow.* New York, NY: The New Press.

Collins, P. (2005). The Meaning of Motherhood in Black Culture and Black Mother-Daughter Relationships. In M. Baca Zinn, P. Hondagneu-Sotelo, & M. A. Messner (Eds.), *Gender through the Prism of Difference* (3rd ed., pp. 285–295). Oxford University Press

Davis, G. Y., & Stevenson, H. C. (2006). Racial socialization experiences and symptoms of depression among Black youth. *Journal of Child and Family Studies, 15*(3), 293–307.

Elmore, C. A., & Gaylord-Harden, N. K. (2013). The influence of supportive parenting and racial socialization messages on African American youth behavioral outcomes. *Journal of Child and Family Studies, 22*(1), 63–75.

Feagin, J. R. (2006). *Systemic racism.* New York, NY: Routledge.

Grills, C., Cooke, D., Douglas, J., Subica, A., Villanueva, S., & Hudson, B. (2016). Culture, racial socialization, and positive African American youth development. *Journal of Black Psychology, 42*(4), 343–373.

Hill, R. (1972). *The strengths of Black families.* New York: Emerson Hall.

Hughes, D., Rodriguez, J., Smith, E. P., Johnson, D. J., Stevenson, H. C., & Spicer, P. (2006). Parents' ethnic-racial socialization practices: a review of research and directions for future study. *Developmental Psychology, 42*(5), 747–770.

Jones, J. M. (2003). TRIOS: A psychologcial theory of the African legacy in American culture. *Journal of Social Issues, 39*(1), 217–242.

Lesane-Brown, C. L. (2006). A review of race socialization within Black families. *Developmental Review*, *26*(4), 400–426.

Lesane-Brown, C. L., Brown, T. N., Caldwell, C. H., & Sellers, R. M. (2005). The comprehensive race socialization inventory. *Journal of Black Studies*, *36*(2), 163–190.

Mendoza-Denton, R., Downey, G., Purdie, V. J., Davis, A., & Pietrzak, J. (2002). Sensitivity to status-based rejection: Implications for African American students' college experience. *Journal of Personality and Social Psychology*, *83*(4), 896–918.

Neblett Jr, E. W., Terzian, M., & Harriott, V. (2010). From racial discrimination to substance use: The buffering effects of racial socialization. *Child Development Perspectives*, *4*(2), 131–137.

Neblett, E. W., White, R. L., Ford, K. R., Phillip, C. L., Nguyen, H. X., & Sellers, R. M. (2008). Patterns of racial socialization and psychological adjustment: Can parental communications about race reduce the impact of racial discrimination? *Journal of Research on Adolescence*, *18*(3), 477–515.

Romano, R. (2003). *Race mixing: Black– White marriage in postwar America*. Cambridge: Harvard University Press.

Rumbaut, R. G. (1994). The crucible within: Ethnic identity, self-esteem, and segmented assimilation among children of immigrants. *International Migration Review, 28*(4), 748–794.

Saleem, F. T., & Lambert, S. (2016). Differential effects of socialization messages for African American adolescents: Personal versus institutional racism. *Journal of Child and Family Studies*, *25*, 1385–1396.

Silverstein, J. (2019). The 1619 project: Introduction. *The New York Time Magazine*, p. 4.

Smith, E. P., Walker, K., Fields, L., Brookins, C. C., & Seay, R. C. (1999). Ethnic identity and its relationship to self-esteem, perceived efficacy and prosocial attitudes in early adolescence. *Journal of Adolescence*, *22*(6), 867–880.

Spencer, M. B. (1983). Children's cultural values and parental child rearing strategies. *Developmental Review*, *3*(4), 351–370.

Stack, C. B. (1974). *All our kin: Strategies for survival in a black community*. Basic Books. New York, NY.

Steele, C. M., & Aronson, J. (1998). Stereotype threat and the test performance of academically successful African Americans. In C. Jencks & M. Phillips (Eds.), *The Black– White test score gap* (pp. 401–427). Brookings Institution Press.

Stewart, E. C., & Bennett, M. J. (1991). *American cultural patterns: A cross-cultural perspective*. Boston, MA: Nicholas Brealey Publishing.

Stevenson, B. (2014). *Just Mercy* New York, NY: Spiegel & Grau.

Stevenson, H. C. (1993). Validation of the scale of racial socialization for African American adolescents: A preliminary analysis. *Psych Discourse, 24*, 12.

Stevenson, H. C. (1994). Validation of the scale of racial socialization for African American adolescents: Steps toward multidimensionality. *Journal of Black Psychology*, *20*(4), 445–468.

Stevenson, H. C. (1995). Relationship of adolescent perceptions of racial socialization to racial identity. *Journal of Black Psychology*, *21*(1), 49–70.

Stevenson, H. C. (1998). Theoretical considerations in measuring racial identity and socialization: Extending the self-further. In R. Jones (Ed.), *African American identity development: Theory, research, and intervention* (pp. 227–263). Hampton, VA: Cobb & Henry.

Stevenson, H. C., Herrero-Taylor, T., Cameron, R., & Davis, G. Y. (2002). Mitigating instigation: Cultural phenomenological influences of anger and fighting among "big-boned" and "baby-faced" African American youth. *Journal of Youth and Adolescence, 31*(6), 473–485.

Stevenson, H. C., Reed, J., Bodison, P., & Bishop, A. (1996). Kinship social support and adolescent racial socialization beliefs: Extending the self to family. *Journal of Black Psychology, 22*(4), 498–508.

Stevenson, H. C., Reed, J., Bodison, P., & Bishop, A. (1997). Racism stress management racial socialization beliefs and the experience of depression and anger in African American youth. *Youth & Society, 29*(2), 197–222.

Stevenson, H. C., & Renard, G. (1993). Trusting ole' wise owls: Therapeutic use of cultural strengths in African-American families. *Professional Psychology: Research and Practice, 24*, 433–442.

Thomas, A. J., & Speight, S. L. (1999). Racial identity and racial socialization attitudes of African American parents. *Journal of Black Psychology, 25*(2), 152–170. doi: 10.1177/0095798499025002002

Thompson, C. E., & Carter, R. T. (2013). *Racial identity theory: Application to individuals, group, and organizational interventions.* New York, NY: Routledge.

Thornton, M. C., Chatters, L. M., Taylor, R. J., & Allen, W. R. (1990). Sociodemographic and environmental correlates of racial socialization by Black parents. *Child Development, 61*, 401–409.

Vera, H., & Gordon, A. (2003) Screen *saviors: Hollywood fictions of Whiteness.* New York: Rowman and Littlefield.

Wang, M.-T., Henry, D. A., Smith, L. V., Huguley, J. P., & Guo, J. (2020). Parental ethnic-racial socialization practices and children of color's psychosocial and behavioral adjustment: A systematic review and meta-analysis. *American Psychologist, 75*(1), 1–22. doi: 10.1037/amp0000464

Wang, M. T., Smith, L. V., Miller-Cotto, D., & Huguley, J. P. (2020b). Parental ethnic-racial socialization and children of color's academic success: A meta-analytic review. *Child Development, 91*(3), e528–e544.

Webber, T. L. (1978). *Deep like the rivers: Education in the slave quarter community, 1831–1865.* New York, NY: W.W. Norton.

Chapter 6

The Community and Its Value

We have reviewed the cultural processes associated with racial identity and racial socialization, and how the two are related. Both aspects of Black culture could not exist without the value placed on community, and the integral role it played in Black life. This cultural value stands out in that it is contrary to the American cultural preference of individualism. In fact, scholars have construed the Black preference for the Black racial and cultural reference group as a form of collectivism, which as we will show, it is not.

The constructs of collectivism and individualism have been popular areas of research across cultural groups both internationally and within the context of the United States. This research has focused on contrasting racial and ethnic groups against White Americans (Vandello & Cohen, 1999). Collectivism has been defined as a cultural value system, which focuses on an interdependent sense of self, where social behavior is guided by the norms and expectations of the group. Considering the orientation toward community prevalent in Black culture, it seems reasonable to assume that Blacks in America would exhibit high levels of collectivism and low levels of individualism (Utsey, Ponterotto, Reynolds, & Cancelli, 2000). However, findings have not supported this notion. In an evaluation of theoretical assumptions and a meta-analysis of collectivism-individualism studies, Oyserman, Coon, and Kemmelmeier (2002) found that African Americans emerged as the most individualistic racial group over and above European Americans, Latino Americans, and Asian Americans. Yet these researchers failed to consider the expressive form of individualism described by Black scholars that has evolved among Black people. The expressive form represents a unique version of individualism, which did not divorce one from the good of the group. It is possible that what was found in these studies was this distinct variety of individualism expressed by Blacks.

An examination of tools used to measure collectivism and individualism in the same study revealed that adding some assessment of a participant's valuation of personal uniqueness significantly increased Blacks' endorsement of individualism. Additionally, assessing the valuation of privacy, personal competition, and self-knowledge increased individualism scores for Blacks. This highlights a

DOI: 10.4324/9781003083221-7

limitation of using collectivism as a cultural value in Blacks in America. While the constructs of individualism and collectivism generally speak to differences across international cultures, they may not fully capture differences among racial groups within the United States. Specifically, there seem to be distinct differences in individualism and collectivism among Blacks versus other American racial groups. Because of this, using collectivism to capture the orientation of Black Americans toward their communities is not sufficient.

A construct employed to specifically and accurately describe the cultural value of the community for Blacks has been called "communalism." Boykin, Jagers, Ellison, and Albury (1997) described communalism as the social interdependence of Black people. It is the belief that the success of the individual and the group are inseparable. Boykin (1984) defined communalism as an Afrocultural concept that

> denotes awareness of the [fundamental] interdependence of people. One's orientation is social rather than being directed toward objects. One acts in accordance with the notion that duty to one's social group is more important than individual privileges and rights. Sharing is promoted because it signifies the affirmation of social interconnectedness; self-centeredness and individual greed are disdained.
>
> (p. 345)

Boykin et al. (1997) went on to explain some of the complexity of communalism, describing five main components. These core components were (a) primacy of social existence, (b) sanctity of social bonds and relations, (c) transcendence of group duties and responsibilities over individual concerns, (d) anchoring of individual identity in the group, and (e) an emphasis on sharing and contributing in support of the group. These components reveal the complexity of this cultural orientation for Blacks. Jagers and Mock (1995) found that a measure of communalism dovetailed with, but was not identical to a Collectivism Scale. Although communalism was positively associated with collectivism and negatively associated with individualism, the construct seems to add something substantive to the study of this cultural orientation in Blacks.

The value of community that we present as a critical aspect of Black culture should not be thought of as something that operates today or just in the recent past, but rather as something that has also been a hallmark of African culture and came with enslaved people when they were brought to the New World. There are many instances and examples that have been documented in history to support this claim. We will report a few, touching on various historical eras and situations to illustrate the manner in which community was held as a value and used for the preservation and advancement of Black American people.

During Slavery

Webber (1978) described community as one cultural theme endemic to the slave community. The core of the community was family, which was uniquely defined. For Black people community involved many components including extended family, peers, educational leaders, and church members. In fact, it is apparent that Blacks engaged in considerable efforts to build and develop community through organizations and institutions. Bennett (1988) tells about such efforts prior to the American revolution and later among free and enslaved people. He states that, on

> Thursday, April 12, 1787... one month before the first session of the U.S. Constitutional Convention and two years before the election of George Washington... eight [Black] men sat down in a room in Philadelphia and created a black social compact... called the African Society. The founding of this seminal organization was only one wave in the tide of institution-building that rolled over the North in the 1780's and 1790's.
>
> (pp. 55–56)

Other groups and organizations were formed in other states as well. In addition, Blacks formed independent churches, lodges, schools, and social organizations. Behind these efforts were, according to Bennett (1988), two driving forces:

> a sense of identity and peoplehood that rejected black subordination and exclusion. The negative current... was a campaign to exclude black Americans from the national social contract...
>
> (p. 56)

> [In response] blacks turned inward and formed their own social institutions and, in the process, created themselves... This [act] of self-generation created a community out of a collective of isolated individuals...
>
> (p. 77)

Much of the activity of building and forming organizations and communities was undertaken by the small percentage of Blacks who were not slaves at the time, but many were former slaves. The Free African Society established by the eight Black men included a church, a society for aid to other Blacks, a political foundation for activism, and the seeds for a Black insurance company.

The first organizations were followed by others in different cities in the North, and the memberships grew to encompass larger numbers of members. It is significant that these organizations were linked and connected to each other, "through the medium of these organizations, blacks exchanged information, ideas, and programs... they began to see their lives in a time-line extending from

Africa to the Day of Judgement they believed would vindicate them" (Bennett, 1988, p. 80). The movement to develop Black churches started in the 1770s with the creation of the first African Baptist churches in states like Georgia, Virginia, and South Carolina. The churches helped Blacks establish social and fraternal organizations, the first of which, an African Lodge, was started in Boston in 1787. These various organizations helped fuel the early efforts to promote Black equal rights.

Following the efforts to organize was the clear need to educate its people and so, Black leaders set out to establish Black schools. "All the while, on another level of existence, black leaders were pressing an increasingly sophisticated campaign against discrimination and segregation" (Bennett, 1988, p. 83).

In the South where the majority (90%) of Blacks resided and were less able to move about and participate in organizations, we still find that the community was at the center of Black people's lives. Much of the slave's life, day in and day out, was devoted to labor. From the morning horn (around 4 am) until midnight, they labored either in the fields, or the main house, or in attending to their own needs and homes. Bennett (1988) notes that this regimen was supposed to crush the slave's spirit and will. Yet he notes that in fact the opposite was true:

> For the slaves, in the most astonishingly creative act in our history, transcended their environment, creating a new structure of meaning and putting their oppressors and the world in their debt. No one can read the record of that transcendence without a sense of awe at the audacity of the slaves' hope. This hope was clearly visible in the concentric circles of community that started in the family and radiated in larger and larger circles that enveloped the whole of the Slave Row. From that community came the rhythmic, spiritual, and psychic piles that bottomed the new synthesis called Black America. The results---the spirituals, the blues, the rhythmic tonality of Black America----point to and guarantee the medium, which was a community of passion and creativity. The community was a product of the plantation, but was neither defined nor contained by the plantation. On the contrary, it was defined by difference, by the fact that it contradicted and called into question the values and institutions of the plantation. The fundamental difference was orientation. The community of the slaves was a communal entity characterized by a collective orientation stemming partly from the African past and partly from the exigencies of the situation. Unlike the slaveholders community, it was oriented toward freedom, toward freedom of the body and soul, which were not defined as two different things but as two aspects of the same thing.

(p. 96)

Bennett (1988) contends that the slave community mirrors communities of today and the recent past, in that it is not defined by geographic boundaries, since it was part of the person and not the situation or location. Each community had selected leaders from among their own and they also looked to the elders for guidance. Moreover, the community and its structure operated around several other interrelated cultural elements such as spirituality:

> The first, of course was the axis of the spirit. In this realm, as in others the slaves reinterpreted white patterns, weaving a whole new universe around biblical images and giving a new dimension and new meaning to Christianity... infusing it with African-oriented melodies and rhythms and adding new patterns, such as the ring shout, ecstatic seizure and communal, call-and-response patterns.
>
> (Bennett, 1988, p. 99)

The Africans and their descendants arranged to worship in private by stealing away into the woods or swamps. In this setting they developed their own manner of worship and connection to one another. Their beliefs were twofold, one in God and the other in spirits, who had power over the living; the second set of beliefs were visible in the use of taboos, charms, and other practices that were contrary to White Christian worship. Yet, as Bennett (1988) points out, the religious element was a part of a more complex set of beliefs and practices.

The second communal element was expressed in music, improvisation, and rhythm. Recall that, according to Jones (2003), rhythm is a core aspect of Black culture. For Bennett and other historians (e.g., Horton & Horton, 2005), music was a central aspect of Black people's lives both in and out of slavery. Bennett (1988) describes it this way: music, improvisation, and rhythm,

> was characterized by the so-called "blues" tonality and a rhythmic, collective and emotional orientation. The same elements are evident in slave [Black] folk lore and philosophy, especially the Brer Rabbit, Brer Fox and Old John cycles. The expression of this orientation was as varied as the people and included cries, hollers, work songs, devil songs, spirituals and blues... The third [communal element] was the extended family. In interpersonal relationships, as in the fields of music and religion, the slaves [Black people] triumphed by transcending and transforming the institutions of their oppressors.
>
> (pp. 102–103)

Their process of transformation can be seen in families. There was considerable pressure and restrictions imposed by the oppressors to conform, and the slave's family was not recognized nor had any legal status, since husband, wife, and children were all the property of the "owners" and could be separated at their will. Moreover, following the outlawing of the importation of slaves into the United States in 1808, multiple mates were often encouraged or forced for the purpose of breeding and market sales. During the brutal system of slavery, the enslaved established a way to mate and marry that helped them to manage their lives and grow (Bennett, 1988). One mechanism that was created and used, outside of the master's view and knowledge, was jumping the broom to marry. Bennett notes that how these marriages occurred revealed that they were based on love and equality, since the woman could end the marriage when she desired, which was not the case for the formal process undertaken by Whites.

It has been suggested (e.g., Stamp, 1956) that Black people were of loose morals and engaged in unrestrained sexual behavior with no sense of family or kinship obligations. However, a comprehensive study by Gutman (1976) about the Black family both free and enslaved revealed that family units, many of which were headed by males, consisted of long-term marriages (30 or more years), and fathers were highly regarded and often important and respected members of the family system. Perhaps because they lived near one another, there was more openness about sex, in particular when it happened before marriage and pregnancy was the result, but for Black people, there was the expectation of marriage in the event of a pending birth. There was also the notion that once married, people would not stray. Lastly, marriage was often supported by an extended family network with and without blood relations, during and after slavery.

As we can see, the family was an important component of the community. The value of communalism persisted through time as well. There is evidence of its presence from before the founding of the nation through the Jim Crow era, and into the present. It is also apparent that communalism consisted of several components. The belief in spirit as reflected in religious belief and practice, and the unique use of music and rhythm all contributed to Black peoples' sense of and the value placed in community. So, while being group-focused may have been fostered, in part, by their circumstances, it is also something that was handed down from their African ancestors.

The Jim Crow Era

As time passed, Black people, or Negros as they were called during the Jim Crow era, were exposed to various experiences including serving the country in World War I (1914–1918) and World War II (1939–1945) both in combat and as workers in military related industries. While their contributions were not recognized at home, the changing times sparked the great migration from the South to the North, which occurred between 1900 and 1970, and these events altered the racial landscape and set the stage for social change and the movement for Civil Rights (Wilkerson, 2010). Slowly, Blacks began to openly reject their second-class status, and collectively they acted to gain the dignity and civil rights that were denied them as American citizens.

It is important to restate the circumstances in which Black Americans acted and to comprehend the weight of what they achieved. It is known that for 250 years, Blacks, whether free or slave, lived in a racial caste system in that they were segregated and held outside the mainstream of society with few exceptions. What is harder to understand is the extent of the domination that they endured. By the mid-20th century, in the 1950s, they took collective action. It was almost 100 years after the Civil War and after they had been freed from slavery, yet they were still held in a racial caste system that involved almost total domination. Morris (1984) notes that the three parts of racial oppression were, and to some extents are, economic, political, and personal.

Blacks were limited regarding where and what type of work they were permitted to have, and as a result, they "were heavily concentrated in the lowest-paying and dirtiest jobs the cities had to offer" (Morris, 1984, p. 1). This meant they held jobs as porters', cooks, laborers and so forth, while less than a quarter of Whites held such jobs. About half of Black women were domestics mostly in the South, a position that 1% of Whites held. If women were not domestics, they also held service-related positions, and overall Blacks earned close to 50% less than Whites. In addition to low wages and physical labor, Blacks' behavior and actions were controlled by Whites to a large extent. Whites were their supervisors and bosses and had considerable authority over them. Blacks accepted the situation because the alternative was not to work at all and to be unable to provide for their families. So, they endured, as had been true in the past. Compounding the economic oppression was the lack of political participation, which was imposed or blocked, as "blacks were systematically excluded from the political process" (Morris, 1984, p. 2). Blacks held no political offices in cites or states where they lived, and there were poll taxes and other obstacles that needed to be overcome for them to be politically active. This is in contrast to the decade of Reconstruction, from 1865 to 1877, when Blacks did in fact hold elected offices in towns, cities, and states, and some worked at the federal level. So, they were in fact capable and able. In the political context, Whites controlled the resources of cities, towns, counties, and states and Whites dominated these positions and oversaw law enforcement as well. Morris (1984) notes that "it was common for law officials to use terror and brutality against blacks. Due process of law was virtually nonexistent because the courts were controlled by white judges and juries, which routinely decided in favor of whites" (p. 2).

Blacks were oppressed also on a personal level in that they were segregated and as such had few personal freedoms. The system of racial segregation marked Blacks as inferior and socially worthless. Because of their low status Black people, by law, were forced to use separate facilities, such as restrooms, water fountains, housing, health care, and so forth. Being separated was not enough. Black people were required to behave in specific ways in relationship to White people or be subject to arrest or death. Whites had to be addressed by formal titles. And Blacks were not allowed to meet Whites' glaze and make eye contact. They had to lower their eyes when meeting White people, women in particular. They had to move aside when a White person walked in the same path. This system of oppression operated in cities as well as in rural areas throughout the country.

And more importantly, rules and laws existed that backed the system of racial oppression, and left Blacks in what seemed to be a helpless situation. Here again, as was the case before the American Revolution, the effort to exclude Blacks was fuel for Blacks to build and develop their own organizations and institutions. Morris (1984) notes:

> Ironically,… segregation… had some positive consequences. It facilitated the development of black institutions and the building of close-knit communities when blacks, irrespective of education and income were forced to live in close proximity and frequent the same social institutions… Cooperation between the various black strata was an important collective resource for survival… within these compact segregated communities' blacks began to sense their collective predicament as well as their collective strength.
>
> (pp. 3–4)

As was true in the past, various institutions served Blacks' interests and goals. Historically Black colleges, universities, and the church served the needs of Blacks. The church was a place where people were not oppressed and they could engage in the cultural activities that nourished them such as listening to sermons, singing, telling stories, and praying. They were also able to gather their resources and discuss any efforts to organize acts of collective resistance. Recall the value of songs and storytelling among Black people: it was in the church that this tradition could be expressed and strengthened since it was one of the few resources Blacks had that they built and supported on their own, and as such, was their institution alone. Morris (1984) argues:

> The black church filled a large part of the institutional void by providing support and direction for the diverse activities of an oppressed group. It furnished outlets for social and artistic expression; a forum for the discussion of important issues; a social environment that developed, trained, and disciplined potential leaders from all walks of life; and meaningful symbols to engender hope, enthusiasm, and a resilient group spirit… the black church has served as the organizational hub of black life…
>
> (p. 5)

The church was an organization headed by its ministers, who through personal qualities were entrusted to lead the congregation. He or she was supported by groups and committees that attended to a range of church activities. The church leaders gave voice to the core values of Black people when they spoke of dignity, integrity, and the struggle for freedom. By stating these values Black leaders were able to stir and grow a desire on the part of Black people to strive for social change. The various churches and leaders were not always of one mind and there were differences and conflicts within and among the various churches.

Yet, they also had some things in common that fostered the combined power of the churches as a force among and by Black people.

As we noted previously, other social organizations also came to being during this time, such as the National Association for the Advancement of Colored People (NAACP), a group created in the North in 1909–1910 by White and Black activists to advocate for equal rights. Its founding was accomplished by middle- and upper-middle class people, and it was not, like the church, rooted in the Black masses. Morris tells the story of the NAACP's origins and its connections to Black people. What should be noted here is that they elected to use legal action and advocacy to achieve their goals of racial equality. In addition, several other groups that organized and fought for civil rights were started in this era (e.g. Congress of Racial Equality, CORE; Southern Christian Leadership Conference, SCLC; etc.).

Transmission of Communalism through the Black Family and Community

Communalism as a core cultural value is rooted in the activity of the groups we have discussed as well as in the families and individuals who were socialized in Black family networks. Since our focus in this book is clinical application and treatment that uses and emphasizes the Black cultural strengths we review and describe, it is important to illustrate how individuals reflect the inculcation of the Black sense of spirit, the value of the group, and how people's actions reflected this cultural value.

All groups are composed of a collection of individuals, as are families. All people come from a family and or parents and reside in a location among other people and families. For many people, our strongest bond and connection during our formative years and early childhood is with our mothers and fathers or caregivers. From these significant relationships, we internalize our understating of the world. Whether we use lessons from our parents as guides of what we do not want to do or as models we wish to emulate, our parents or caregivers and families play powerful roles in shaping who we are and how we view, understand, and interact with the world around us.

Individuals interpret their experiences from their unique vantage point and perspective. That is, they see the world and others through their eyes and senses. Our predispositions and ways of being come from us and are shaped by others and the circumstances we encounter in our lives. As we have noted previously, social and cultural groups take different positions on how we should interact with the world and what principles we should use to guide our society and culture. Some may hold that we should shape our world, while others may believe that we should seek to be one with the world, and others might hold that we are the subjects of the world around us. Some may believe that we should focus on the wishes of the individual, or follow the wisdom of the authorities and elders, or find guidance in thoughtful group-based decisions or the collective good. There are options that one can select from.

In the collection of narratives that Webber (1978) used in his study of the slave community, the theme of the connection to one's parents was quite strong and persistent. The mother was held in extremely high regard and fathers also held an important place in their children's minds and hearts. Family also went beyond the parents and blood relations as we have noted previously. Whether the world is hostile or not, parents and families have the responsibility and the obligation to educate and socialize their offspring. Some assume this role, and others may not fully embrace the task. Nevertheless, children are dependent on the adults around them and as such are taught both directly and indirectly. In particular, children learn how to live in the circumstances into which they were born. Regardless of status, whether living as a slave or segregated or as a free person, in their respective community, the situation meant, for some, that family and community were often the same and few hard lines were drawn to distinguish between the two. Webber (1978) observes that for Blacks,

> Mother was the central figure in the… family's educational role. From the time she first suckled her child at her breast, rocked him to her lap, or sang him to sleep, she began the process of transmitting values, beliefs, feelings, that would be reinforced later more deliberately. As a baby the black child… learned that comfort and security were to be found in black arms; that nurture came from black breast; that drowsy tranquility accompanied the sounds of black music; that love was the caress of a black hand or the singing of a black voice.
>
> (p. 159)

In their narratives, former slaves often recalled their early years when the child was comforted by the songs and warmth of their mother's body. Songs served many purposes; some taught about spiritual beliefs and others about a mother's love. As the child aged, lessons grew in number and frequency. Much of the early lessons were centered around self-care and how to care for others in the family that were younger. They were taught how to wash clothes, how to feed and watch out for infants, and how to comb hair. Other activities were imparted, like how to sew, spin, iron, clean, and stuff a mattress, how to make candles, and to cook, and so on.

> More important, perhaps, than her teaching of household skills, was the role which mother played in the transmission of religious beliefs, a longing for freedom, a desire to learn, a way of viewing and dealing with white people, and a sense of identification and solidarity with the other members of the… community… In families without grandparents, it was frequently the role of mother to transmit the stories of Africa, and the folklore and songs of the community which she had learned from her own parents or grandparents. These

stories… served not merely to transmit values and attitudes to each new generation but, by linking children to their ancestors, helped cement family ties.

(Webber, 1978, pp. 162–163)

Respect for the elders and obeying were also important lessons for Black children.
The rules were strictly, and sometimes harshly, enforced. As the child aged, the
role of fathers became more pronounced and important. Some would provide extra
food and clothes and those that were capable made furniture and other items for
the home and taught their children how to do the same. Fathers also taught how
to hunt and fish and were able at times to earn extra money for the family in these
endeavors. Those fathers that had skills and were artisans passed on what they
knew as well. Like mothers, fathers told and taught through stories and sang songs.
Lessons about race were also taught by mothers and fathers when time permitted. From their parents children learned about relationships and family bonds. The
domestic slave trade meant that families were often separated from one another.
When fathers and mothers were not able or present, grandfathers and grandmothers would assume their roles and teach the children. And when other family members were not around or able, members of the community stepped into the roles
described. Older brothers and sisters in the Black family also made an important
and critical contribution to raising younger siblings. As is apparent, the community
and its members were vital in the survival of its members. The entire community,
in the form of parents, extended family, peers, and leaders all identified with one
another and functioned to nurture, protect, discipline, and educate one another.

Similar practices were undertaken after the Civil War when Black people were
free from slavery, but the restrictions and oppression simply took different forms
and methods. The emergence of Black Codes and Jim Crow laws meant that racial
oppression was legal and Blacks had to live in a state of constant fear and hostility,
with little to no protection from authorities. Their status as second-class citizens
was codified in these new laws that dictated they be separate from the mainstream
White society. Once again, their situation meant that they needed to create institutions and organizations and family systems that helped them maintain their human
dignity. Blacks relied on similar values and beliefs to weather the new storms of
racial oppression. They banded together and families were, as before, the center of
the community. While Black people were no longer property, they were nevertheless dependent as poor sharecroppers or laborers working for little and often even
less. In this circumstance, they still managed to hold their heads high and establish
accepted codes of behavior and decorum for themselves and their children. Chafe,
Gavins, and Korstad (2001) observe:

Seeking to overcome this legacy of inhumanity, freed people and their pos-
terity created and sustained fundamental relationships, building families and
kinship networks, forming supportive communities and organizing economic,
educational, political and religious institutions. Self-help and mutual aid in

raising of children, caring for the sick and helping the destitute were crucial for the survival and advancement of individuals, families, and communities. The spirit of responsibility quickened as African Americans were denied equal citizenship and were all but excluded from access to mainstream financial institutions. In the face of oppression, they forged a moral economy, creatively fostering racial solidarity, progress, and equality.

(p. 89)

For instance, consider the story of David Mathews who was born in 1920 in Mississippi. He tells about his recollections growing up:

I grew up in a rural community. My mother and father were Christians, and they were laborers. We were sharecroppers (…) We had high moral values in that they taught us against stealing, robbing, or taking anything that was not ours (…) They also taught us to do a day's work for a day's pay and be honest with people as we go from day to day.

(cited in, Chafe et al., 2001, p. 108)

There were the brothers Dixie, who recalled some aspects of how they worked in collaboration with one another in the community to share and support each other in spite of limited resources:

A.I (…) and Samuel Dixie were bothers [who] talked about the role of lodges and other organizations during their time. I joined the [the Order of Emancipated Americans] in the [19] thirties (…) See, you paid 75 cents a month [and they] give you $200 in cash when you die (…) if you were a farmer and your mule died and you belonged to the (…) Order, everybody that had a mule had to give you a day's work until they could get you another mule. And if your house get burned down, they would chip in and help you get shelter.

(cited in, Chafe et al, 2001, pp. 108–109)

Parents and other family wanted their children to do better than them and a high value was placed on education and going to school. So, through time, the group functioned as an interdependent whole and passed on the value of the group to each new generation. The shape and form of the cultural values changed across time and circumstances. Yet, we contend that the value of communalism has been retained by Black people across the centuries.

Communalism Research Evidence

Our purpose is to document the areas of cultural practice undertaken by Blacks that contribute to their well-being and psychological health. In that sense we are putting forth, as others have done, a form of Black cultural strength that is grounded not in deprivation or oppression, but rather in beliefs, emotions, and actions that aided in Black people's ability to live through harsh and brutal treatment in American society. As Nobles (1991) notes,

> African Americans derive their most fundamental self-definition from several cultural and philosophical premises which we share with most West African "tribes"... In exploring the character of these premises, which are basic conceptions of the nature of man [humans] and his relation to other men [humans] and his environment, we hope to establish a foundation upon which a black psychology can be constructed. Thus, it will be contended that black psychology is something more than the psychology of so-called underprivileged peoples, more than the experience of living in ghettos, or of having been forced into dehumanizing conditions of slavery. It is more than the "darker" dimensions of general psychology. Its unique status is from the positive features of basic African philosophy which dictates the values, customs, attitudes and behavior of Africans in Africa and the New World.
>
> (p. 47)

For Nobles, African people had in common two core beliefs that guided their lives and religions. The first, common ethos (i.e., subconscious spiritual disposition), was the idea that people had to live with nature and be in harmony with its rhythms. It was vital that people be one with nature. The second vital core belief is the survival of one's people. According to this core belief, a person must act to the benefit and for the good of the "tribe" or their people; the community is paramount. Nobles (1991) notes,

> A great number of beliefs and practices were and can be found in African society. However, these beliefs and/or traditions were handed down from father to son for generations upon generation. As such, and in accordance with the prevailing *oral tradition,* (...) the acts were communal.
>
> (p. 49)

Nobles' observations laid the foundation for the research efforts tied to demonstrating the existence of the cultural value of communalism in present day Black people. This work was reported in studies by Jagers and Mock (1995) and Boykin, Jagers, Ellison, and Albury (1997).[1] Boykin and colleagues defined communalism and developed a measure to assess its presence. They began their paper by noting that Black Americans' cultural legacy is characterized by

> spirituality, which suggests a focus on the vitalistic, shared essence of all things; the oral tradition, which places a premium on the spoken word; rhythmic-movement expressiveness; and communalism, which highlights the social interdependence of people... the essence of the communal

orientation… is that individuals view themselves as being inextricably linked with others in their social milieu. There exists an emphasis on social bonds and mutual interdependence such that the good of the individual is closely intertwined with the good of the group.

(Boykin et al., 1997, pp. 409–410)

The communal orientation is expressed in the extended family system, in goal-oriented activities, and in preferences for cooperative learning settings. Boykin et al. used the following definition of the Black American construct or cultural value of communalism to construct their measure:

Communalism denotes awareness of the fundamental interdependence of people (…) There is overriding importance attached to social bonds and social relationships (…) one's identity is tied to group membership rather than individual status and possessions. Sharing is promoted because it affirms the importance of social interconnectedness…

(Boykin et al., 1997, p. 411)

Boykin et al., conducted two studies to determine the validity and psychometric properties of the communalism instrument, and found, using four samples, that the instrument was reliable and had face validity. They also reported convergent validity as well as finding that the scale was related to the social orientation of study participants. Jagers and Mock (1995) examined whether the Communalism Scale would be related to collectivism and inversely related to individualist preferences. They did not confirm the communal and collective relationship but did find that there was an inverse relationship to individual preferences. They also reported that communalism was related to what they call prosocial values (i.e., equality and social justice), and they found that participants felt that their views were similar to those of their parents and extended family.

The study of communalism in Blacks provides strong and consistent evidence of the implications of this cultural orientation for the overall well-being of Blacks. Scholars in education have shown that, for Black children and adolescents,' communalism is positively associated with academic performance, and positive attitudes toward task engagement, and is negatively associated with gang-related activity (Jagers and Mock, 1993; Jagers, 1996; Albury, 1993; Jagers & Mock, 1995; Dill & Boykin, 2000). In addition, there is evidence to suggest that communalism leads to increased moral reasoning, engagement in volunteerism, and decreased violence in Blacks (Humphries, Parker, & Jagers, 2000; Woods and Jagers, 2003; Mattis et al., 2000; Jagers, Sydnor, Mouttapa, & Flay, 2007). Gooden (2013) found that communalism was positively associated with thriving in youth, a construct that indicates positive emotions, motivation, and purpose. Additionally, researchers found communalism to be a strong positive predictor of prenatal emotional health over and above other factors such as ethnicity and economic status (Abdou et al., 2010).

Similar to the study of racial socialization, a main limitation of these findings is that many study samples are made up of children and adolescents. In addition, researchers have primarily studied communalism as a cultural value without pairing it with other Black values. Communalism is a byproduct of the racial socialization and racism-related coping processes. As we have discussed, racial socialization is aimed at orienting the child to the Black racial group. Therefore, while not commonly discussed in racial socialization research, an inclination toward a communalistic social perspective may be an implicit part of this process, taking place mostly through modeling and vicarious learning. The strength of communalism in the Black American community is even displayed through consideration of the role of other members besides the parent(s) or primary caregiver(s) in racial socialization research. To date, only a few investigators have examined communalism with other Black cultural values.

Jagers, Smith, Mock, and Dill (1997) conducted two studies. The first examined the endorsement and associations between communalism, spirituality, and affect, and the importance of emotional receptivity and expressiveness. The authors found high endorsement of and moderate positive associations between the three cultural values. In addition, this Afrocultural social ethos significantly predicted both a cooperative academic attitude and competitive academic attitude. In the second study, the social ethos made up of communalism, affect, and spirituality significantly predicted both empathy and views of human nature. However, in some post-hoc analyses, only one cultural value was found to be a significant predictor of the outcome variables. For instance, the affective orientation was found to be the only significant predictor of philosophies of human nature.

These studies provide some support for the usefulness of examining cultural values as interrelated rather than as isolated variables. However, there were numerous limitations in these studies including the use of measures with low internal consistencies, and both studies were with children and adolescents. The meaning and significance of the cultural ways communicated by family and community are likely to change as children grow into adulthood, possibly becoming more aware of the inequalities for Blacks in many domains of their lives. It is imperative that parents, caregivers, and other adults be studied and understood, as they are the primary vehicles for the transmission of cultural values.

Despite the lack of research with adults, some researchers have linked communalism with other Black cultural values. Brown et al.'s (2013) examination of parental attachment, communalism, and racial identity provides evidence of the need to look at cultural values together rather than separately. The authors found a strong positive association between communalism and the later stages of racial identity development in a sample of Black college students. In 2010, the same authors found evidence of the predictive value of communalism for student self-efficacy and self-esteem (Tyler et al., 2010). In other studies, communalism has been positively associated with increased resilience, violence reduction, subjective well-being, community engagement, and thriving (Constantine, Alleyne, Wallace, & Franklin-Jackson, 2006; Grayman-Simpson & Mattis, 2017; Wallace, McGee, Malone-Colon, & Boykin, 2018).

These studies show that communalism has a positive impact on Black people's growth, development, and overall well-being, and it has a generally positive impact on the functioning of Blacks. In addition, communalism may be indicative of the more implicit communications in the racial socialization process. Communalism, while tending to the needs of the larger group, also seems to have individual psychological rewards for Blacks. Related to communal life, as has been described, is what is referred to as cultural spirituality, or a foundational sense of connection with forces beyond the human. We transition to a discussion of what Mbiti (1970) called, as part of African philosophy, a "spiritual disposition... a faith in a transcendental force and a sense of vital solidarity" (p. 148). Religion, for Black Americans, is the most observable expression of spirituality (Jones, 1980). To be human was to be religious.

Note

1 Research on communalism is based on the conceptual and scale development study of Boykins et al (1997), which was followed by Jagers and Mock (1995), even though the publication dates do not reflect this. Jagers and Mock cite the Boykin, et al paper, so there must have been some publication lag.

References

Abdou, C. M., Dunkel Schetter, C., Campos, B., Hilmert, C. J., Dominguez, T. P., Hobel, C. J., ... & Sandman, C. (2010). Communalism predicts prenatal affect, stress, and physiology better than ethnicity and socioeconomic status. *Cultural Diversity and Ethnic Minority Psychology, 16*(3), 395–403.

Albury, A. (1993). Social orientations, learning conditions and learning outcomes among low-Income Black and White grade school children. Unpublished doctoral dissertation, Howard University, Washington, DC.

Bennett, L. Jr. (1988). *Before the Mayflower: A history of Black America* (6th ed.). Chicago. IL: Johnson Publishing Co.

Boykin, A. W. (1984). Reading achievement and the social-cultural frame of reference of Afro-American children. *The Journal of Negro Education, 53*(4), 464–473.

Boykin, A. W., Jagers, R. J., Ellison, C. M., & Albury, A. (1997). Communalism: conceptualization and measurement of an Afrocultural social orientation. *Journal of Black Studies, 27*(3), 409–418.

Brown, C. L., Love, K. M., Tyler, K. M., Garriot, P. O., Thomas, D., & Roan-Belle, C. (2013). Parental attachment, family communalism, and racial identity among African American college students. *Journal of Multicultural Counseling and Development, 41*(2), 108–122.

Chafe, W. H., Gavins, R., & Korstad, R. (2001). *Remembering Jim Crow*. New York, NY: The New Press.

Constantine, M. G., Alleyne, V. L., Wallace, B. C., & Franklin-Jackson, D. C. (2006). Africentric cultural values: Their relation to positive mental health in African American adolescent girls. *The Journal of Black Psychology, 32*(2), 141–154. doi: 10.1177/0095798406286801

Dill, E. M., & Boykin, A. W. (2000). The comparative influence of individual, peer tutoring, and communal learning contexts on the text recall of African American children. *Journal of Black Psychology, 26*(1), 65–78.

Gooden, A. S. (2013). *Individual and community factors associated with thriving among African American adolescents in the context of stressors* (unpublished doctoral manuscript). DePaul University, Chicago, IL.

Grayman-Simpson, N., & Mattis, J. S. (2017). Communalism Scale 2015 cultural validity study. *Journal of Pan African Studies, 10*(3), 163–172.

Gutman, H. G. (1976). *The Black family in slavery and freedom, 1750–1925* (p. 385). New York, NY: Blackwell.

Horton, J. O., & Horton, L. E. (2005). *Slavery and the making of America*. New York, NY: Oxford University Press.

Humphries, M. L., Parker, B. L., & Jagers, R. J. (2000). Predictors of moral reasoning among African American children: A preliminary study. *Journal of Black Psychology, 26*(1), 51–64.

Jagers, R. J. (1996). Culture and problem behaviors among inner-city African–American youth further explorations. *Journal of Adolescence, 19*(4), 371–381.

Jagers, R. J., & Mock, L. O. (1995). The Communalism Scale and collectivistic-individualistic tendencies: some preliminary findings. *Journal of Black Psychology, 21*(2), 153–167.

Jagers, R. J., & Smith, P. (1996). Further examination of the Spirituality Scale. *Journal of Black Psychology, 22*(4), 429–442.

Jagers, R. J., & Mock, L. O. (1993). Culture and social outcomes among inner-city African-American children: An Afro-graphic exploration Journal of Black Psychology, 19(4), 391–405.

Jagers, R. J., Smith, P., Mock, L. O., & Dill, E. (1997). An Afrocultural social ethos: Component orientations and some social implications. *Journal of Black Psychology, 23*(4), 328–343.

Jagers, R. J., Sydnor, K., Mouttapa, M., & Flay, B. R. (2007). Protective factors associated with preadolescent violence: Preliminary work on a cultural model. *American Journal of Community Psychology, 40*(1–2), 138–145.

Jones R.L. (1980). Black Psychology (2nd ed.). New York, N.Y.: Harper & Row Publishers.

Jones, J. M. (2003). TRIOS: A psychologcial theory of the African legacy in American culture. *Journal of Social Issues, 39*(1), 217–242.

Mattis, J. S., Jagers, R. J., Hatcher, C. A., Lawhon, G. D., Murphy, E. J., & Murray, Y. F. (2000). Religiosity, volunteerism, and community involvement among African American men: An exploratory analysis. *Journal of Community Psychology, 28*(4), 391–406. https://doi.org/10.1002/1520-6629(200007)28:4<391::AID-JCOP2>3.0.CO;2-A

Mbiti, J. S. (1970). African religions and philosophy. Portsmouth, NH: Heinemann.

Morris, A. D. (1984). *The origins of the civil Rights movement: Black communities organizing for change*. New York, NY: The Free Press.

Nobles, W. W. (1991). African Philosophy: Foundations of Black psychology. In R. L. Jones (Ed.). *Black psychology* (3rd ed.) (pp. 47–64). Berkeley, CA.: Cobb & Henry Publishers.

Oyserman, D., Coon, H. M., & Kemmelmeier, M. (2002). Rethinking individualism and collectivism: evaluation of theoretical assumptions and meta-analyses. *Psychological Bulletin, 128*(1), 3–72.

Stamp, K. M., (1956). The peculiar institution. New York, N.Y.: Vintage Books.

Tyler, K., Love, K., Brown, C., Roan-Belle, C., Thomas, D., & Garriott, P. O. (2010). Linking communalism to achievement correlates for Black and White undergraduates. *International Journal of Teaching and Learning in Higher Education, 22*(1), 23–31.

Utsey, S. O., Ponterotto, J. G., Reynolds, A. L., & Cancelli, A. A. (2000). Racial discrimination, coping, life satisfaction, and self-esteem among African Americans. *Journal of Counseling & Development, 78*(1), 72–80.

Vandello, J. A., & Cohen, D. (1999). Patterns of individualism and collectivism across the United States. *Journal of Personality and Social Psychology, 77*(2), 279–292.

Wallace, C. M., McGee, Z. T., Malone-Colon, L., & Boykin, A. W. (2018). The impact of culture-based protective factors on reducing rates of violence among African American adolescent and young adult males. *Journal of Social Issues, 74*(3), 635–651.

Webber, T. L. (1978). *Deep like the rivers: Education in the slave quarter community, 1831–1865.* New York, NY: W.W. Norton.

Wilkerson, I. (2010). *The warmth of other suns: The epic story of America's great migration.* New York, NY: Random House.

Woods, L. N., & Jagers, R. J. (2003). Are cultural values predictors of moral reasoning in African American adolescents? *Journal of Black Psychology, 29*(1), 102–118.

Chapter 7

Cultural Spirituality and Racism-Related Coping

We contend that Black Americans integrated many of their traditional African customs into their new lives and cultural practices in North America. Contrary to what some would have us believe, Blacks had a culture and sense of community. Black cultural spirituality is often expressed in religious practices, but it can be expressed in other ways as well. In this chapter, we define religion and spirituality, discuss how these pertain to Black Americans in greater detail than has been touched on in previous chapters, and explore the connection between racism-related coping and spirituality.

Meaning of Religion and Spirituality

There is often confusion about the distinction between religion and spirituality, with the terms used interchangeably. Dyson, Cobb, and Forman's (1997) review of the literature on the meaning of spirituality contends that religion refers to socially based organizations in which a group of people participate, and thus they argue that religion is focused on systems of practices and beliefs for the social group. Some scholars believe that the central element of spirituality is the way that one conceives of the relationship between oneself, God and others, and in this way, spirituality is community oriented. The activity involved in spiritualty is the search for meaning in life, and the search also provides for hope, the sense that things will unfold in a positive way, and that hope is often found in others. More than anything else, the interdependence on others and one's relationship to God and others is central to the concept of spirituality. These same elements characterize Black Americans' cultural spirituality. Being both religious and spiritual involves a set of beliefs about God that helps shape one's values (Dyson et al., 1997). Dyson and colleagues (1997) note that religious expression is narrower than spirituality, in that broader forms of spiritual expression seem warranted (Mervaiglia, 1999).

Mattis and Jagers (2001), offer the following definitions: they define religion as

> a shared system of beliefs, mythology, and rituals associated with a god or gods. Religiosity… is defined as an individual's degree of adherence to

DOI: 10.4324/9781003083221-8

the beliefs, doctrines and practices of a religion... spirituality refer(s) to an acknowledgement of a non-material force that permeates all affairs, human and non-human.

(p. 522)

Hill and Pargament (2003) point out that religion is becoming fixed as a system of ideas and commitments, that deemphasizes the personal aspects of faith, while spiritual refers often to the personal and subjective aspects of religious experience. For these authors,

Religion and spirituality represent related rather than independent constructs... spirituality can be understood as a search for the sacred, a process through which people seek to discover, hold on to, and when necessary transform whatever they hold sacred in their lives.

(p. 65)

The sacred can be the divine, God, or ultimate reality. Taylor and Chatters (2010) also present definitions of religiosity and spiritualty, in which, religion is defined as

a multidimensional construct encompassing public and private behaviors, attitudes and beliefs, organized around a structural system of tenets, practices, and ritual and is characterized as community-focused, formal, and behaviorally oriented... Spirituality in contrast, is subjective, individualistic, and informal, and is seen as a means of establishing relationships to the sacred and search for answers to fundamental life questions... Viewed in this way, spirituality is a separate and distinct construct from religiosity...

(p. 282)

Spirituality is thought of as a higher-order endeavor with individual agency that allows for greater personal expression, benefits, and outcomes. This is a perspective that reflects how Africans and their descendants report their spiritual and religious ideas and behaviors. Other scholars who have explored the distinctions between spirituality and religion have also suggested different definitions for the two constructs (Hill & Pargament, 2008). For instance, Burkhardt (1989) suggests that spirituality is about discovering meaning and purpose in life, harmony in relationship to others, self, and a higher being, and inner strength, and contends that religion is a form of spiritual expression. Similarly, Emblen (1992) believes that religion is the worship practices and beliefs an individual engages in, while spirituality is a personal life principle having to do with one's relationship to God or the person's notion of the creator or of nature, and as such spirituality is seen as encompassing religion. Dyson and colleagues (1997) had similar ideas about the themes of spirituality noting that it includes life's meaning, hope, and relatedness.

Because our concern is the mental health of the individual, it is helpful to also present definitions of the constructs from a mental health perspective. Fukuyama and Sevig (1999) define religion as an organized system of worship, traditions, and rituals. For these scholars, religion has several elements: (1) ritual, which refers to acts which occur in a prescribed order; (2) doctrine, which outlines how the person is related to the sacred; (3) emotion, for example fear, love etc.; (4) knowledge about the writings and principles of ones' beliefs; (5) ethics, or rules for proper behavior, and what is good and what is not; and (6) community, the group that shares one's beliefs.

While Fukuyama and Sevig argue that religion and spiritualty are interrelated, they also suggest that the term "spirituality" refers to "a universal concept," and "religion tends to define a more concrete expression" (p. 7). More importantly, it is their position that the two concepts be understood within the context of culture. "To extend the discussion about universal versus culture-specific approaches to multicultural counselling … we suggest that spirituality describes universal qualities and religion the culture-specific expression of spirit" (Fukuyama & Sevig, 1999, p. 7). From the various definitions reviewed, while religion is the mechanism through which a relationship with God and one's community is cultivated, spirituality describes one's orientation to a higher force or being that includes life's meaning, hope, harmony, inner strength, and interconnectedness with others.

As discussed, communalism is the social orientation of Black Americans. It spans from African ancestry and has been maintained in present day Black American life through institutions such as the Black church. Even theories of racial socialization and coping with racism include the importance of spirituality for Black people (Stevenson, 1994; Forsyth & Carter, 2012). Nantambu (1998) writes that spirituality represents a direct connectedness/inter-relatedness with nature, the cosmos, the universe, and that spirituality is about the God-force, Amen-Ra, "the giver of life." While many Black Americans are religious, spirituality stretches beyond religious practices and manifests in one's orientation toward everyday life. Thus, *cultural spirituality* characterizes the religious expression of Black Americans. We have pointed out that many academics and citizens believed that Blacks were primitive people with no pre-determined set of beliefs or practices grounded in their native cultures, while others have argued that the opposite is true. Nevertheless, it is clear that Black Americans hold onto a set of principles that constitutes their *cultural spirituality*. We also argue that Blacks' racism-related coping strategies are reflected in part in their spiritual principles. Before we turn to that discussion, we review some of the core propositions of *cultural spirituality*.

It is clear that belief in God and/or a Supreme Being is at the center of Black people's spiritual foundation and religious expressions. What that belief means and where it came from is the subject of considerable debate among social scientists (e.g., Bennett, 1988; Dodson, 2002; Horton & Horton, 2005). We, however, believe that there are cultural behaviors, beliefs, and emotions that have been retained over the centuries that contribute to Black people's psychological health and demonstrate strength in their cultural practices (Johnson & Carter, 2020). One is *cultural spirituality*. It is not just religious faith or practice per se. We argue, as do others (Belgrave & Allison, 2019), that spirituality is intertwined with religion, it is/was related to a sense of hope, reflects connections with the natural world and the spirit world, and helps cement family and community bonds. The form and function of this cultural value has changed and shifted over time as have the other cultural practices we present in other chapters. We acknowledge the strong and persistent religious adherence many Black people have and still exhibit (Taylor and Chatters, 2010). At the same time, we contend that undergirding Blacks' religious behavior and emotion is a cultural practice and value this is shared and operates to bind the group into a larger community, and that transcends mere church going. In our view, cultural spirituality has to do with a set of beliefs about how a people view the world around them and how they interact with it.

We use cultural spirituality to denote a Black American orientation to the world and universe that is different from Western religious practice and belief in which one's faith or beliefs are separate from one's day to day life. Jagers and Smith (1996) contend that Black American spirituality reflects the belief that all things contain and house a life force and this force has a governing roles in one's life. In addition, the authors state that a belief in a life force comes with a sense of connection with one's African ancestors.

Religion and Spirituality in Africa, During Slavery, and Beyond

Historians note that prior to the arrival of Europeans on the West coast of Africa, Africans there and in other locations on the continent practiced many religions, which included Christianity, Islam, and traditional African religions.

> At the beginning of the sixteenth [century] (1500's), the royal house of Kongo, converted to Christianity, Catholicism, in various syncretic forms, infiltrated the posts along the Angolan coast and spread northward. Islam filtered in from the north. Whatever the sources of the new religions, most converts saw little cause to surrender their own deities. They incorporated Christianity and Islam to serve their own needs and gave Jesus, Mohammad a place in their spiritual pantheon of new religious practices. Polities, and theologies, emerged from the mixing of Christianity, Islam, polytheism, and animism.
>
> (Berlin, 1998, p. 21)

So, while accepting the basic tenets of other religions, prior to being captives, Africans blended their core spiritual beliefs with that of established religions like

Christianity and Islam. Blassingame (1979) observed that there were similarities in European and African cultures such that it was possible to blend or recreate aspects of the African ways. In this way, Africans were able to use European forms to serve African customs, "Most Africans believed in a Creator, or all-powerful God whom one addresses directly through prayers, sacrifices, rituals, songs, and dances" (Blassingame, 1979, p. 20). He continues, stating that,

> Christian forms were so similar to African religious patterns that it was relatively easy for early slaves to incorporate... with their traditional practices and beliefs. In America, Jehovah replaced the Creator, and Jesus, the Holy Ghost, and Saints replaced lesser gods. The Africans preserved many of their sacred ceremonies in the conventional Christian ritual and ceremonies...
> (Blassingame, 1979, p. 21)

The retention of African forms appears in songs and burial practices. In particular, spirituals created by slaves contained African elements and evoked strong emotions as they were intended. "Not only did Southern slaves decorate graves like their African ancestor, they also retained the practice of celebrating the journey of the deceased to his 'home' by dancing, singing, and drinking" (Blassingame, 1979, p. 45). The Bible and Koran contained similarities that got the attention of slaves and made it possible for them to align themselves with the less structured denominations, especially since churches had taken up the cause of teaching about Christ to the so-called heathens from the primitive African continent (Blassingame, 1979; Harding, 1981; Genovese, 1974).

Mintz and Price (1976) contend that Africans began to transform their cultural beliefs and practices from the moment they became captives, in the marches to the ocean, in the factories where they were held before being taken on ships, and during the middle passage. Unlike other scholars who thought that these experiences made it impossible for Africans to hold on to much of their past knowledge or beliefs, Mintz and Price (1976) contend that "the beginnings of what would later develop into 'African-American cultures' must date from the very earliest interactions of the newly enslaved men and women on the African continent itself" (p. 42).

They point to the cooperative efforts of the captives that sowed the seeds for new cultural patterns. They go on to observe, "Just as the development of new social ties marked the initial enslavement experience, so also new *cultural systems* were beginning to take shape" (Mintz & Price, 1972, p. 44), such as the start of Black American religions. Acknowledging the diversity and variety of African religions, they note that some general principles marked and set apart Blacks' beliefs about God and religion:

> Most... African religions seem to have shared certain fundamental assumptions about the nature of causality and the ability of divination to reveal

specific causes, about the active role of the dead in the lives of the living, about the responsiveness of (most) deities to human actions, about the close relationship between social conflict and illness or misfortune and many others.

(Mintz & Price, 1972, p. 45)

Dodson (2002) writes regarding African religious beliefs:

The enslaved Africans who survived the Middle Passage and settled in the Americas came from diverse religious backgrounds. Though these religions numbered in the thousands, they frequently shared a number of common ideas about the nature of God and the universe and their relationships to the temporal and spiritual worlds. Most believed in an all-powerful God, the Supreme Being to whom they could speak directly through prayer, sacrifices, rituals, songs and dances (...) Ancestors formed a part of their spiritual worlds and they too could be summoned through prayer, rituals, and sacrifices to intervene on their behalf... Spirts also dwelt on the land, in the trees, and on the rocks of the kinship group community as well as in the sky above and the waters that flowed through. God and the spirits were everywhere, and religion was so pervasive in traditional African life that it was present in all aspects of social, cultural, and political life. Religion was not simply a part of life, religion was life-so much so that there generally was no distinction in traditional African life between the sacred and the secular.

(p. 133)

Many Africans in other parts of the New World adapted their religions and were able to use much of their traditional African religious and spiritual beliefs, in many cases, continuously through organized religions to the present day. Because they outnumbered Whites, slaves in many parts of South America and the Caribbean were able to practice and use their traditional customs without constant suppression. However, scholars have argued that in North America the situation was very different (Hazzard-Donald, 2013; Raboteau, 2004). Whereas countries in the rest of the Americas had an influx of both slaves and free Africans into the early 19th century who were able to continually infuse New World religious practices with traditional African spirituality, the importation of slaves to most of North America slowed progressively starting after the American Revolution in the late 18th century. In North America there was a greater focus on breeding slaves and trading them domestically. As such, the vast majority of slaves in the colonies were native-born (Raboteau, 2004). In North America, Whites were the majority, most slaves lived on small plantations where there were less than 20 slaves, and slaves were under constant control and surveillance. As a result, they argue, Blacks in North America did not have the advantage of numbers that allowed them to practice their African rites and rituals, as was the case in South America or the various Caribbean Island nations (Raboteau, 2004).

Furthermore, whereas slaves in Catholic countries, such as Brazil and Cuba, were able to syncretize the worship of traditional West African deities onto Catholic saints, there were virtually no opportunities for the syncretic transfer of African deities in North American Protestantism (Hazzard-Donald, 2013).

Nevertheless, there is evidence that over generations, enslaved Africans in North America adapted and adjusted certain West and Central West African religious and spiritual traditions, and that some of these practices continue to be integrated into modern day Black American religious and spiritual practices, as well as secular music and dance (Hazzard-Donald, 2013; Raboteau, 2004). These practices evolved over time into *Hoodoo*, "the indigenous, herbal, healing, and supernatural-controlling folk tradition" (Hazzard-Donald, 2013, p. 4). The Hoodoo system preceded the Black church and

> was known to all in the slave community and was part of the psychic structure of every individual enslaved there. It was a glue that held the slave community together. It included folk wisdom and advice. It addressed the needs of the slave community and, later, the free African American community; it integrated psychological support, spiritual direction, physical strength, and medicinal treatment.
>
> (p. 15)

Hazzard-Donald (2013) argues that eight components of traditional West and Central African religions, that were likely shared by the various ethnic groups represented among Black American slaves, were integrated and formed the basis of Hoodoo: (1) counterclockwise sacred circle dancing; (2) spirit possession; (3) the principle of sacrifice; (4) ritual water immersion; (5) divination; (6) ancestor reverence; (7) belief in spiritual cause of malady; and (8) herbal and naturopathic medicine. Along with these African elements, Hoodoo was also influenced by Native American spiritual beliefs, Protestantism, and European folk beliefs. The two most notable examples of West African religious traditions that were continued in North America during slavery and even after Emancipation were the Ring Shout and root work or conjuring, elements of which continue into the present day.

White slave owners were initially very resistant to the conversion of slaves to Christianity as they believed that doing so would lead slaves to perceive themselves as equal to Whites and ultimately require that they emancipate them. This fear predominated to such an extent that by 1706, legislation had been passed in six colonies declaring that baptism did not equate with emancipation (Raboteau, 2004). During early efforts to convert slaves, Whites sought to teach the "heathen Africans" proper Christian ideals, such as: that they were meant to be slaves, and that they should obey their masters and not create any disruptions. Blassingame (1979) notes that these efforts to teach Blacks what to believe or to shape Christianity to their viewpoint failed to sway Black people who rejected such teachings and led to fewer converts. "Continued stress on obedience discouraged slaves [Blacks] from going to church, caused them to shift to other denominations, or led to complete rejection of Christianity" (p. 86). It turns out that of the different denominations available in North America, only a few of them appealed to enslaved Black people. In going to church, the slaves took pleasure in singing and liked the degree of autonomy allowed in that they were able to exercise their religious learnings.

While most Southern and Northern slave holders had many reasons to not want religious teaching for slaves, as time passed, the majority did employ such teaching. We have already noted the content and message of these efforts to civilize Africans and American Blacks. In turn, Blacks were active in dismissing the religious instruction as false and amoral, nor did they accept the Bible as taught by the preachers and ministers provided by the slave owners or White religious leaders. Webber (1978) notes that the slaves knew and believed that "Christianity revolved around the complementary principles that God intended all men (women) to be free and that, therefore, slavery was wrong" (p. 82).

Historians have documented what they describe as the "Great Awakening," which according to Dodson (2002), was a period during the mid- to late-1700s in the colonies, prior to the revolutionary conflict with the British, when Blacks and colonists, many poor and working class, were introduced to Christian beliefs and practices. Many converts in the North were taken into the Episcopal, Presbyterian, Methodist, and Congregational churches. Evangelical ministers were touring the country and seeking to bring salvation to all the people who could be reached. Dodson (2002) notes that "African Americans remolded Christianity's content and structure for their own cultural and spiritual needs" (p. 135). White Christians wanted Blacks to learn from scripture that they should be submissive and obedient and accept their status as slaves. Slaves in essence rejected the messages from Whites when they taught them to accept their lot. Dodson (2002) writes that beginning in the 18th century,

> Allies of the slaveholders in their attempts to 'civilize the heathen' Africans and make them better, more loyal servants... tried to teach the enslaved that they were born to be slaves, that they should work and serve their masters faithfully, and that they should never disobey their master or lie or steal.
>
> (p. 138)

Of the various denominations presented to Blacks, the ones that offered more autonomy had the greatest appeal. For instance, Catholicism's structure and process removed the worshiper from direct communication with God and the spirit world, a situation that was contrary to Blacks' spiritual preferences and beliefs, but Baptists, Methodists, and Episcopalians offered a religion that allowed Africans to

> invent their own Afro-Christian religious practices. Fusing remnants of their traditional African worship... with their own interpretations of the Christian

faith, these praise meetings became unique New World African religious experiences. African-American oratory, music, and religious and theological worldviews are all rooted in the African Christian religious experience invented by enslaved Africans during the era of slavery.

(Dodson, 2002, p. 138)

As a result, many Blacks in the South and other parts of the country elected to participate in the Baptist, Methodist, and Presbyterian churches.

The unique elements of the Africans' belief system are what makes it stand apart from traditional forms of Christianity. For instance, the conviction that the people and community were regularly interacting with the spirit world, and that the spirits were also part of daily life, was one of their core spiritual principles. Observers attributed Blacks' beliefs to primitive superstition and witchcraft; Africans' beliefs were considered to be a "perversion of the natural revelations of God" (Dodson, 2002, p. 141). Dodson notes that the

Black faith that evolved from the coming together of diverse religious influences became … something distinctly different from any of its major contributors. Both the slave congregations of the South – "the invisible institutions" (religious meetings held away from Whites, often in hidden locations) and the more or less free black churches of the North developed a religion that masked a subliminal outrage balanced with patience, cheerfulness, and a boundless confidence in the ultimate justice of God.

(Dodson, 2002, p. 147)

Belgrave and Allison (2019) point out that while free and enslaved Africans adopted Christian beliefs, nevertheless, their perspectives on their faith were formed mostly by their African-based spiritual convictions and principles. The slaves' religious activities outside the reach of Whites allowed them to incorporate many of their African cultural religious ideals and perspectives and to retain their views of the Supreme Being, nature, as well as the power of the ancestors and spirits. They were also able to establish independent institutions in the North, and later in the South, that went beyond just tending to the people's souls. By the mid-1800s, a number of Black religious leaders had broken away from White churches and formed independent Black churches and denominations, and in the late-1800s as the Civil War ended, many sent missionaries to the south to encourage Black people to leave White churches and join Black churches (Lincoln & Mamiya, 1990). After emancipation, the Black church only increased in importance and influence. Writing about the Jim Crow years (1876–1964), Chafe, Gavins, and Korstad (2001) observe that

churches were vital centers of African-American culture… they ministered to the spiritual and temporal needs of the community and were places for affirmation and celebration... In churches many young people met the men and women whom they later courted and married. Churches also were safe places for political activities...

(p. 90)

In this same vain, Taylor and Chatters (2010) state:

Black churches have a long tradition of spearheading social, educational, and health services, to their congregations and surrounding communities, including youth programs, economic development initiatives, programs for the elderly and their caregivers, income maintenance and job training, to name a few. These programing efforts reflect a particular worldview of African American religious traditions and emphasizes the communal nature of worship, the collectivity of the church, and the role of the Black church in mediating the broader social environment.

(p. 280)

The central proposition in Blacks' beliefs system expressed in their religious practice is contained in their certainty in the spiritual, and the link between the living, the spirits, and the group. The unique character of Black American spirituality was captured in research conducted generations after the Civil Rights Movement. Mattis (2000) found that Black women's characterizations of their spirituality was consistent with universal themes in research on spirituality, including a sense of connection to a higher power that is both internal and external; consciousness of meta-physicality; life purpose and meaning; understanding and accepting the self; and positively influencing relationships with others. But Black spirituality was unique in its emphasis on facilitating efforts to manage and cope with adversity, guidance, life instruction, and peace. In a concept analysis of 20 studies of African American spirituality in nursing, psychology, and sociology, Newlin, Knafl, and Melkus (2002) found that many of the dimensions of African American spirituality were consistent with spiritual dimensions identified in research on mainstream White spirituality such as benevolence and transcendence, a personal connection with God or a higher power, and a sense of supportive and altruistic interconnectedness with others. As in Mattis' study of Black women, they found that across all 20 studies they reviewed, African American spirituality had two dimensions, which were defining characteristics that distinguished it from those found in research on spirituality among White people. These dimensions were what they describe as a consoling dimension, wherein spirituality provides, "a liberating source of peace, compassion, love, protection, warmth, and comfort" and a transformative dimension through which spirituality was "a source of healing, personal growth, liberation, strength, guidance, meaning, purpose, coping, hope, renewal, and interpretation of experience" (p. 66). They also found that African American spirituality contributed to heightened interpersonal connectedness and emotional equilibrium, and empowered change (i.e., "active coping, personal growth, positive interpretation of life events, and better physical health", p. 66).

Research has found that spirituality is consistently positively associated with indicators of psychosocial health among Black Americans such as marital satisfaction, academic success, achieving sobriety, existential well-being, psychological well-being, and relational health (Balkin, Neal, Stewart, Hendricks, & Litem, 2022; Fincham, Ajayi, & Beach, 2011; Krentzman, Farkas, & Townsend, 2010; Reed & Neville, 2014; Wood & Hilton, 2012). It has also been found to moderate the impact of racial stress on well-being (Bowen-Reid & Harrell, 2002), suggesting that cultural spirituality not only contributes to psychosocial health but also is an important mechanism that has been used by Black Americans across generations to cope with the racial oppression they encounter.

Cultural Spirituality and Racism-Related Coping

Scholars contend that traditional African religious and spiritual beliefs established a center around which Black American culture and identity formed, and that African beliefs in "spiritual forces… ideas about death, the afterlife, and transmigration proved crucial in the development of slave resistance and revolt" and "strengthened a community ethic of resistance that made large-scale slave rebellion possible" (Young, 2012, p. 3). There is evidence that root work and conjuring were a form of spiritual resistance that was directly used to protect and empower slaves, particularly in the context of slave rebellions (e.g., the role of the conjurer Gullah Jack in Denmark Vesey's insurrectionary plot of 1822; Young, 2012).

Over time, from the early colonial days to the present, the church became one of the central institutions in the Black American community. Black churches served many functions in the Black community. One was the struggle against racism and racial oppression. The church nurtured leaders who led the fight against racial discrimination and inequality. Berry and Blassingame (1982) stated:

> The institution black people developed in the period before the Civil War and perpetuated thereafter provided shelter from American racism. The two most important institutions, the family and church, sustained blacks through slavery, segregation, violence, and oppression. Within the family and church, self-realization and a sense of community worth and pride developed.
>
> (p. xviii)

Over four centuries in the United States, Black Americans have developed myriad strategies to respond to, manage, deal with, and resist racial oppression. In psychological research, the strategies Black people use to struggle against racism have mostly been examined through the concept of coping. As we have shown in earlier chapters, there are consistent racial disparities in health, social status, and mental health found when Blacks are compared to Whites and other groups. Research suggests that racial discrimination and racism may be directly and indirectly implicated in the development of psychological distress and physical illness in Black Americans (Carter & Pieterse, 2020). The prevalence of racism is high for Blacks, with between 40% and 98% of samples reporting exposure to racial discrimination (e.g., Carter & Pieterse, 2020). Studies have found associations between racial discrimination and/or race-related-stress and lower life satisfaction and well-being (e.g., Deitch et al., 2003), increased distress (e.g., Broman, Mavaddat, & Hsu, 2000), negative emotional reactions (Carter & Reynolds 2011; Carter & Forsyth, 2010), and psychological symptoms (e.g., Carter et al., 2019).

Although many decades of research provide support for the notion that racism is experienced as a unique stressor for African Americans and that the psychological and physiological impact of exposure is negative, race-related stress or discrimination typically accounts for only a small percentage of the variability in mental health outcomes in many studies (Carter & Johnson, 2019; Pascoe & Richman, 2009). As a result, scholars have examined a variety of other factors that could explain the variability in psychological reactions to race-related stress. Racism-related coping is a potential moderating variable that has received attention in the research literature.

Coping is defined as cognitive, emotional, and behavioral efforts to manage external or internal demands that exceed a person's resources (Folkman & Moskowitz, 2004). Investigations of coping have tended to focus on how predominantly White samples cope with generic stressors (i.e., death of loved ones, loss of employment, divorce). Fewer studies have examined coping with generic stressors among Black Americans, and even fewer have focused on how Black people cope with race-related stressors. Scholars have also increasingly explored emotion regulation, a construct that overlaps with coping, in understanding Black Americans' responses to racism (see Jacob et al., 2023 and Wilson & Gentzler, 2021 for a review). Emotion regulation focuses on ways that individuals manage negative and/or positive emotions before, during, and after an incident or event. It includes strategies to downregulate (i.e., decrease emotions) or upregulate (i.e., increase) emotions, and common strategies examined in research on coping with racism include cognitive reappraisal and expressive suppression (Wilson & Gentzler, 2021).

A recent review of quantitative and qualitative studies focused on coping and emotion regulation strategies used by Black adults to cope with racism published between 1996 and 2021 identified 35 different strategies across the 26 studies reviewed (Jacob et al., 2023). Though the majority of studies reviewed did not examine the effectiveness of coping strategies, the authors grouped the strategies into eight categories, which they characterized as either functional, ambiguous, or dysfunctional. Functional strategies included social support (such as venting, humor, therapy, participating in support groups, and seeking support from friends and family), direct strategies (such as confrontation, problem-solving, covert resistance, and speaking out), identity affirmation (such as Africultural strategies, spirituality and religion, positive self-statements, and art), and activism (such as community and civic engagement, educating others, and public resistance). Ambiguous strategies, that could be either functional or dysfunctional depending on the situation, included cognitive strategies (such as processing the event, positive reframing, acceptance, meaning making, and planning) and physical strategies (such as engaging in physical activity, working harder to prove oneself worthy, i.e., John Henryism, and resisting retaliation). Dysfunctional strategies included avoidance (such as assimilation, ritual-centered coping, distancing, disengagement, cognitive emotional debriefing, and self-blame and accepting responsibility) and substance abuse. In their analysis of the articles, they found that problem-focused coping (i.e., active individual efforts to confront a stressor to eliminate, modify, or reduce it), social support (i.e., seeking support from formal groups or talking with friends and family), and religious coping (attending church, using prayer, or leveraging spirituality) were used most frequently in general. But social support and religious coping were more common among women, whereas passive strategies, such as ignoring, were more common among men. They also found a general preference for active rather than passive strategies, suggesting that doing something, no matter how small, likely leads to a sense of agency in the face of racism.

Among the studies that have examined how Black people cope with racism and racial discrimination, only a limited number of quantitative studies have examined the effectiveness of coping strategies in reducing negative mental health symptoms, and even fewer have examined their effectiveness in contributing to well-being. The coping studies that have examined outcomes have, for the most part, examined the influence of approach coping (i.e., problem-focused strategies that focus on changing, removing, navigating, or managing the stressor) and avoidant coping (i.e., emotion-focused strategies that focus on reducing negative emotional reactions/responses to the stressor), and the results have been mixed. In some studies, avoidant strategies were associated with poor outcomes, including lower life satisfaction (Utsey, Ponterotto, Reynolds, & Cancelli, 2000), reduced quality of life (Merluzzi, Phillip, Zhang, & Sullivan, 2015), negative emotions (Hyers, 2007), depression (Hill & Hoggard, 2018), and distress (Smith, Stewart, Myers, & Latu, 2008). In at least one study, avoidant strategies were associated with better outcomes in the form of decreased psychological symptoms (Sanders Thompson, 2006), while approach coping was associated with poor outcomes in the form of increased psychological symptoms (Sanders Thompson, 2006). The inconsistency in these results likely reflect differences that arise from the use of coping measures to assess situational (i.e., strategies used to cope with a specific incident or situation) as compared to dispositional (i.e., strategies that are used habitually by a person regardless of the situation) coping styles, and the influence of unmeasured moderating variables. They may also reflect the use of generic coping measures that were created to measure strategies used to deal with general life stressors (Forsyth & Carter, 2012; Thomas, Witherspoon, & Speight, 2008). Just as scholars have argued that race-related stress is different from general stress, a number of scholars have suggested that generic coping measures cannot adequately capture the range of specific race-related coping strategies Blacks used to deal with racism (e.g., Brondolo, ver Halen, Pencille, Beatty, & Contrada, 2009; Harrell, 2000; Scott, 2003a; Smith et al., 2008).

Studies have found differences in the strategies Black people use to cope with non-racial and racial stressors (Brown, Phillips, Abdullah, Vinson, & Robertson, 2010; Plummer & Slane, 1996), and differences in the strategies Blacks use to cope with racial discrimination as compared to Whites and Asian Americans (Sanders Thompson, 2006). Some studies have attempted to address the limitations inherent in the use of generic coping measures by conducting factor analyses of a generic coping measure (the COPE) with Black American samples to construct scales considered to be more culturally congruent for Blacks (e.g., Greer, Ricks & Baylor, 2015; Greer & Cavalhieri, 2019; Lewis, Williams, Peppers, & Gadson, 2017; Pearson et al., 2014; Williams & Lewis, 2019). These studies have generally found that avoidant strategies are associated with increased symptoms. Other studies have used the Africultural Coping Systems Inventory (ACSI; Utsey et al., 2000), a measure developed to assess the specific coping strategies Blacks in America have developed over time to deal with a variety of stressors including racism (e.g., Greer, 2011; Greer, 2021; Greer, 2024; Shahid, Nelson, & Cardemil, 2018; Thomas et al., 2008). To date, even these studies have had mixed results. Furthermore, both studies using the COPE Scale and the ACSI have generally found that spiritual coping was associated with increased psychological symptoms such as anxiety and interpersonal sensitivity (Greer, 2011; Greer & Cavalhieri, 2019), and lower academic self-concept (Greer, 2021).

The mixed, and in some cases counterintuitive findings, are likely because while the adaptations of the COPE measure and the ACSI do a better job of capturing the ways the Black Americans cope with generic stress, they still fail to capture the full range of responses that are specific to coping with racism. It is important to note that race-related stressors are different from generic life stressors to which all people regardless of race are exposed. Race-related stressors reflect an endemic power differential that is often outside of one's ability to control or safely intervene. They occur on multiple levels (e.g., interpersonal, intragroup, institutional, cultural, structural), and in and across every stage of life from infancy to old age. Race-related stress influences access to essential resources such as housing, education, work, wealth, and health care, and constrains and limits access to opportunities. Race-related stressors are often interlocking, persistent, and have a cumulative effect on health and well-being, and as such they require a different set of coping strategies that is distinct from the generic strategies assessed in standard coping measures. For example, both historically and currently, Black Americans have coped with and resisted racism using collective healing as well as collective action such as boycotts, protesting, civic engagement, and participating in Black organizations, and/or through legal means of filing complaints or taking legal action. While some aspects of collective healing strategies (e.g., social support and religious or spiritual coping) are captured in generic or Africultural coping measures, none of the collective action strategies are. Over the years a number of descriptive and qualitative studies have examined how Blacks in particular cope with racism (e.g., Benkert & Peters, 2005; Daly, Jennings, Beckett, & Leashore, 1995; Evans, 1997; Feagin, 1991; Shorter-Gooden, 2004; see Jacobs et al., 2023 for a review). These studies do a better job of capturing the unique strategies that Black Americans use to resist, manage, and deal with racism, including behaviors such as code switching for example, that are either not adequately captured or not captured at all in generic, and even the Africultural, Coping Scales.

In a review of 56 studies on coping with various forms of stigmatization and discrimination, the authors found that only 13 studies used measures designed to specifically assess strategies used to cope with stigma/discrimination, and only 2 of the measures used were designed to assess coping with racism (Partow, Cook, & McDonald, 2021). Only one measure, the Racism-Related Coping Scale (RRCS; Forsyth & Carter, 2014), currently exists to assess the specific racism-related coping strategies that Black Americans use to deal with racism. The RRCS was developed to assess the situational coping behaviors used to deal with and resist racism. Developed based on an initial pool of 127 items derived largely from qualitative studies of coping with racism and historical accounts of resistance against racism, factor analyses identified eight types of racism-related coping: (1) *Bargaining*, which consists of mostly cognitive actions focused on efforts to make sense of the experience, to examine one's own responsibility in bringing the incident about, and to change one's behavior in order to manage others' perceptions; (2) *Hypervigilance*, which is characterized by increased caution and sensitivity in interactions with others who are not Black, the use of avoidant behavior to evade future racially charged interactions, and cognitive preoccupation with the incident; (3), *Social support*, which comprised a range of behaviors and cognitions intended to seek and provide support to one self and to others; (4) *Confrontation*, which involves direct expression of anger and/or communication with the perpetrator of the incident; (5) *Empowered Action*, which reflects the channeling of community and/or legal resources to make those involved accountable for their actions; (6) *Spiritual actions*, which includes seeking support from religious institutions and religious books, engaging in self-soothing, or using spiritual practices such as meditation, prayer and singing; (7) *Racial Consciousness*, which includes efforts to connect with or express one's cultural heritage and history and to take action against racism; and (8) *Constrained Resistance*, which includes both passive (e.g., work slowing strategies, use of drugs and alcohol) and active (e.g., use of intimidation) individual-level efforts to resist racism.

In a study with 233 Black American adults ranging in age from 18 to 72 years old, Forsyth and Carter (2012) found that the majority of the incidents reported by participants took place in a service setting such as a restaurant, store and other places of business, at work or at school, and were committed by service employees, a workplace superior, colleague, or a stranger. The vast majority of those perpetrating the racial mistreatment incidents were White. Analysis of the characteristics of the incidents reported by the participants indicated that the different incident characteristics (location, perpetrator's relationship to the target, harassment vs. discrimination) were not associated with differences in psychological responses. Investigation of where the incident took place and the types of racism-related coping found that participants used spiritual strategies to cope with racial mistreatment at work more often than in service settings, and used bargaining to cope with incidents that took place at school more often than those that took place in service settings. Participants relied on hypervigilant strategies to cope when the perpetrator was their boss (or other workplace superior) or colleague more often than they did when the perpetrator was a service employee, and used hypervigilance, social support, and spiritual coping more often when the perpetrator was their boss than when s/he was a stranger. They used empowered action to cope with mistreatment from a security or police officer more often than with a stranger, and used bargaining to deal with mistreatment by a colleague more often than mistreatment by a service employee. A series of regressions indicated which coping types were predictive of psychological distress or well-being. First, hypervigilance and constrained resistance significantly predicted psychological distress, while empowered action and spiritual coping strategies were inversely related to psychological distress. Empowered action and spiritual coping strategies predicted well-being, and hypervigilance and constrained resistance were negatively related to well-being.

These results show that when Blacks rely on asserting their rights, harnessing resources, and actively engaging the situation, as well as when they rely on spiritual practices and beliefs, these types of responses are associated with positive mental health outcomes. On the other hand, when Blacks use passive (e.g., work slowing strategies, use of drugs and alcohol) and active efforts to resist racism (e.g., use of intimidation), employ increased caution and sensitivity in interactions with others who are not Black, or use avoidant strategies to evade future racially charged interactions, and become cognitively preoccupied with the incident, these types of responses are associated with greater psychological distress (Forsyth, 2010). These results are consistent with more recent research that has explored mindfulness, as well as activism, civic engagement, and race-related vigilance as coping strategies that are unique to coping with racism.

While most studies of spiritual coping with racism among Black Americans have found poor outcomes, at least three studies have found that mindfulness moderates the relationship between racism and anxious arousal (Graham,

West, & Roemer, 2013) and depressive and anxious symptoms (Zapolski, Faidley, & Beuttlich, 2019), and moderates the relationship between both discrimination and race-related vigilance and depressive symptoms (Watson-Singleton, Hill, & Case, 2019) among African Americans. The positive outcomes from mindfulness as contrasted with the poor outcomes in studies using measures of spiritual and religious coping highlight the multidimensionality of cultural spirituality. Though the studies of mindfulness use measures that assess non-religious mindfulness practices or traits, these practices and traits are likely enhanced through aspects of religious belief and practice such as prayer and meditation. The disparate results further suggest that the failure to find consistently positive outcomes for spiritual coping reflects that the scales used in research may not capture the multidimensionality of cultural spirituality, which includes participation in religious organizations, communities, and activities, as well as individual beliefs and practices.

Studies have found that high support for the Black Lives Matter movement moderated the relationship between racial discrimination and depressive symptoms (Watson-Singleton, Mekawi, Wilkins, Hill & Case, 2020), and that civic engagement buffered the impact of neighborhood discrimination on aggressive behavior for adolescents (Francois, Wu, Doe, Tucker, & Theall, 2023), suggesting that engaging in low-risk collective actions may benefit both community and individuals. At the same time, research has found that engaging in anti-racist activism can increase levels of stress, anxiety (Hope, Velez, Offidanti-Bertrand, Keels & Durkee, 2018), and anticipatory racism-related stress (i.e., worrying about and anticipating future race-related encounters; Hope, Volpe, Briggs, & Benson, 2022). Additionally, studies have found associations between increased racism-related vigilance, a type of anticipatory racism-related stress that includes anticipating and preparing for future racism, and increased stress (Himmelstein, Young, Sanchez, & Jackson, 2015), depression (LaVeist, Thorpe, & Pierre 2014; Watson-Singleton et al., 2019), and poor sleep (Hicken, Lee, Ailshire, Burgard, & Williams, 2013).

One reason for the mixed results in research on the effectiveness of different strategies to cope with racism is that there are a variety of situational (i.e., aspects of the racial experience itself) and individual(i.e., racial identity, personality, interpersonal communication skills)-level factors that influence every aspect of the coping process from how an incident is appraised and reappraised, what strategies are leveraged, and whether a specific strategy is functional or adaptive for a given person in a particular situation. A number of recent developmental reviews of coping with racism across the lifespan (Jones et al., 2020; Neblett, 2023; Wilson & Gentzler, 2021) have emphasized the central role of racial identity, racial socialization, and spirituality as resilience factors that are essential in the development of one's ability to accurately recognize, appraise, reappraise, and develop and effectively use the adaptive coping skills necessary to successfully navigate and negotiate stressful encounters with a variety of forms of racism, resulting in the maintenance of psychological well-being (Jones et al., 2020).

A small number of quantitative studies have assessed the influence of psychosocial variables such as racial identity (e.g., Greer, 2011; Lewis et al., 2017; Neville, Heppner, & Wang, 1997; Utsey, Bolden, Lanier, & Williams, 2007: West, Donovan, & Roemer, 2010; Williams & Lewis, 2019; see Neblett, 2023), racial socialization, and cultural orientation (e.g., Scott, 2003a, 2003b; see Neblett, 2023), and level of acculturation (e.g., Brown et al., 2011) on the dispositional coping styles and situational strategies used to cope with racism among Black Americans. These studies have generally found that positive racial identity, racial socialization, and being more oriented toward one's culture was associated with the use of more adaptive or functional coping strategies and improved outcomes.

Only one study has examined the combined effects of racial identity and the specific racism-related strategies Black Americans use to cope with racism. Forsyth and Carter (2012) found a complex interplay between racial identity and coping strategies on psychological symptoms and well-being. Their findings suggested that those who had a more stable and positive racial identity seemed to be able to appraise race-related stress situations as a challenge rather than a threat, were less likely to internalize negative racial experiences, and were able to effectively leverage a focused set of coping strategies including confrontation, empowered action, constrained resistance, and spirituality.

Overall, the research suggests that coping with racism is a complex process that is influenced by a variety of factors, and as such no coping strategy can be expected to be effective across all situations and for all people (Jacob et al., 2023; Wilson & Gentzler, 2021). The strategies Black people choose to use in coping with racism depends on the type of racism they encounter, the specifics of the situation, appraisal of the level of physical and psychological threat, as well as cultural, racial, and individual factors such as personality, racial identity, level of acculturation, and gender. For example, Black women may have more leeway to engage in active and confrontation strategies than men as Black men may be perceived as more threatening and are therefore more likely to encounter harsh or violent reactions to active coping strategies (Jacob et al., 2023). The types of racial stressors Black people are exposed to as well as the strategies they use to cope with racism evolve and change over the life course (Jones et al., 2020). It is possible that a variety of strategies do contribute to well-being, even if they do not attenuate symptoms, though most studies have focused only on symptoms. Furthermore, many of the strategies that are most effective in managing or regulating emotions and alleviating stress and symptoms on the individual level in the short term may not be effective in working toward the collective struggle against systemic and structural racism in the long term (Jacobs et al., 2023).

Most quantitative research considers the effectiveness of a specific strategy, or the influence of certain individual difference variables on the effectiveness of certain strategies, but few consider the way these factors work together to influence well-being. Although they didn't explicitly consider experiences of racial discrimination, Johnson and Carter (2019) found that when considered together, racial identity, racial socialization, communalism, cultural spirituality, and racism-related coping contributed to psychological health and well-being for Black Americans. Their study reveals that the cultural practices Blacks employ that contribute to their psychological health should be considered a set of practices that, in combination, work to shield Blacks from the potential and well-established damage of racial oppression and racial discrimination. Together, we propose that the range of cultural values and propositions that we have identified as Black cultural strengths coalesce to form a barrier to mental illness and serve as a wall of strength for Black people, and are related to overall psychological health.

In the chapters up to this point, we have provided a review of the development and current status of research and theory on Black cultural strengths in the areas of spirituality, communalism, racism-related coping, racial identity and racial socialization. Moving forward, we now turn to the application of these cultural strengths in mental health care for Black Americans through reviewing research and outlining ways in which Black cultural strengths can be integrated into clinical care, training of mental health professionals, and policy decisions that govern mental health practice.

References

Balkin, R. S., Neal, S. A., Stewart, K. D., Hendricks, L., & Arañez Litam, S. D. (2022). Spirituality and relational health among Black Americans. *Journal of Counseling & Development, 100*(4), 412–420.

Benkert, R., & Peters, R. M. (2005). African American women's coping with health care prejudice. *Western Journal of Nursing Research, 27*(7), 863–889. doi: 10.1177/0193945905278588.

Belgrave, F. Z., & Allison, (2019). *African American psychology: From Africa to America (4th Ed.)*. Los Angles, CA.: Sage

Bennett, L. Jr. (1988). *Before the Mayflower: A history of Black America* (6th ed.). Chicago. IL: Johnson Publishing Co.

Blassingame, J. W. (1979). *The slave community: Plantation life in the antebellum south.* New York, NY: Oxford University Press.

Berlin, I.,(1998). *Many thousands gone: the first two centuries in north Americs*. Cambridge, MA.: The Belknap Press of Harvard University Press.

Berry, M. F., & Blassingame, J. W. (1982). *Long memory: The Black experience in America*. New York, NY: Oxford University Press.

Bowen-Reid, T. L., & Harrell, J. P. (2002). Racist experiences and health outcomes: An examination of spirituality as a buffer. *Journal of Black Psychology, 28*(1), 18–36.

Broman, C. L., Mavaddat, R., & Hsu, S. (2000). The experience and consequences of perceived racial discrimination: A study of African Americans. *Journal of Black Psychology, 26*(2), 165–180.

Brondolo, E., ver Halen, N., Pencille, M., Beatty, D., & Contrada, R. (2009). Coping with racism: A selective review of the literature and a theoretical and methodological critique. *Journal of Behavioral Medicine, 32*, 64–88.

Brown, T. L., Phillips, C. M., Abdullah, T., Vinson, E. & Robertson, J. (2010). Are the coping strategies African Americans use different for general versus racism-related stressors? *Journal of Black Psychology, 37*(3), 311–335.

Burkhardt, M. A. (1989). Spirituality: An analysis of the concept. *Holistic Nursing Practice, 3*(3), 69–77.

Carter, R. T., & Forsyth, J. M. (2010). Reactions to racial discrimination: Emotional stress and help-seeking behaviors *Psychological Trauma: Theory, Policy, Research, and Practice,2*(3), 183–191.

Carter, R. T., & Reynolds, A. L. (2011). Race-related stress, racial identity statuses, and emotional reactions of Black Americans *Cultural Diversity and Ethnic Minority Psychology,17*(2), 156–162.

Carter, R. T., Johnson, V., Kirkinis, K., Roberson, K., Muchow, C., & Galgay, C. (2019). A meta-analytic review of racial discrimination: Relationships to health and culture. *Race and Social Problems, 11*(1), 15–32.

Carter, R. T. & Pieterse, A. (2020). *Measuring the effects of racism: Guidelines for the assessment and treatment of race-based traumatic stress injury.* New York, NY: Columbia University Press.

Chafe, W. H., Gavins, R., & Korstad, R. (2001). *Remembering Jim Crow.* New York, NY: The New Press.

Daly, A., Jennings, J., Beckett, J. O., & Leashore, B. R. (1995). Effective coping strategies of African-Americans. *Social Work, 4*(2), 240–248.

Deitch, E. A., Barsky, A., Butz, R. M., Chan, S., Brief, A. P., & Bradley, J. C. (2003). Subtle yet significant: The existence and impact of everyday racial discrimination in the workplace. *Human Relations, 56*(11), 1299–1324.

Dodson, H. (2002). *Jubilee: The emergence of African-American culture.* Washington, DC: National Geographic.

Dyson, J., Cobb, M., & Forman, D. (1997). The meaning of spirituality: A literature review. *Journal of Advanced Nursing, 26*, 1183–1188.

Emblen, J. D. (1992). Religion and spirituality defined according to current use in nursing literature. *Journal of Professional Nursing, 8*(1), 41–47.

Evans, K. M. (1997). Wellness and coping activities of African-American counselors. *Journal of Black Psychology, 23*(1), 24–35.

Feagin, J. R. (1991). The continuing significance of race: Antiblack discrimination in public places. *American Sociological Review, 56*, 101–116.

Fincham, F. D., Ajayi, C., & Beach, S. R. (2011). Spirituality and marital satisfaction in African American couples. *Psychology of Religion and Spirituality, 3*(4), 259.

Folkman, S., & Moskowitz, J. T. (2004). Coping: Pitfalls and promise. *Annual Review of Psychology, 55*, 745–774.

Forsyth, J. M. (2010). *The influence of racial identity and racism-related coping on mental health among Black Americans.* Unpublished Doctoral Dissertation. Teachers College, Columbia University.

Forsyth, J., & Carter, R. T. (2012) The influence of racial identity status attitudes and racism-related coping on mental health among Black Americans, *Cultural Diversity and Ethnic Minority Psychology, 18*(2), 128–140.

Forsyth, J., & Carter, R. T. (2014). The development and preliminary validation of the racism-related Coping Scale. *Psychological Trauma: Theory, Policy, Research, and Practice, 6*(6), 632–643.

Francois, S., Wu, K., Doe, E., Tucker, A., & Theall, K. (2023). The influence of racial violence in neighborhoods and schools on the psycho-behavioral outcomes in adolescence. *Research in Human Development, 20*(1–2), 48–64.

Fukuyama, M. A., & Sevig, T. D. (1999). *Integrating spirituality into multicultural counseling.* Sage Publications.

Genovese, E. D. (1974). *Roll Jordon, roll: The world the slaves made.* New York, NY: Vintage Books.

Graham, J. R., West, L. M., & Roemer, L. (2013). The experience of racism and anxiety symptoms in an African-American sample: Moderating effects of trait mindfulness. *Mindfulness, 4*(4), 332–341.

Greer, T. M. (2011). Coping strategies as moderators of the relation between individual race-related stress and mental health symptoms for African American women. *Psychology of Women Quarterly, 35*(2), 215–226.

Greer, T. M. (2021). The moderating role of coping strategies in understanding the effects of race-related stress on academic self-concept for African American students. *The Journal of Negro Education, 90*(2), 224–235.

Greer, T. M. (2024). African-Centered spirituality as a buffer of psychological symptoms related to specific forms of racism for African Americans. *Journal of Black Psychology, 50*(2), 165–193.

Greer, T. M., & Cavalheri, K. (2019). The role of coping strategies in understanding the effects of institutional racism on mental health outcomes for African American men. *Journal of Black Psychology, 45*(5), 405–433.

Greer, T. M., Ricks, J., & Baylor, A. A. (2015). The moderating role of coping strategies in understanding the effects of intragroup race-related stressors on academic performance and overall levels of perceived stress for African American students. *Journal of Black Psychology, 41*(6), 565–585.

Harding, V. (1981). *There is a river: The Black struggle for freedom in America.* San Diego, CA: A Harvest Book.

Harrell, S. P. (2000). A multidimensional conceptualization of racism-related stress: Implications for the well-being of people of color. *American Journal of Orthopsychiatry, 70*(1), 42–57.

Hazzard-Donald, K. (2013). *Mojo Workin': The old African American Hoodoo system.* Springfield: University of Illinois Press.

Hicken, M. T., Lee, H., Ailshire, J., Burgard, S. A., & Williams, D. R. (2013). "Every shut eye, ain't sleep": The role of racism-related vigilance in racial/ethnic disparities in sleep difficulty. *Race and Social Problems, 5,* 100–112.

Hill, P. C., & Pargament, K. I. (2003). Advances in the conceptualization and measurement of religion and spirituality. *American Psychologist, 58*(1), 64–74.

Hill, P. C., & Pargament, K. I. (2008). Advances in the conceptualization and measurement of religion and spirituality: Implications for physical and mental health research. *Psychology of Religion and Spirituality, S*(1), 3–17.

Hill, L. K., & Hoggard, L. S. (2018). Active coping moderates associations among race-related stress, rumination, and depressive symptoms in emerging adult African American women. *Development and Psychopathology, 30*(5), 1817–1835.

Himmelstein, M. S., Young, D. M., Sanchez, D. T., & Jackson, J. S. (2015). Vigilance in the discrimination-stress model for Black Americans. *Psychology & Health, 30*(3), 253–267.

Hope, E. C., Velez, G., Offidanti-Bertrand, C., Keels, M., & Durkee, M. I. (2018). Political activism and mental health among Black and Latinx college students. *Cultural Diversity and Ethnic Minority Psychology, 24*(1), 26–39.

Hope, E. C., Volpe, V. V., Briggs, A. S., & Benson, G. P. (2022). Anti-racism activism among Black adolescents and emerging adults: Understanding the roles of racism and anticipatory racism-related stress. *Child Development, 93*, 717–731.

Horton, J. O., & Horton, L. E. (2005). *Slavery and the making of America.* New York, NY: Oxford University Press.

Hyers, L. (2007). Resisting prejudice every day: Exploring women's assertive responses to anti-Black racism, anti-semitism, heterosexism, and sexism. *Sex Roles, 56*, 1–12.

Jacob, G., Faber, S. C., Faber, N., Bartlett, A., Ouimet, A. J., & Williams, M. T. (2023). A systematic review of Black people coping with racism: Approaches, analysis, and empowerment. *Perspectives on Psychological Science, 18*(2), 392–415.

Jagers, R. J. & Smith, P. (1996). Further examination of the Spirituality Scale. *Journal of Black Psychology, 22*(4), 429–442.

Johnson, V., & Carter, R.T., (2020) Black cultural strengths and psychological well-being: An empirical analysis with Black American adults. *Journal of Black Psychology, 46*(1), 55–89.

Jones, S. C. T., Anderson, R. E., Gaskin-Wasson, A. L., Sawyer, B. A., Applewhite, K., & Metzger, I. W. (2020). From "crib to coffin": Navigating coping from racism-related stress throughout the lifespan of Black Americans. *American Journal of Orthopsychiatry, 90*(2), 267–282.

Krentzman, A. R., Farkas, K. J., & Townsend, A. L. (2010). Spirituality, religiousness, and alcoholism treatment outcomes: A comparison between black and white participants. *Alcoholism Treatment Quarterly, 28*(2), 128–150.

Lewis, J. A., Williams, M. G., Peppers, E. J. & Gadson, C. A. (2017). Applying intersectionality to explore relations between gendered racism and health among Black women. *Journal of Counseling Psychology, 64*(5), 475–486.

Lincoln, C. E., & Mamiya, L. H. (1990). *The Black church in the African American experience.* Durham, NC: Duke University Press.

Mattis, J. S. (2000). African American women's definitions of spirituality and religiousity. *Journal of Black Psychology, 26*(1), 101–122.

Mattis, J. S., & Jagers, R. J. (2001). A relational framework for the study of religiosity and spirituality in the lives of African Americans. *Journal of Community Psychology, 29*(5), 519–539.

Merluzzi, T. V., Philip, E. J., Zhang, Z., & Sullivan, C. (2015). Perceived discrimination, coping, and quality of life for African-American and Caucasian persons with cancer. *Cultural Diversity and Ethnic Minority Psychology, 21*(3), 337–344.

Neblett, E. W., Jr. (2023). Racial, ethnic, and cultural resilience factors in African American youth mental health. *Annual Review of Clinical Psychology, 19*, 361–379. https://doi.org/10.1146/annurev-clinpsy-072720-015146

Mervaiglia, M. C. (1999). Critical analysis of spirituality and its empirical indicators. *Journal of Holistic Nursing, 17*(1), 18–33.

Mintz, S. W., & Price, R. (1976). *The birth of African-American culture: An anthropological perspective.* Boston, MA: Beacon Press.

Nantambu, K., (1998). Pan-Africanism versus Pan-African nationalism: An Afrocentric analysis. *Journal of Black Studies, 28,* (5), 561–574.

Neville, H. A., Heppner, P. P., & Wang, L. F. (1997). Relations among racial identity attitudes, perceived stressors, and coping styles in African American college students. *Journal of Counseling & Development, 75*(4), 303–311.

Newlin, K., Knafl, K., & Melkus, G. D. E. (2002). African-American spirituality: A concept analysis. *Advances in Nursing Science, 25*(2), 57–70.

Partow, S., Cook, R., & McDonald, R. (2021). A literature review of the measurement of coping with stigmatization and discrimination. *Basic and Applied Social Psychology, 43*(5), 319–340.

Pascoe, E. A., & Smart Richman, L. (2009). Perceived discrimination and health: A meta-analytic review. *Psychological Bulletin, 135*(4), 531–554.

Pearson, M. R., Derlega, V. J., Henson, J. M., Holmes, K. Y., Ferrer, R. A., & Harrison, S. B. (2014). Role of neuroticism and coping strategies in psychological reactions to a racist incident among African American University students. *Journal of Black Psychology, 40*(1), 81–111.

Plummer, D. L., & Slane, S. (1996). Patterns of coping in racially stressful situations. *Journal of Black Psychology, 22*(3), 302–315.

Raboteau, A. J. (2004). *Slave religion: The "invisible institution" in the antebellum south.* New York, NY: Oxford University Press.

Reed, T. D., & Neville, H. A. (2014). The influence of religiosity and spirituality on psychological well-being among Black women. *Journal of Black Psychology, 40*(4), 384–401.

Shahid, N. N., Nelson, T., & Cardemil, E. V. (2018). Lift every voice: Exploring the stressors and coping mechanisms of Black college women attending predominantly White institutions. *Journal of Black Psychology, 44*(1), 3–24.

Sanders Thompson, V. L. (2006). Coping responses and the experience of discrimination. *Journal of Applied Social Psychology, 36*(5), 1198–1214.

Scott, L. D. (2003a). The relation of racial identity and racial socialization to coping with discrimination among African American adolescents. *Journal of Black Studies, 33*(4), 520–538.

Scott Jr, L. D. (2003b). Cultural orientation and coping with perceived discrimination among African American youth. *Journal of Black Psychology, 29*(3), 235–256.

Shorter-Gooden, K. (2004). Multiple resistance strategies: How African American women cope with racism and sexism. *Journal of Black Psychology, 30*(3), 406–425.

Smith, V., Stewart, T., Myers, A., & Latu, I. (2008). Implicit coping responses to racism predict African Americans' level of psychological distress. *Basic and Applied Social Psychology, 30,* 246–277.

Stevenson, H. C. (1994). Validation of the scale of racial socialization for African American adolescents: Steps toward multidimensionality. *Journal of Black Psychology, 20*(4), 445–468.

Taylor, R. J., & Chatters, L. M. (2010). Importance of religion and spirituality in the lives of African Americans, Caribbean Blacks and non-Hispanic Whites. *Journal of Negro Education, 79*(3), 280–294.

Thomas, A. J., Witherspoon, K. M., & Speight, S. L. (2008). Gendered racism, psychological distress, and coping styles of African American women. *Cultural Diversity and Ethnic Minority Psychology*, *14*(4), 307–314.

Utsey, S. O., Adams, E. P., & Bolden, M. (2000). Development and initial validation of the Africultural Coping Systems Inventory. *Journal of Black Psychology*, *26*(2), 194–215.

Utsey, S. O., Bolden, M. A., Lanier, Y., & Williams III, O. (2007). Examining the role of culture-specific coping as a predictor of resilient outcomes in African Americans from high-risk urban communities. *Journal of Black Psychology*, *33*(1), 75–93.

Utsey, S. O., Ponterotto, J. G., Reynolds, A. L. & Cancelli, A. A. (2000). Racial discrimination, coping, life satisfaction, and self-esteem among African Americans. *Journal of Counseling & Development*, *78*(1), 72–80.

Utsey, S. O., Payne, Y. A., Jackson, E. S., & Jones, A. M. (2002). Race-related stress, quality of life indicators, and life satisfaction among elderly African Americans. *Cultural Diversity and Ethnic Minority Psychology*, *8*(3), 224.

Watson-Singleton, N. N., Hill, L. K. & Case, A. D. (2019). Past discrimination, race-related vigilance, and depressive symptoms: the moderating role of mindfulness. *Mindfulness*, *10*(9), 1768–1778.

Watson-Singleton, N. N., Mekawi, Y., Wilkins, K., & Jatta, I. F. (2020). Racism's effect on depressive symptoms: Examining perseverative cognition and Black Lives Matter activism as moderators. *Jorunal of Counseling Psychology*, *68*(1), 27–37.

West, L. M., Donovan, R. A., & Roemer, L. (2010). Coping with racism: What works and doesn't work for Black women? *Journal of Black Psychology*, *36*(3), 331–349.

Williams, M. G., & Lewis, J. A. (2019). Gendered racial microaggressions and depressive symptoms among Black women: A moderated mediation model. *Psychology of Women Quarterly*, *43*(3), 368–380.

Wilson, T. K., & Gentzler, A. L. (2021). Emotion regulation and coping with racial stressors among African Americans across the lifespan. *Developmental Review*, *61*, 100967.

Wood, J. L., & Hilton, A. A. (2012). Spirituality and academic success: Perceptions of African American males in the community college. *Religion & Education*, *39*(1), 28–47.

Young, J. (2012). African religions in the early south. *Journal of Southern Religion* 14. Retrieved from https://jsreligion.org/issues/vol14/young.html.

Zapolski, F., & Beuttlich, Marcy R. (2019). The experience of racism on behavioral health outcomes: the moderating impact of mindfulness. *Mindfulness*, *10*(1), 168–178.

Chapter 8

Review of the Black Cultural Strengths Clinical and Research Literature

In this chapter, we review the clinical and research evidence for the presence of Black Americans' cultural strengths. We build from the foundation of the previous chapters, which have indicated some of the cultural values and practices Blacks employed overtime. We review select theoretical, clinical, and research literature that focused on using Black cultural strengths in practice and tested its effectiveness. We focus on cultural variables that scholars regarded as health-promoting and beneficial to individuals and Black Americans as a whole. We have elucidated some specific aspects of Black American culture that enabled survival in North America for Black Americans. The review begins with research and clinical literature from the 1980s and moves to the present, as it denotes what researchers and scholars have written about this topic. We sought out empirical investigations as well, that validate the perspectives of clinicians and scholars who advocated for the use of mental health interventions grounded in the strengths of Black Americans.

Empirical support for Black cultural values was presented early by a number of researchers (e.g., Carter & Helms, 1987; 1990; Jones, 2003). Carter and Helms (1990) used the Intercultural Values Inventory and racial identity measures to explore whether Whites and Blacks had different cultural value preferences when compared to one another. The model of cultural value orientations was presented by Kluckhohn and Strodtbeck (1961) and the Intercultural Values Inventory (ICV, Carter, & Helms, 1990) used these existential propositions and alternatives in a survey format to compare distinct groups' cultural preferences. Group members select one of three alternatives for each proposition or value orientations. There are five orientations that reflected the groups cultural foundation or worldview. These consisted of groups': view of: human nature (evil/good/mixed); relationship to nature (harmony/master/subjugation); temporal focus (past/future/present); preferred form of social relationships (lineal or follow elders/collateral or group-based/individual); and preferred form

DOI: 10.4324/9781003083221-9

of self-expression (emotional/ or being contemplative or being-in-becoming/ action-oriented or doing, Carter & Helms, 1987; Carter 1991).

Carter's (1990) analyses were designed to determine if Whites and Blacks had the same or different cultural value preferences when compared to one another. The racial group comparison showed that Blacks and Whites differed on 8 of the 15 value orientation alternatives, but the findings were not consistent with theory about how Blacks, in relation to Whites, would look in terms of values. In the comparisons, Blacks preferred significantly more than Whites five of the eight options. Whites had significantly higher mean scores than Blacks on three of the alternatives. Blacks had higher means on evil for the Human Nature orientation; subjugation for the Person-Nature orientation; and past for the Temporal orientation. Blacks endorsed being-in-becoming for the Self-expression orientation, while Whites endorsed being. For the Social Relationships orientation, Blacks opted for lineal or following authority, whereas Whites endorsed the individual and collateral alternatives. Overall, he found empirical evidence to show that Whites and Blacks exhibited meaningful differences in their cultural values preferences. Yet, Carter and Helms (1987) and Carter (1990) expected that within-group analyses using racial identity would reveal a different set of relationships than when the racial groups were compared.

In a separate study, Carter and Helms (1987) used within-group analyses, wherein racial identity attitudes indicated differences within both racial groups. The within-group analyses for Blacks, revealed that racial identity was a component of self, and was related to Blacks' cultural values preferences. Carter and Helms (1987) reported that

> racial identity attitudes predicted three of the five Afro-centric value alternatives (Harmony with Nature, Doing Activity, and Collateral Social Relations and none of the Euro-centric based on Euro-American philosophy) alternatives. Immersion-Emersion and Internalization attitudes significantly predicted belief in Collateral Social Relations… (meaning that Social Relations are governed by the will of the group over the wishes of individuals). In addition, … Internalization attitudes were also predictive of a belief in Harmony with Nature and Doing Activity orientations … empirical support for Boykin's (1982) and Nobles (1980) contentions that vestiges of African philosophy beliefs have been retained by Afro-American culture and are expressed by the self-actualizing Afro-Americans.
>
> (p. 193)

Additionally, Carter (1990) reported that the analysis of Whites' value orientations and their racial identity attitudes, showed that the three racial identity attitudes of Contact, Disintegration and Reintegration were more often related to their cultural value preferences, "suggesting that these lower-stage racial identity attitudes may be strongly predictive of White cultural characteristics then higher ... attitudes" (Carter, 1990, p. 116).

The investigation revealed several important discoveries about cultural values and racial differences and similarities. Both Whites and Blacks shared cultural values that were related to being American. However, when psychological and social variables were taken into account, differences did emerge, which seemed to be related to their socio-cultural and racial contexts. So, the effort to establish empirical evidence for distinct Black cultural values was successful, yet more complex than was realized.

Jackson and Sears (1992) advise that employing an Afrocentric worldview would result in effective stress reduction for Black women. These scholars point out that due to stress-related exposure, Black women have higher rates of illness and poorer health outcomes such as high blood pressure. They contend these higher rates come about due to both biological and social factors. What seemed clear was that social factors related to poverty and stress contributed to the causes of high stress levels for Black women. Yet in this area, as with others we have outlined in this volume, despite the high levels of stress women and Black people experience they have evolved ways to deal with these stressors. Black women employed a range of coping mechanisms, such as seeking social support and indirect help, and using prayer and direct action. Jackson and Sears (1992) content that since cognitive appraisal is central to dealing with stress, how an individual views the world would influence their appraisal of possible stressors, and guide the course of action that could be considered. They also argue that the cultural differences between Whites and Blacks was ignored or dismissed or seen as pathology, and as such when Blacks tried to be part of the mainstream, they also took on the cultural ways of Whites and lost connection with their African roots. Jackson and Sears (1992) state that

> because of the African ancestry of African Americans and the isolation they have experienced in the United States ... remnants of an African worldview still exist among them and aided them in adapting to life in the United States.
>
> (p. 186)

Elements of that worldview includes: spirituality; communalism, or being group-oriented, cooperative and interdependent; living in harmony with nature; placing high value on self-knowledge; being present- and past-oriented; believing in the union of opposites (i.e., both-and vs. either-or); and valuing goals that are achieved through human and spiritual means rather than by using technology. Jackson and Sears (1992) provide a few empirical studies that support these cultural ways. They go on to note that these African-centered values mediate stress. They state, "An Africentric worldview has the potential to counter the negative images that African American women experience through racism and sexism" (Jackson & Sears, 1992, p. 186). They also note empirical evidence that shows a strong relationship between an Africentric worldview and psychological functioning.

Stevenson and Renard (1993) contend that Black cultural strengths can be used effectively in clinical work with Black families. "Without acknowledging and confronting oppression for many African-American clients, professional psychology becomes another societal institution of illegitimate and abusive power" (p. 434). These authors point to cultural strengths such as racial socialization as a central feature of Black teachings and socialization. Like Jackson and Sears, they outline specific aspects of Black culture that set it apart from European-American cultural systems. Some of these have been noted such as spirituality and community, past/present time or social time, harmony with nature, and they add orality (as reflected in preference for speaking and interacting). Other additions included Verve, which has to do with movement that is novel and lively, not routine and sequential; Affect, which "represents the interrelationships of feelings, thoughts and actions, and suggests that expression of emotions is a healthful exercise, not an example of poor impulse control" (Stevenson & Renard, 1993, p. 435); Expressive individualism, which refers to the unique style a person may adopt, which sets them apart, while not disconnecting them from the group, and allows for spontaneity, personal signature, and creative artistry as opposed to systemic planning and mechanical operations. These authors go on to discuss obstacles and recommended strategies that can be used with Black families. One that is illustrated is called gift-giving. They use a clinical case example to demonstrate how giving family members a gift from the therapist can raise his/her credibility with the participants in the therapy process. A critical element of working with Black families is their experiences with racism and oppression, which could result in considerable distrust of people in authority, Stevenson and Renard (1993) state regarding this mistrust

> that therapist and supervisors may do well to view the distrust of persons in authority roles as adaptive and survivalistic, to acknowledge the [Black] family's worldview and self-perception as valid, and to accept unique cultural expressions as strengths that can enhance the effectiveness of therapy if used.
>
> (p. 440)

Frame, Williams, and Green (1999) focus on the use of spirituality in working with Black women in therapy. They draw on similar historical and social issues that such women encounter and advocate for the use of employing spiritual practices in the effort to promote healing. They describe several activities that they contend are helpful in getting women to address their particular distress.

Hines and Boyd-Franklin's (2005) and Chavis' (2004) articles about Black families outline some strengths like kinship bonds and extended family systems, flexible gender roles, religion and spirituality, work, and education as well proposing the use of a multisystem treatment approach, which includes more than considerations of personal issues and adds social, political, economic, and environmental factors as well. These authors note the range of things that cause Blacks to distrust therapy and how to avoid these pitfalls. Chavis (2004) argues that genograms could be employed to document strengths in families such as religion and spirituality as well as the nature of the kinship networks that extend across generations (see, Waites, 2009).

Other investigators (e.g., Christian & Barbarin, 2001; Thomas, Davidson, & McAdoo, 2008; Utsey, Giesbrecht, Hook, & Stanard, 2008) have sought to validate the benefits of Black cultural strengths, in various ways. Christian and Barbarin (2001) examined the effects of spirituality and racial attributions on children's psychological adjustment and disordered behavior. They explored whether engaging in religious activity as a coping tool and providing racial explanations of negative events would result in less frequent behavior and emotional disruptions from their children. These researchers found that regularly attending church was related to fewer reports of problems or conflicts with adults or peers, less depression and obstinate acting out, and less immature behavior from young children. However, external attributions of racism did not lessen behavioral or emotional issues in young children. These researchers noted:

> Parents in this study derived comfort from participating in religious activities such as attending church, reading the Bible, and praying. Therefore, it is clear that religious and spiritual resources are already present in a large number of African American families: the present study merely would support the notion that nourishing and supporting continuation of these resources is a good idea. Also, it is important to keep in mind that religiosity may not be a key factor – it may be the case that spirituality, which is different is the factor.
>
> (Christian & Barbarin, 2001, p. 61)

Brown (2008) examined whether racial socialization and social support provided protection to Black people, and contributed to their ability to adapt and cope with hardships and oppression. This researcher notes that some Black people are taught how to overcome various obstacles and barriers. Brown's contention is that aspects of Black culture provide a buffer from the reality of racism. Brown defines racial socialization as a

> process, families [use to] shape a child's beliefs and attitudes of race status, as it relates to personal and group identity and how they fit into this context … These forms of racial socialization can include modeling of behaviors; specific messages; exposure to specific context, objects or environments [research] found that two out of three Black parents indicted that they provided their child with some type of racial socialization.
>
> (p. 33)

Brown (2008) observes further that social support functions as a cultural pattern that contributes to Blacks' ability to overcome adversity, a view that research evidence supports. So, the study sought to build on previous evidence by studying both racial socialization and social support together in African American adults. The expectation of the research was to determine if these two cultural elements would predict resiliency. Participants were 152 men and women who completed instruments designed to access social support, racial socialization, and resiliency.

The findings indicated that receiving racial socialization messages and feeling that one was supported was related to one's sense of resiliency. The study focused on a variety of messages that could have been transmitted. There were particular types of messages that were more strongly related to being resilient. In fact it was messages about cultural pride and learning about Black American heritage that were most significantly related to being resilient. Support systems also had a similar relationship. However, the support need not be from family, but support that was provided from community and related sources were as valuable. Evidence cited in the article noted that racial socialization messages from people outside the family were more frequent and more related to instilling positive messages about racial pride and African and Black American culture.

Thomas et al. (2008) explored whether a school-based intervention designed for young females could promote what they called cultural assets, namely ethnic or racial identity, a collective orientation, racial awareness, and liberatory activism. The experiment was conducted in a public high school with control and intervention groups. The intervention was administered over a ten week period twice a week. The results of the intervention showed a stronger ethnic identity, greater sense of community, and awareness of racism, as well as more activism. In a related study, Utsey et al. (2008) examined whether cultural values reduced the distress from exposure to racism. They suggested that cultural and psychological resources would reduce the distress associated with general life stress and race-related stress. Their study confirmed that psychological resources had a negative effect on psychological distress and that race-related stress had a positive and direct effect on less psychological distress. These researchers found that racial pride and religiosity functioned as cultural resources and were related to family cohesion and adaptation (sociofamilial resources). Thus, they contend this shows the importance of family and social support in the process of developing positive racial identity. Moreover, racial socialization occurs within the family system and within the community, thus it is the context for considerable Black cultural learning.

Related intervention studies have also been conducted, for instance, Davis et al. (2009) report on the Grady Nia Project, which is an intervention designed to aid abused and suicidal Black women. The intervention is notable because it was strength-based and participants found the intervention to be of value and helped them handle their abuse and lessen subsequent thoughts of self-harm. Risk factors decreased and protective ones increased, after the intervention.

Another intervention described by Watson, Washington, and Stepteau-Watson (2015) designed to foster positive development in young Black males and to reduce violence, and criminal justice contact. Provided mentoring and exposure to Afrocentric cultural arts and tools. It was found that the youth improved their behavior and committed fewer or no violent acts after the project. The participants noted that they learned to make better decisions and felt better about themselves. Bell-Tolliver, Burgess, and Brock (2009) reported on a study of 30 family therapists, who were interviewed about how they used Black cultural strengths in their practices. The researchers were able to identify several themes and specific strengths that were used and addressed while working with their Black families. The themes aligned with Hill's work regarding unique strengths of Black families. These were kinship bonds; religious orientation in the form of spiritualty and faith, which families used to solve their problems; and flexible family roles in dealing with racism families encountered. The families exhibited work and educational achievement foci such that they pushed one another to get ahead and to do better in the society irrespective of obvious obstacles. Families also were found to be willing to seek and use professional help when needed.

The participants reported also how they incorporated these strengths in their treatment processes. They noted that one way to help these families was to accept and honor their family structure and its lines of authority. They indicated the importance of building trust with family members, by being honest and providing encouragement and validation. They highlighted the need to listen and learn how families used their strengths, by drawing on the families victories and using the vehicle of storytelling, and allowing members to share their own particular stories. Therapists pointed out that it was essential that family members be able to use the word of God and related spiritual beliefs in the helping process with Black families. Therapists observed that as families participated in the process with acceptance of their strengths, they were able to grow more effective in communicating and problem-solving, and exhibited higher levels of confidence in their abilities. Recognizing that the obstacles and difficulties families faced were not related to them as individuals was important in healing and getting through the presenting issues (Bell-Tolliver et al., 2009).

Gaylord-Harden, Burrow, and Cunningham (2012) and Grills, Cooke, Douglas et al. (2016) contend that using Black cultural strengths can promote positive and stress reducing development for youth and children. They argue that building upon Africentric values and racial socialization can enhance prosocial behavior and move youth and children to engage in political, community oriented and justice/equity mindsets and actions. Grills, Cooke, Douglas et al. (2016), found that "cultural and group consciousness variables were…significant predictors of African American positive youth development" (p. 361).

By relying on certain Black cultural practices such as racial socialization and particular strengths, youth, adults, and children's development and lives can be improved and the impact of stressors can be reduced. Many clinicians and scholars describe interventions and programs that either seek to understand learn how Blacks define their experiences or how programs to reduce stress and draw on traditional and often overlooked assets of Black life. This perspective was behind a study by Oney, DePaulo, Lewis, and Sellers (2015), who investigated whether particular cultural attitudes would be related to eating behaviors in Black men and women. These researchers explored Jones' TRIOS variables employing an instrument developed to assess multiple dimensions of Black culture: time, rhythm, improvisation, orality, and spirituality. It was found that time orientation was related to eating, in that the more future oriented participants were, focused the more dieting they undertook while improvisation was associated with less bulimic eating. The authors concluded that participants used flexible problem-solving in the face of stress. Improvisation was also related to lower levels of food control. The researchers state that "high levels of improvisation are linked to more active coping mechanisms and less reliance on manipulation of food intake when dealing with stressful situations" (p. 6). Spiritual orientation was related to less bulimic eating, which suggests that Black people, use spiritual beliefs and practices such as praying, meditating and reading religious material as ways to cope with distress associated with eating. Some gender differences were reported as well, where men were more oriented to the past and women were more spiritual. Regardless, the study provides empirical evidence for the health promoting features of Black cultural practices and beliefs.

Researchers and scholars have shown the importance of the Black Church in the lives of Black Americans, yet it is not clear if the church also aids people in seeking professional help with psychological and emotional distress. Harris and Wong (2018) examined whether the church, which is often the preferred choice for seeking help with mental stress could be an effective resource. Harris and Wong used a focused group with 10–12 participants to explore these questions for Black should be church-going college students. The interviews were analyzed using phenomenological methods to generate critical themes from the data. The researchers found two primary themes, culture and help-seeking. Participants reported that the church was a critical aspect of their cultural development, in that it contributed to their identity as children and youth. It was experienced as part of their extended family system, it provided healthy and constructive images of the Black family, and offered role models. Their experiences in the church were described as foundational in that it was a source of spiritual connection, social support, and cultural validation and identity. Many noted that their church-going was unique and they felt that what it provided in terms of worship and spiritual connection could not be found elsewhere. In regard to seeking help inside or outside of the church, participants noted that they felt encouraged to cope with emotional issues through spiritual means, and that there was more attention given to physical health then mental. Seeking professional help was an act of last resort, when all else had failed. It seems that professional helpers are still not the first or preferred sources of help. Family, church, and related systems were tapped first and were seen as preferable for the young adults in the study.

Anderson, McKenny, and Stevenson (2019) report on the EMBRace program that was designed to develop racial socialization and reduce racial stress and enhance racial coping. They contend that racial socialization, the messages delivered to young people both directly and indirectly within families, should be considered a cultural strength that is associated with positive outcomes. They note that traditional coping mechanisms fail to function for Black people and families, since most people in general do not need to cope with continuous racial discrimination and racism as social stressors in their lives.

Racial socialization functions as a protective factor in that it allows parents and family members to teach their young how to manage and understand and limit the negative and adverse effects of racism. This is done by teaching about cultural history and instilling pride and esteem in the young by letting them know what his/her ancestors achieved and how they lived and what they valued. The young are also taught not to trust people from other racial groups. Anderson et al. (2019) describe a seven-week intervention aimed at youth to aid in their parents and the youths learning about how to "Engage, Manage, and Bond." The engagement involves helping the participants interact and talk to one another about race and stress, how to employ effective coping, and to make the connections between parents and children stronger.

Researchers also have pointed out that it would be beneficial to learn how Black people might define aspects of their lives, since it is possible that how they see or define health or well-being may not be consistent with popular or mainstream definitions. Alagaraja and Hooper (2022) assume that well-being involves emotional stability and positive relationships. This definition was assumed to apply to Black people with little effort to document whether that was an accurate assumption or not. They point out the deficit perspective that dominates the health and clinical literature and how, as we have pointed out, the deficit thinking about Black people often leads to mistreatment, misconceptions, and inaccuracies, that led to underdiagnosing which hampers optimal care.

Their qualitative study explored how community-based Black people defined well-being from their perspective. They discovered that many of the ways that their study participants referenced well-being did not conform to what was found in the existing literature. Thirty-five adults were interviewed and themes extracted from them, in which they discussed what well-being meant to them, which was "feeling good," as in having a pain-free life, or enjoying family relationships and activities, having a belief in God and strong faith. Also, being involved in church and religious and spiritual activities felt good. And having a constructive state of mind, which included several things such as learning to let go of worries, drama, and stress. They learned also to avoid negative energy, to be focused on accomplishments and resolve problems, to look for the good in situations, and to be at peace with your community, all these contributed to their well-being. Self-care also mattered which was contrary to what was known, as Alagaraja and Hooper (2022) stated "wellbeing research is typically grounded in psychological perspectives, where wellbeing is viewed as an individual-level experience…The study participants identified intergenerational family ties and community networks (e.g., involvement in church activities) as mechanism that foster wellbeing" (p. 2068). They noted further that the literature is devoid of relevant information about Black people that is grounded in their experiences and history, and that using what is known about White Americans should not be used to aid Blacks.

Other clinical scholars (e.g., Coard, Wiley, & Evans, 2021; Harper, James, Curtis, & Ramey, 2021) present information about programs and interventions aimed at fostering behavioral, and social competence in Black children by helping parents learn effective strategies and to rely on their own cultural strengths. Coard et al. (2021) employed a community prevention program for Black parents, in which they expected participants, to have higher regard for universal and culturally sanctioned practice, and they expected to observe fewer child-related issues in behavior and to see an increase in social competence, lastly they thought that the participants would report high levels of satisfaction and attendance with the program. Although their findings did not confirm all their assumptions they did note an increase in parents' use of proactive racial socialization and the program was highly and positively rated by participants. Harper et al. (2021) describe a community-involved culture-specific intervention model aimed at promoting positive youth development.

Griffin and Armstead (2020) investigated how Black adults responded to racial stress in a sample of 74 adults between 30 and 55 years of age. They used eight focus groups and qualitative methods to capture how Blacks coped with stressful racial encounters, the participants were. Narrative dialogue was coded and analyzed for themes and subthemes. The researchers noted evidence of various types of strategies to cope with racial stress. They stated:

Blacks within our sample utilized a complex and context-embedded range of coping styles to deal with racism. These coping strategies were not guided by emotional responsiveness, but by behavioral, emotional, and cognitive adaptations to the context of the Black experience.

(p. 618)

Griffin and Armstead (2020) reported seven coping responses to racism: avoidance coping, which consisted of denial and rejection of the racial nature of what occurred; humiliation, where the person felt shame and disrespected by the encounter; physical reactivity, involved physical symptoms like chest pains and stomach distress; overall distrust of Whites, meaning that the person lacks confidence that White people can be relied upon for support; problem-solving coping, meant the person looked for ways to challenge the racial situation, by seeking emotional support, or demanding respect, or documenting the incident and going to people in authority with the violation; cultural assimilation; meant accepting that Whites are right in their actions; and emotional coping which included negative reactions of fear, anxiety, anger, and distress. Those that did not problems solve were left with physical and emotional symptoms of distress.

Balkin, Neal, Stewart, Hendricks, and Litam (2022) explored the extent to which spirituality could preserve wellness in Black adults. These authors note that there is a distinction between religion and spirituality, in that religion is considered the divine elements of life that are shared with others, while spirituality refers to being aware that life has sacred dimensions. The two, they contend, are linked in many ways and that spiritualty is a core aspect of wellness. For instance, prayer and meditation had been shown to have a positive impact on mental health. Also, positive styles of coping can buffer distress that then protects the person from harm. Relational health, refers to the positive outcomes from engaging in heathy, growth-fostering relationships that include experiences of zest, empowerment, clarity, self-worth, and connection. Such elements function to provide protection from sources of psychosocial stress. The study involved some 233 participants, and measures of spiritualty and relational health. It was found that relational health, specifically, mentor and community relationships, was positively related to spirituality. This result highlights the benefits and importance of communalism and collective identity within Black spiritualty. Balkin et al. (2022), stated that "Black Americans maybe socialized to adopt certain elements of individualistic culture, but they may retain and place high value on these elements of African culture passed down through generations" (p. 417).

Johnson and Carter (2017) used a complex statistical model to test whether a group of Black cultural values were related to one another and if as a group would reveal Black cultural strengths and psychological well-being. It was hypothesized that higher levels of Black cultural strengths would be associated with increased psychological well-being and life satisfaction. The study included 486 Black, middle-class, American adults with an average age of 31. Findings indicated that cultural patterns were related to psychosocial health (i.e., life satisfaction and psychological well-being). In particular, health promoting aspects of racial identity (i.e., racial centrality, Internalization attitudes); racial socialization (i.e., racial pride and cultural socialization); racism-related coping (i.e., confrontation); as well as higher levels of communalism and spirituality combined would indicate one latent (or not measured directly) factor, Black cultural strength. These researchers also predicted that Black cultural strengths would, in turn, predict psychosocial health. Johnson and Carter's (2020) analyses found that Black cultural strength comprising levels of mature racial identity, positive racial socialization, effective racism-related coping, and high levels of both cultural spirituality and communalism was positively associated with psychosocial health.

Empirical evidence provides support for a set of Black cultural values that are interrelated (Bediako & Harris, 2017; Forsyth & Carter, 2012; Jagers, Smith, Mock, & Dill, 1997) and positively associated with psychological well-being, life satisfaction, quality of life, and other pro-social variables such as self-esteem and optimism, and negatively related to depression and posttraumatic stress disorder (PTSD) (Hughes, Kiecolt, Keith, & Demo, 2015; Forsyth & Carter, 2014). However, scholars studied these relationships between the cultural values and practices in isolation.

Johnson (2017) and Johnson and Carter's (2020) used multiple instruments to capture the complex variables that they thought comprised Black cultural strengths; they also believed that these strengths work together and as a group functioned to aid psychosocial health and well-being. For instance, Mature Black Racial Identity was measured using the private regard (i.e., one's positive or negative feelings toward Blacks and being Black) and centrality (i.e., the importance of being Black to oneself) subscales from the Multidimensional Inventory of Black Identity (MIBI; Sellers, 2013) and the internalization (i.e., belief in the value of ones' racial group) subscale was used from Black Racial Identity Attitudes Scale. Effective coping with racism assessed an individual's use of racism-related coping skills with the Racism-Related Coping Scale (*RRCS*; Forsyth & Carter, 2014). In their study, only four of the eight scales were used: Confrontation, Empowered Action, Spiritual, and Constrained Resistance coping. Communalism was measured with two scales: The Communalism Scale (Boykin, Jagers, Ellison, & Albury, 1997) that assesses the degree to which respondents are socially interdependent and adhere to a group orientation. The African American Collectivism Scale (*AACS*; Lukwago et al., 2001) is designed to assess collectivism in African Americans. Cultural spirituality was measured with two scales; The Spirituality Scale (*SS*; Jagers & Smith, 1996) which assesses Africultural spirituality, and the Daily Spiritual Experiences Scale (*DSES*; Underwood & Teresi, 2002) that assesses one's spiritual experiences in daily life. Positive Racial Socialization was measured with subscales of the Racial Socialization Scale. Namely, the preparation for bias and Cultural Socialization Scales were used in the study. The measure assesses the types of racial socialization messages an individual has been the recipient of. Psychosocial health was measured using two scales: The Satisfaction with Life Scale is a measure that assesses one's self-reported general satisfaction with their life, and The Mental Health Inventory, which assesses mental health emotions and symptoms, the Global Psychological Well-Being Scale was used in their study. Johnson and Carter's findings illustrate the interdependence of Black cultural strengths.

Communalism was most strongly predicted by Black cultural strength, followed by mature racial identity, cultural spirituality, positive racial socialization, and lastly, effective racism-related coping. This pattern of least to strongest indicators speaks to how these values interact with one another. First, one's level of connectedness with other Blacks may be an essential part of Black cultural strength, in that without a communalistic orientation, one's ability to develop a mature racial identity, recognize and then learn to effectively cope with racism, and absorb racial socialization messages could be compromised. Alternatively, communalism could be considered a byproduct of other Black cultural values or practices. For instance, as one is socialized as a Black person, part of that process may involve teachings about how one can and should rely on other Blacks, even those outside of their immediate family or social network.

It is not surprising that mature racial identity would also strongly predict Black cultural strength. It has been associated with most of the other Black cultural practices including racism-related coping and racial socialization. One's understanding of race in their lives and their regard toward the Black racial group is an essential component of Black cultural strength, and certainly impacts the way that parents socialize their children, and thus how Black cultural values are passed intergenerationally (Thomas & Speight, 1999).

Positive racial socialization and effective racism-related coping were additional correlates in the model speaking to the possibility that some racial socialization messages, particularly those geared toward preparation for bias, may also include recommendations about how to effectively cope with racism. If this is true, perhaps racial socialization messages are focused on effective strategies and other coping tools (i.e., bargaining, hypervigilance) that are not necessarily learned strategies, but results of emotional distress related to the racial incidents. Without the communalistic nature of Black culture, individuals may face distressing race-based incidents, pursue coping methods, and be faced without sufficient social support in the aftermath.

The Black cultural strength model fits into the larger context of findings about the state of psychological health within the Black community. Scholars have found that when compared to other People of Color, Blacks did better in terms of psychological and physical health correlates of racism (Carter, Lau, Johnson, & Kirkinis, 2017). This is not to say that Black Americans do not suffer from racial oppression. Rather, Black cultural strengths may mitigate these effects.

Johnson and Carter's (2020) findings point to cultural values that should be promoted and reinforced for Black American clients in therapy. Clients may be facing pressures to conform to White cultural values in a variety of settings (e.g., academic). Clinicians should consider ways in which the Black clients could be helped or guided to regain (if it was lost) their sense of communalism, even within an institution which does not reflect their own cultural values. A therapist may suggest the client consider joining Black organizations.

Clinicians may serve the role of additional racial socializers, and suggest racism-related coping strategies that have been empirically proven to be effective. For instance, a clinician may find that a client relies heavily on cognitive racism-related coping. The clinician may suggest that the client "get out of their head" and confront the parties involved. Further, a clinician can rely on their knowledge of the client's spirituality to suggest they also utilize spiritual coping strategies as well (e.g., praying). Even if the individual does not regularly engage in formalized religious practices, clinicians should be aware they may endorse high levels of spiritual coping.

The research suggests that the application of Black cultural strengths could have important implications for both the process and mental health interventions among Black Americans as well as outcomes associated with these interventions. We will discuss ways in which Black cultural strengths can be integrated in mental health interventions utilized with Black Americans.

References

Alagaraja, M., & Hooper, L. M. (2022). Wellbeing among Black American adults living in low-resourced communities. *Journal of Community Psychology, 50*(5), 2058–2071.

Anderson, R. E., McKenny, M. C., & Stevenson, H. C. (2019). EMBR ace: Developing a racial socialization intervention to reduce racial stress and enhance racial coping among Black parents and adolescents. *Family Process, 58*(1), 53–67. https://doi.org/10.1111/famp.12412

Balkin, R. S., Neal, S. A., Stewart, K. D., Hendricks, L., & Litam, S. D. A. (2022). Spirituality and relational health among Black Americans. *Journal of Counseling & Development, 100*(4), 412–420.

Bediako, S. M., & Harris, C. (2017). Communalism moderates the association between racial centrality and emergency department use for Sickle Cell disease pain. *Journal of Black Psychology, 43*(7), 659–668. doi: 10.1177/0095798417696785.

Bell-Tolliver, L., Burgess, R., & Brock, L. J. (2009). African American therapists working with African American families: An exploration of the strengths perspective in treatment. *Journal of Marital and Family Therapy, 35*(3), 293–307. https://doi.org/10.1111/j.1752-0606.2009.00117.x

Boykin, A. W., Jagers, R. J., Ellison, C. M., & Albury, A. (1997). Communalism: Conceptualization and measurement of an Afrocultural social orientation. *Journal of Black Studies, 27*(3), 409–418. https://doi.org/10.1177/002193479702700308

Boykin, W. A. (1982). On the academic performance of Afro-American children. In J. T. Spence (Ed.), *Assessing achievement.* San Francisco: W.B. Saunders.

Brown, D. L. (2008). African American resiliency: Examining racial socialization and social support as protective factors. *Journal of Black Psychology, 34*(1), 32–48.

Carter, R. T. (1990a). Cultural value differences between African Americans and White Americans. *Journal of College Student Development, 31*(1), 71–79.

Carter, R. T. (1990b). The relationship between racism and racial identity among White Americans: An exploratory investigation. *Journal of Counseling and Development, 69*, 46–50.

Carter, R. T. (1991). Cultural values: A review of empirical research and implications for counseling. *Journal of Counseling and Development, 70*, 164–173.

Carter, R. T., & Helms, J. E. (1987). The relationship of Black value-orientations to racial identity attitudes. *Measurement and Evaluation in Counseling and Development, 19*, 185–195.

Carter, R. T., & Helms, J. E. (1990). The intercultural values inventory. In *Test in microfiche test collection.* Princeton, NJ: Educational Testing Service.

Carter, R. T., Lau, M. Y., Johnson, V., & Kirkinis, K. (2017). Racial discrimination and health outcomes among racial/ethnic minorities: A meta-analytic review. *Journal of Multicultural Counseling and Development, 45*(1), 232–259. doi: 10.1002/jmcd.12076.

Chavis M. A. (2004). Genograms and African American families: Employing family strengths of spirituality, religion, and extended family network. *Michigan Family Review, 9*(1), 30–36.

Christian, M. D., & Barbarin, O. A. (2001). Cultural resources and psychological adjustment of African American children: Effects of spirituality and racial attribution. *Journal of Black Psychology, 27*(1), 43–63.

Coard, S. I., Wiley, K. C., & Evans, A. G. (2021). The Black Parenting Strengths and Strategies Program–Racialized Short (BPSS-RS): "Real-world" dismantle, implementation, and evaluation. *Adversity and Resilience Science, 2*, 235–245.

Davis, S. P., Arnette, N. C., Bethea, K. S., Graves, K. N., Rhodes, M. N., Harp, S. E., Dunn, S. E., Patel, M. N., & Kaslow, N. J. (2009). The Grady Nia Project: A culturally competent intervention for low-income, abused, and suicidal African American women. *Professional Psychology: Research and Practice, 40*(2), 141–147. doi: 10.1037/a0014566

Eyerman, R. (2001). *Cultural trauma: Slavery and the formation of African American identity.* Cambridge: Cambridge University Press.

Forsyth, J., & Carter, R. T. (2012). The relationship between racial identity status attitudes, racism-related coping, and mental health among Black Americans. *Cultural Diversity and Ethnic Minority Psychology, 18*(2), 128–140. doi: 10.1037/a0027660.

Forsyth, J. M., & Carter, R. T. (2014). Development and preliminary validation of the Racism- Related Coping Scale. *Psychological Trauma: Theory, Research, Practice, and Policy, 6*(6), 632–643. doi: 10.1037/a0036702

Frame, M. W., Williams, C. B., & Green, E. L. (1999). Balm in Gilead: Spiritual dimensions in counseling African American women. *Journal of Multicultural Counseling and Development, 27*(4), 182–192.

Griffin, E.K., Armstead, C. (2020). Black's Coping Responses to Racial Stress. *Journal Racial and Ethnic Health Disparities*, *7*, 609–618. https://doi.org/10.1007/s40615-019-00690-w

Grills, C., Cooke, D., Douglas, J., Subica, A., Villanueva, S., & Hudson, B. (2016). Culture, Racial Socialization, and Positive African American Youth Development. *Journal of Black Psychology*, *42*(4), 343–373. https://doi.org/10.1177/0095798415 578004

Harper, E. A., James, A. G., Curtis, C., & Ramey, D. (2021). Using the participatory culture-specific intervention model to improve a positive youth development program for African American adolescent girls. *Journal of Educational and Psychological Consultation*, *31*(1), 61–81.

Harris, A., R. J., & Wong, C.D., (2018). African American college students and the Black church and counseling. *Journal of College Counseling, 21,* 15–28.

Hines, P. M., & Boyd-Franklin, N. (2005). African American families. *Ethnicity and Family Therapy*, *3*, 87–100.

Hughes, M., Kiecolt, K. J., Keith, V. M., & Demo, D. H. (2015). Racial identity and well-being among African Americans. *Social Psychology Quarterly*, *78*(1), 25–48. doi: 10.1177/0190272514554043.

Jackson, A. P., & Sears, S. J. (1992). Implications of an Africentric worldview in reducing stress for African American women. *Journal of Counseling and Development, 71*, 184–190.

Jagers, R. J., Smith, P., Mock, L. O., & Dill, E. (1997). An Afrocultural social ethos: Component orientations and some social implications. *Journal of Black Psychology*, *23*(4), 328–343. doi: 10.1177/00957984970234002.

Johnson, V. E. (2017). Testing a Model of Black Cultural Strength Using Structural Equation Modeling. Dissertation Abstracts international.

Johnson, V., & Carter, R. T. (2020) Black cultural strengths and psychological well-being: An empirical analysis with Black American adults. *Journal of Black Psychology, 46(1),* 55–89. doi: 10.1177/0095798419889752.

Jones, J. M. (2003). TRIOS: A psychological theory of the African legacy in American culture. *Journal of Social Issues*, *59*(1), 217–242.

Kluckhohn, F. R. & Strodtbeck, F. L. (1961). *Variations in value orientations*. Evanston, IL: Row, Peterson.

Mikle, K. S., & Gilbert, D. J. (2020). A systematic review of culturally relevant marriage and couple relationship education programs for African-American couples. *Rethinking Social Work Practice with Multicultural Communities*, 50–75.

Nobles, W. E. (1980). African philosophy: Foundations for Black psychology. In R. L. Jones (Ed.), *Black Psychology*(2nd ed.) (pp. 23–36). New York: Harper & Row *27(4):1–18* . doi: 10.1007/s12111-023-09638-1.

Oney, C., DePaulo, D., Lewis, R., & Sellers, R. (2015). Eating behaviors and related cultural attitudes of African American men and women. *Health Psychology Open, 2*(2), Article 2055102915605974. https://doi.org/10.1177/2055102915605974

Paris, D. (2021, July). Culturally sustaining pedagogies and our futures. *The Educational Forum*, *85*(4), 364–376.

Stevenson, H. C., & Renard, G. (1993). Trusting ole'wise owls: Therapeutic use of cultural strengths in African-American families. *Professional Psychology: Research and Practice*, *24*(4), 433.

Thomas, A. J., & Speight, S. L. (1999). Racial identity and racial socialization attitudes of African American parents. *Journal of Black Psychology*, *25*(2), 152–170. doi: 10.1177/0095798499025002002.

Travis Jr, R., & Leech, T. G. (2014). Empowerment-based positive youth development: A new understanding of healthy development for African American youth. *Journal of Research on Adolescence*, *24*(1), 93–116.

Underwood, L.G., & Teresi, J.A., (2002). The Daily Spiritual Experience Scale. *Annals of Behavioral Medicine, 24*(1), 1, 22-33. doi: 10.1037/t01587-000

Utsey, S. O., Giesbrecht, N., Hook, J., & Stanard, P. M. (2008). Cultural, sociofamilial, and psychological resources that inhibit psychological distress in African Americans exposed to stressful life events and race-related stress. *Journal of Counseling Psychology, 55*(1), 49–62. doi: 10.1037/0022-0167.55.1.49.

Waites, C. (2009). Building on strengths: Intergenerational practice with African American families. *Social Work, 54*(3), 278–287.

Watson, J., Washington, G., & Stepteau-Watson, D. (2015). Umoja: A culturally specific approach to mentoring young African American males. *Child and Adolescent Social Work Journal, 32*, 81–90.

Chapter 9

Clinical Considerations in the Application of Black American Cultural Strengths to Mental Health Care

The counseling and psychotherapy literature has routinely referenced lower utilization of mental health services among Black Americans with barriers to treatment including stigma, factors associated with the clinician and therapeutic practices, affordability, availability, and accessibility (Cooper-Patrick et al. 1999; Snowden, 1999; Planey et al., 2019). Among clinician and therapeutic practices, the notion of cultural mistrust has been identified as an important consideration. Located in the history of racial oppression, and the manner in which psychological and psychiatric practice have been complicit in the oppression of Black Americans (Torres, 2023; Haeny et al., 2021), the expectation that treatment might not be helpful, and in fact could be harmful, is captured by a study that reported Black American endorsement of the following statements: "White professionals could not understand the problems of African American families" and "I am suspicious that White professionals would not treat my child as well as s/he would treat a White child" (Planey et al., 2019, p. 193). Indeed, some scholars have referenced cultural mistrust as a healthy cultural paranoia, given the history of racial oppression and subjugation experienced by Black Americans within the United States (Turner et al., 2019). Given the manner in which specific racial experiences might influence the engagement in mental health care among Black Americans, integrating racial cultural patterns and worldview, and race-related experiences could be an important approach to provide more culturally consistent and relevant care, thereby increasing the participation of Black Americans in counseling and psychotherapy.

Consider the following clinical scenario: A clinician meets a Black American female for an intake session. The presenting concerns center around a history of unhealthy romantic relationships, a suspicion that she might have an undiagnosed attention deficit and hyperactivity disorder (ADHD), and the stress of working as a Black woman in corporate America. During the session, the client indicates that she has had prior experience in counseling; however, none of the treatments were sustained – partly due to her perception that the clinicians did

DOI: 10.4324/9781003083221-10

not understand her cultural experiences as a Black woman. Note the following exchange:

Therapist: "Earlier you mentioned that you felt previous therapists were not understanding your experience as a Black woman…what made you think this?"

Client: "Well, they never spoke to me about it … they never spoke with me about being a Black woman."

The salience of race in this vignette both directly and indirectly provides an urgent reminder of the need to incorporate race-related factors directly into the mental health care of Black Americans (Cuevas et al., 2016; Boyd-Franklin, 2013). The preponderance of Eurocentric conceptualizations of mental health (Kerney et al., 2024), the hesitancy and inability of many therapists to attend to race and racism in the therapeutic encounter (Stoute, 2020), and the lack of integration of cultural strengths as a therapeutic approach (Jones et al., 2020) provides an important context for the documented lower levels of utilization of professional mental health care among Black Americans. Research has noted that the incorporation of culturally consistent and resonant mental health interventions likely increase both the efficacy of treatment and the utilization of clinical services among Black American adults (Lateef, Nartey, Amoako, & Lateef, 2022).

In the prior chapters, we have identified cultural variables that serve as a source of strength and positivity for Black Americans. These include cultural patterns that pre-date enslavement and have been passed down generationally including spirituality, communalism, orality as a way of communicating and the centrality of rhythm. Additionally, cultural patterns that have emerged from the experience of racial oppression include racism-related coping and racial socialization. We now turn to an application of these cultural variables within the mental health care of Black Americans.

Spirituality and Mental Health

Religious beliefs and spirituality have been described as a "central component of the cultural heritage of African Americans" (Boyd-Franklin, 2010, p. 997). Stemming from an African cultural tradition that views the psyche and the spirit as the same construct (Mbiti, 1990), Jones (2004) notes that spirituality can be considered "forces beyond human beings act with effect in the world of human beings*"* (p. 168). In this regard, Jones describes spirituality as dealing with Gods, Spirits, and Human Beings and notes that spirituality "pervades the essence of humanity and that individuals cannot live beyond its sphere" (p. 168). For many Black Americans, spiritual practices are located within organized religion such as the church. For the Black community, the church has been noted to serve a few important functions, including a place for emotional expression, providing a sense of meaning and purpose, and facilitating a communal experience. Many Black Americans, in particular those with heritage from the Caribbean diaspora, may practice versions of or incorporate aspects of traditional West African predominantly Yoruba religions into their spiritual practice. Many of these religions have been practiced continuously in the diaspora since slaves were brough to the New World. These religions are referred to as Orisha/Shango (Trinidad and Tobago), Obeah (most English-speaking Caribbean islands), Voodun (Haiti), Quimbois (Francophone islands), Lucumi (Cuba), Candomblé (Brazil), and Santeria (Puerto Rico, Dominican Republic, and Cuba) (Curry, 2020). We have previously documented that cultural spirituality is a consistent African value. Although the enactment of spirituality has shifted over the centuries with enslavement having a significant impact on how Black Americans engaged their spiritual existence, the central theme of recognition of a Supreme Being that could be accessed through rituals such as prayer, dance, song, and sacrifice is a central Black/African cultural value (Dodson, 2002).

When considering spirituality as a cultural strength, we need to ask how spirituality contributes positively to the life experience of Black Americans, and what function it serves in regard to psychological well-being. Many Africentric scholars would resonate with the perception of Myers and colleagues (2000) when they note that for Black Americans, spirituality is an essential element in wellness. Furthermore, recent research indicates that Black Americans view spirituality as a core component of mental health. Kerney et al. (2024) interviewed 60 Black American adults in order to assess their perceptions of factors that constitute mental health. Many participants reflect on the role of spirit, noting a dynamic balance between the spirit and psyche with a participant stating, "Mental health is the interconnected nature of psychological, emotional, physical, and spiritual well-being" (p. 12). Beyond including spirituality as a core part of mental health, it appears that for Black Americans, spirituality is also a mechanism toward mental health. The Black church, a central vehicle for the enacting of spirituality, has been an integral part of the Black American experience for centuries providing a space for community, spiritual expression, and liberation. During enslavement, the Black church – informal gatherings for spiritual expression – served as an instrument for support, hope, and dreams of liberation. It is well-known that the church played a central role in the civil rights movement with many leaders allowing the church to be a place where messages of equal rights were proclaimed and activism was nurtured and nourished. More recently, beyond the spiritual and religious aspects of church life, the church has been a place to champion the improvement of Black Americans in areas of education, health, and financial literacy (Avent & Cashwell, 2015; Rowland & Isaac-Savage, 2014; Stephens et al., 2020). Spirituality is a core aspect of the TRIOS model offered by Jones (2004), which includes cultural and philosophical aspects of Time, Rhythm, Improvisation, Orality, and Spirituality. Note, Jones contends:

> TRIOSic qualities that consist of staying focused in the present, employing creative and flexible problem-solving strategies in unpredictable and threatening situations, utilizing oral communication to transmit cultural values and political self-protective courses of action, and sustaining the human spirit through connection to a higher being and the natural rhythms of nature and the soul operate for the adaptation and coping of African Americans.
>
> (p. 241)

In sum, spirituality is a core component of the Black American experience. In regard to health and well-being, we see spirituality as both a constituent and determinant of well-being. Furthermore, adjunctive benefits of spirituality include communalism as evidenced by the Black Church, activism, the provision of a counter-narrative to perceptions of inferiority, and the facilitation of spiritually based coping strategies to deal with the ongoing adversity of racial oppression (Jacob et al., 2023; Hayward & Krause, 2015).

Clinical Applications of Spirituality

Incorporating spirituality as an important consideration in psychotherapeutic work with Black Americans has been noted in the counseling and psychotherapy literature (Mattis & Natasha-Grayman, 2013), "it is very important for psychologists working with African American clients to not limit appropriate inquiries to religion or religious beliefs but to expand the subject to include whether spirituality or spiritual beliefs are a part of their lives" (Boyd-Franklin, 2010, p. 979).

Dominant models of psychology that stem from a European/White worldview tend to view psychological and spiritual processes as separate domains; however as we have already indicated for Black Americans, the spirit and psyche are viewed as deeply connected. As such, the clinical applications of spirituality may take different forms. Boyd-Franklin (2010) notes that for some Black Americans, psychological distress may be expressed in spiritual terms thereby highlighting the need for the clinicians to inquire as to the role and salience of spirituality in the individual's life. Here the clinician displays a cultural attunement and a communication of interest in understanding the client as they experience the world. A simple and effective spiritual assessment has been offered by Hodge (2004, p. 38), which includes the following questions:

1 I was wondering if you consider spirituality or religion to be a personal strength?
2 In what ways does your spirituality help you cope with the difficulties you encounter?

3   Are there certain spiritual beliefs and practices that you find particularly helpful in dealing with problems?
4   I was also wondering if you attend a church or participate in some other type
of spiritual community?
5   Do resources exist in your church community that might be helpful to you?
6   Are there any spiritual needs I can help you address?

For the Black American client, it could be helpful to place these questions in the
context of their racial and cultural experience, recognizing the cultural role of
spirituality and religion (Dodson, 2002). Additional applications of spirituality
in mental health practice with Black Americans include understanding the role
spirituality plays for the individual, in the family context dynamic, and as part
of being connected to the larger community. In Bell-Tolliver and Wilkerson's
(2011) study in which African American therapists were asked to identify aspects
of a strength-based approach for working with Black Americans, 95% of the participants highlight the connection between family ties referred to as kinship, religious orientation, and spiritual practice. These therapists emphasized the need
to inquire, understand, and incorporate religion and spirituality as important
aspects of kinship networks, and identified spirituality and religious orientation
as important strengths within the Black American community. Boyd-Franklin
(2010) describes ways in which the Black Church operates as a source of adjunctive support and encourages clinicians, with their client's permission, to actively
seek out ways to connect the client with church-based resources, writing that
Black churches "are a natural base for mental health interventions in the African
American community" (p. 994). Additionally, Queener and Martin (2001) present a framework in which clinical services and life skills are promoted through
partnerships with Black churches and congregations. In this framework, church
pastors and other administrators promote mental health treatment and support
through sermons, referrals, distribution of brochures, and participation in other
church-related programming.

As a reminder that one cannot divorce religious and spiritual orientation from
other aspects of identity for Black Americans, Mattis and Grayman-Simpson
(2013) report that those Black Americans who endorse high levels of subjective
religiosity also report pride in the racial group, while others who are affiliated
with more social justice-oriented faith traditions see faith as a tool for "liberation
and social transformation (p. 549).

Spiritual and religious-based practices are widely seen as instrumental in
facilitation of effective coping with racism and other life adversities associated
with being Black in America. As such, assisting Black American clients in identifying the specific faith-based practices (prayer, reading of scripture – Bible,
Quran, meeting in religious congregations, etc.), spiritual-based practices
(meditation, drumming, maintaining a sense of connection with and/or honoring one's ancestors), and spiritual/religious-based values that inform approaches

to relationships, that account for meaning-making and sense of purpose, and that provide a framework in which to understand human existence should be identified, supported, and affirmed as pathways to mental health and subjective well-being.

Communalism and Mental Health

There are many examples of organizations within the Black American community that are grounded through a shared cultural identity and the historical experience of the racial oppression of Americans of African Descent. Perhaps the most visible of these organizations is the National Association for the Advancement of Colored People (NAACP). Rooted in a mission to achieve "equity, political rights and social inclusion," the NAACP is driven by the experience of Black Americans as a collective community. Whether they're cultural or political groups across the social and political spectrum (e.g., Black Panther Party, United Negro Fund, 100 Black Men, 100 Black Women, Jack and Jill organization), Black American Associations are grounded in the experience of communalism, described by Boykin et al., as "the social interdependence of Black People" (1997).

In thinking of how communalism is appreciated as a cultural strength, we note a further description and definition by Boykin (1983), which presents the foundational understanding of communalism as a strength for Black Americans that

> denotes awareness of the [fundamental] interdependence of people. One's orientation is social rather than being directed toward objects. One acts in accordance with the notion that duty to one's social group is more important than individual privileges and rights. Sharing is promoted because it signifies the affirmation of social interconnectedness; self-centeredness and individual greed are disdained.
>
> (p. 385)

When reviewing empirical research, we note that that there is evidence to support the notion that communalism should be viewed as a cultural strength among Black Americans. Grayman-Simpson and Mattis (2017) present the results of a validation study of the Communalism Scale (Boykin et al., 1997). This psychometrically valid measure is based on five aspects of communalism, namely: (1) anchoring of individual identity in group; (2) transcendence of group duties and responsibilities over individual concerns; (3) sanctity of social bonds and relations; (4) primacy of social existence; and, (5) emphasis on sharing and contributing in support of the group. Results indicate that, among a sample of African American adults, communalism is positively associated with subjective well-being and community engagement (Grayman-Simpson & Mattis, 2017).

In a study that examined the relationship between communalism, religiosity and thriving among a sample of Black American adolescents, results indicate positive relationships between high endorsement of communalism and high levels of thriving, defined by the authors as "lack of problem behaviors and psychopathology and the presence of positive development and well-being" (p. 119). Of particular importance to the applications of cultural strengths in counseling and clinical work, the reduction or elimination of problem behaviors, recovery from psychopathology, as well as evidence of positive development and well-being are the primary goals of counseling and psychotherapy. Given the findings associated with communalism, it is clear to see how important communalism can be for counseling intervention. We suggest that communalism facilitates a type of cultural congruence and the counseling and psychotherapy literature identifies congruence as a central outcome of effective counseling and psychotherapy (Stephen, 2023).

It is important to note areas of overlap between the various cultural strengths we are addressing in this chapter and this book. In describing the relation between racial identity and well-being, Hughes et al., (2015) report findings indicating that among African Americans a stronger identification with one's racial group is associated with less depressive symptoms and greater self-esteem. As such, clinical work that facilitates a greater sense of connection to one's identity could be associated with a greater sense of communalism, which, in turn, is associated with greater engagement in the community and greater levels of subjective well-being or happiness.

Clinical Applications of Communalism

Earlier in this chapter, we have reviewed ways in which spirituality and religion are cultural strengths and can be incorporated in the clinical process. In doing so, we also spoke to the manner in which spirituality and religion should be understood as a larger communal experience among Black Americans. How then has communalism been used in mental health care with Black Americans that extends beyond the boundaries of spirituality and religion?

In the applied literature, communalism has been viewed as shared responsibility for community and "holistic systems of support." Furthermore, communalism has been identified as a "critical cultural asset among African American youth" (Woods-Jager, Briggs, Gaylord-Harden, Cho, & Lemon, 2021, p. 331). Research suggests that for Black Americans, communalism is associated with a range of positive health-related outcomes, including increased resilience, violence reduction, and subjective well-being (Constantine, Alleyne, Wallace, & Franklin-Jackson, 2006; Grayman-Simpson & Mattis, 2017; Wallace et al., 2018). Wilson and Williams (2013) utilize the Southern African concept of Ubuntu – the notion that our humanness is bound with the humanity of others – as a way of explicating the benefits of communalism for Black Americans. In doing so, they identify five core Black American values, namely humanness, caring, sharing, respect, and compassion as stemming from the cultural tradition of Ubuntu and connect these to aspects of mental health including connectedness, social competency, and social consciousness.

Given that communalism is a core component of African values, and given the heterogeneity that exists among Black Americans in regard to affinity with cultural values and salience of racial identity, it might be helpful for the clinician to undertake an assessment of cultural values as part of the initial intake procedure. Lateef, Gale, Parker, and Frempong (2024) provide a review of psychometrically sound Afrocentric instruments which have both research and practical utility. Measures such as the Africentrism Scale, the Africentric Home Environment Inventory, and the Asante-Based Afrocentricty Scale could serve as useful assessment devices and provide an entry point for discussion of the role of cultural values such as communalism in the lives of Black Americans. Finally, a gender-specific intervention that has implications for both communalism and racial socialization is Rites of Passage (ROP), a range of programming which centers African cultural values in socialization programming for Black make adolescents. Miller and McDaniel (2021) describe ROP as incorporating three primary foci: (1) sense of history, (2) sense of community, and (3) sense of Supreme Being. Programming through ROP is designed to address the following areas: honoring the ancestors (pouring libations); understanding the role of elders (permission from the elders); redefining manhood from an African-centered lens; African/African American history and culture; study skills; understanding racism/White supremacy; discovering and practicing family rituals and traditions; visiting significant African American historical sites; and economic development (money, banking, and finances/entrepreneurship). Research indicates that ROP programming for Black adolescent boys may enhance community engagement, build responsible citizenship, and improve self-perception through the development of positive masculine identity (Kingsman, 2021). Communalism as evidenced in well-being interventions for Black adolescent girls includes adapted rites of passage programming focused on educational and cultural enhancement with evidence suggesting efficacy and noting improvements in self-esteem and racial socialization scores post-programming (Williams-Butler et al., 2024).

Racial Socialization and Mental Health

In Chapter 4, we define racial socialization as "teachings about race relations and protection against racism, as well as the process of learning about how to function as a member of the Black cultural group." Although the literature suggests that racial socialization is primarily a family level variable (Umaña-Taylor & Hill, 2020), there is evidence to suggest that racial socialization can take place in non-family related contexts as well, for example schools (Byrd & Lagette, 2022). The value of racial socialization as a strength is attached to the phenomenon of race-based socialization practices. These include an accurate understanding of the history of one's racial group, the instillation of a sense of pride in one's race, and the understanding of racial discrimination and strategies to manage race in society (e.g., the talk; Anderson et al., 2023).

The denigration and oppression of Black Americans has been most vividly captured by the Transatlantic Slave trade; however, perceptions of the African as uncivilized, savage, and heathen pre-dated the slave trade and to some degree provide an ideological rationale for treating enslaved Africans as less than human (Asante, 2001; Carter & Pieterse, 2005). Indeed, even social problems that Black Americans have experienced have historically been given a biological or genetic explanation. As Oliver (1989) writes:

> Advocates of the genetic inferiority perspective argue that the high rates of social problems among Blacks is a product or expression of Black peoples' innate inferiority to Caucasians and other racial groups. Moreover, advocates of this perspective argue that Blacks possess genetic traits and characteristics that predispose them to engage in problematic behavior at higher rates than Whites.
>
> (p. 15)

Generational effects of subjugation have been noted to have a psychological impact, one being an internalization of the ideology of inferiority where the oppressed accepts the deficit-oriented narrative that has been constructed by the oppressor. Racial socialization as a cultural strength therefore has many benefits – the core benefit being allowing for a resistance of the deficit perspective and in its place facilitating a sense of pride, acceptance, and joy in one's racial group and associated cultural characteristics.

Indeed, there is a substantial body of psychological literature that articulates Black racial socialization as a cultural strength. To illustrate, Grills and colleagues (2016) examined the relationship between cultural orientation, Africentric values, and racial socialization in a large sample of African American adolescents and found a positive relationship between racial socialization/ adherence to African-centered cultural values and positive youth development operationalized as being future-oriented, exhibiting prosocial behavior, being committed to political/community, and having social justice/equality civic mindedness. Furthermore, Wang and colleagues (2020), employing meta-analysis, indicated that racial socialization is associated with less externalizing problems, improved self-perception, greater interpersonal relationship quality, improved academic performance, and higher levels of motivation and engagement (Wang et al., 2020b). It appears therefore that racial socialization acts as a strength by restoring a positive perception, raising critical consciousness associated with how racism functions in society, and therefore allows one to externalize sources of distress as opposed to internalize perceptions of inferiority or damage.

Clinical Applications of Racial Socialization

> Ethnic Racial Socialization (ERS) has the potential to be an innovative and important practice to incorporate into the mental health field. Given the currently mixed findings regarding some dimensions of ERS, however, we suggest that cultural socialization or those messages emphasizing cultural and racial pride be the primary dimension explored for psychotherapy use because the majority of the studies have found support for those messages being associated with positive mental health outcomes. In addition, it should be noted that although the cultural socialization dimension appears to be the most positive, the dimensions of preparation for bias and promotion of mistrust should not be dismissed as being related only to negative outcomes. It is possible that having conversations about ways to cope with discrimination and ways to mistrust certain situations for safety is not only adaptive but also protective for African American families living in highly racially charged environments.
>
> (Reynolds & Gonzalez-Backen, 2017, p. 198)

The above summary statement drawn from a meta-analytic examination of the impact of racial socialization in the psychotherapy process provides a clear articulation of the manner in which racial socialization functions as a strength in counseling and psychotherapy. Cultural and racial pride facilitate positive mental health outcomes and also serve as a type of protection against the harmful psychological consequences of racism. Additionally, research indicates that racial socialization might also promote resilience in the face of racial discrimination and oppression (Neblett, Terzian, & Harriott, 2010; Jones et al., 2021).

To provide further evidence of the clinical efficacy of racial socialization, there are now a number of evidence-based approaches that incorporate racial socialization as a central aspect of treatment. Metzger, Anderson, Are, and Ritchwood (2021) describe the integration of racial socialization in cognitive behavioral therapy (CBT) and provide findings suggesting that racial socialization-based CBT results in improved outcomes for adolescents reporting racial trauma symptoms. Anderson et al. (2019) present a manualized treatment approach for facilitating a reduction in racial stress and improvements in coping entitled Engaging, Managing and Bonding through race (EMBrace), which incorporates the Racial Encounter Coping Appraisal and Socialization Theory (RECAST). The centrality of racial socialization in EMBrace is clearly seen in the content focus and projected outcome for each session. To illustrate, the content focus for Session 1 is cultural pride and the deliverable is affection; the content focus for Session 2 is preparation for bias and the deliverable is protection; the content focus for Session 3 is promotion of distrust and the deliverable is correction; the content focus for Session 4 is egalitarianism and the deliverable is connection; and the content focus for Session 5 is applied skills for effective racial encounter coping (Anderson et al., 2019).

Racial Identity and Mental Health

Racial identity, the psychological relationship one has with one's racial group membership, has been posited to have a positive effect on psychological functioning among Black populations. Recognizing that racial identity is a fluid and contextually driven psychological state, mature racial identity statuses are viewed as serving a protective function in the face of racism or some other threat to self-concept based on racial group membership. Additionally positive racial identity has been associated with such factors as greater sense of mastery, greater self-esteem, fewer depressive and anxiety symptoms, and lower rates of substance abuse (Blassingame et al., 2023; Hughes, Keith, & Demo, 2015; Zapolski et al., 2019).

Research indicates that Black Americans tend of feel positively about their racial group and report higher levels of self-esteem (Twenge & Crocker, 2002). Additionally, racial identity differentially predicts psychological functioning with mature aspects of racial identity (i.e., being able to accept one's own racial group and recognize the value of others) in contrast to immature aspects of racial identity (i.e., negative self-group related concepts and race-related confusion) being associated with greater psychological well-being (Pierre & Mahalik, 2005; McClain et al., 2016). Relatedly, the perception that your racial group is viewed positively is also associated with improved health outcomes (Zapolski, Beutlich, Fisher, & Barnes-Najor, 2019), and stronger group identification has been noted to be associated with more positive feelings about one's racial group, more meaning attached to living, and provides a protective function against suicide (Blassingame et al., 2023).

As a set of cognitive schemas/assumptions and an accompanying set of affective/emotional responses, racial identity is understood as a strength across a range of dimensions. Identity statuses that are affirming and accepting of oneself and one's racial group can facilitate increased coping when faced with racial incidents or racism, and allow an individual to accurately externalize the source of stress. Additionally, given the psychological benefits associated with collective esteem and collective identity (i.e., positive aspects of the self associated with one's affiliation with a larger community of individuals bound by ethnic heritage or racial group membership), positive racial identification might provide a psychological buffer against race-related stress. Indeed, strongly identifying as Black has been noted to be associated with greater well-being and fewer depressive symptoms (Hughes et al., 2015; Lewis et al., 2018). It could be that racial identity is an extension of communally held cultural patterns that existed before enslavement, and which was further forged as a function of enslavement. "African traditional values would refer to those social ideals that pertain to and are indigenous to African people" (p. 208) and have been identified as a sense of community; respect for and authority of elders; sense of time; and intercommunal relations (Columbus, 2014). Therefore, from an African perspective, citizenship is not a function of blind patriotism; however, it is noted to be relational concept designed to strengthen a cultural community (Vickery, 2016).

Clinical Applications of Racial Identity

It is now widely accepted that racial identity both influences Black Americans' perceptions of racism and racial discrimination and can serve as a buffer against psychological injury associated with racial discrimination (Yip, 2021). There is also evidence to suggest that negative or less mature aspects of racial identity exacerbate psychological symptoms associated with racial discrimination (Seaton & Iida, 2019). Finally, research also indicates that racial identity can have an impact on coping strategies when faced with racism. Lewis et al. (2020) provide evidence suggesting that mature racial identity statuses are associated with active coping strategies among Black and Latinx college undergraduate students while immature racial identity statuses were associated with avoidance coping strategies among Asian college students. Given these findings, clinical interventions that focus on developing mature and positive racial identity attitudes among Black Americans have been the focus in the research and clinical literature.

We have noted that racial identity inherently notates heterogeneity among Black Americans, with different racial identity statuses associated with varying psychological constructs (Carter, 1995). As such, strategies to invite discussion about racial identity are considered critical to the facilitation and development of positive racial identity. Barnes, Williams, and Barnes (2014) have described a card sort technique in facilitating clients' reactions to their own racial identity salience. By providing questions associated with multiple aspects of identity (e.g. age, religion, sexual identity, and racial identity), clients are asked to sort the cards according to levels of importance or salience. Guiding questions that accompany this task include "how important is your race to you as a person?"; "What behaviors do you believe people in your racial group share?"; "What things about your racial group are you most appreciative of and what do you abhor." This type of inquiry allows the clinician to enter into a dialogue with a client about a perception and feeling about their racial identity and thereby make an assessment of their racial identity status. Pieterse and Miller (2009) recommend the utilization of racial identity measurement scales as another approach for discussing and introducing racial identity related material to the client. Models of teaching racial identity development in the context of counselor training might also have applicability to psycho-educational practices within counseling and psychotherapy. Utsey, Gernat, and Bolden (2003) review various didactic and experiential approaches to facilitating awareness of oneself as a racial being, the function of racism in society, and building a healthy sense of self in regard to one's racial group membership. Challenger, Duquette, and Pascascio (2020) describe a psychoeducational group in which racial identity is taught through group process and sharing of information. The foci of the psychoeducational racial identity group include making positive choices, speaking one's truth, and developing personal worth.

As with most psychotherapeutic endeavors, the more a clinician knows about the client, the more effective the intervention can be through the conveying of empathic understanding and validation of experience. When working with Black American clients, an exploration of racial identity could be received as an indication of the clinician's willingness to understand the client in their totality, and provide the client permission to speak on subjects that are often met with judgment, shame, and guilt.

Racism-Related Coping and Mental Health

Although the empirical literature has now provided ample evidence of the detrimental impact of racism on the psychological and physical health of Black Americans (Black, Johnson, & VanHoose, 2015; LaFave et al., 2022; Pieterse, Todd, Neville, & Carter, 2012; Pollock, 2021; Williams & Williams-Morris, 2000), experientially Black Americans have understood the relationship between racism and health for centuries (Escott, 1979). An account of enslavement by enslaved individuals in the rich literature broadly described as Slave Narratives documents ways in which Black Americans, individuals and communities, coped with, adapted to, and resisted the physical, social and psychological indignities associated with enslavement (Ernest, 2014). As such, the construct of coping and resistance is appreciated as an important part of the mental health experience of Black Americans (Jones et al., 2023). A review of empirical examinations of coping strategies among Black Americans places the strategies in a continuum from dysfunctional to functional. Notably the functional coping strategies include the following: social support (e.g., collective coping, instrumental support), direct action (e.g., problem solving, speaking out and confrontation), identity affirmation (e.g., positive statements, africultural coping, spirituality/religion), and activism (e.g., public resistance and educating others; Jacob et al., 2023).

In the psychological literature, coping is framed as strategies associated with responding to perceived stress (Lazarus & Folkman, 1984). For Black Americans, racism is viewed as a specific type of stressor with Harrell (2000) describing racism-related stress as "the race-related transactions between individuals or groups and their environment that emerge from the dynamics of racism, and that are perceived to tax or exceed existing individual and collective resources or threaten well-being" (p. 44). There is evidence to support the notion that variation in types of coping is associated with variable outcomes regarding psychological distress and well-being. To illustrate, Greer and colleagues have presented evidence suggesting that some forms of culture-specific coping (e.g., ritual-based), or coping strategies that are self-reliant in nature, contribute to greater levels of psychological distress (e.g., interpersonal sensitivity, anxiety symptoms) among Black Americans. Furthermore, the type of racism being encountered also influences the efficacy of coping strategies being employed (Greer & Cavalhieri, 2019; Greer, 2011). Based on a review of the literature,

Jacob et al. (2023) identify the following pattern of racism-related experiences and effective coping strategies: spiritual-centered coping is effective for interpersonal racism; active coping strategies are effective for institutional racism; and collective coping and social support are effective for cultural racism.

Clinical Applications of Racism-Related Coping

The preceding discussion outlining cultural variables as instrumental in sustaining mental health among Black Americans, and therefore of critical importance in the clinical work with this population, captures the elements associated with the application of racism-related coping in clinical work. Jones and colleagues (2023) encourage clinicians to explicitly address coping with racism. Allowing clients to speak about their experiences of racism, assessing the types of coping strategies employed, and creating a "safe, emotionally facilitative space" (p. 275), both strengthens the therapeutic alliance and allows the client to explore the efficacy of their coping strategies without fear of shame or blame. Additionally, armed with an evidence-based understanding of which coping strategies have been found to be more and less effective, clinicians can provide clients with psycho-education on which coping strategies to employ in response to which racism-related experiences. Jones and colleagues highlight the need to take a developmental approach when understanding and exploring racism-related coping strategies. For Black American children, the family becomes the primary source of coping through racial socialization processes, affirmation of racial group, and provision of cohesion and support. Noting that children recognize race at an early age and studies continue to document Black children's preference for White and lighter skin (Gibson et al., 2015), proactive racial socialization provides an opportunity to challenge the internalization of negative stereotypes and lower self-worth based on racial group membership. In adulthood and later adolescence (emerging adulthood), individuals typically have greater levels of autonomy, which allows for a greater range of racism-related coping behaviors including acts of resistance and more active collective engagement in both resistance and the provision of support. The Association of Black Psychologists (ABPsi) has endorsed the formation of emotional emancipation circles as a self-help group-based experience in which Black individuals can process emotions associated with perceived inferiority and the ongoing devaluation of Black Americans (Grills et al., 2016).

It is important to note several empirically supported interventions designed to foster coping and resilience among Black Americans. These include the Bakari project dealing with six areas of self-mastery among young Black men, namely, self-awareness/spirituality, history, relationship, skill development, leadership, community service, and validation (Parham et al., 2015); the Black Parenting Strengths and Strategies (BPSS, Coard et al., 2007) and the EMBrace model previously described (Anderson et al., 2018), which incorporate parental and family-oriented racial socialization strategies; the Promoting Racial Identity Development in Early Education (PRIDE, University of Pittsburgh) focused on the development of positive racial identity through the use of a parent-child curriculum; and Preventing Long-Term Anger and Aggression in Youth (PLAAY, Stevenson, 2003), designed to use athletics and cultural socialization as a way of facilitating coping and anger management with Black American boys.

At the individual level, racism-related coping strategies used more frequently include religion, emotional support, and instrumental support (Brown et al., 2011; Shahid et al., 2018).

For clinicians seeking to support positive coping strategies, it is important to consider the intersection of coping behavior and other cultural variables such as racial identity and racial socialization. Forsyth and Carter (2012) present an investigation examining coping strategies and racial identity statuses among a sample of 233 Black American adults. Notably, empowerment-based strategies (channeling of community/legal-based strategies to hold perpetrators accountable) in combination with mature racial identity statuses, such as Internalization, were associated with the lowest level of psychological symptoms. This is an important reminder that coping with racism reflects a complex integration of internal psychological resources, racial identity statuses, prior exposure to racial socialization, access to social support, opportunities for emotional expression and debriefing, and participation in religious or spiritually based activities. Collectively, these activities facilitate acceptance of and pride in racial group, connection with ones' community and a sense of solidarity, and decreased affective reactivity through validation and recognition of the emotional harm associated with experiences of racism.

References

Anderson, R. E., Ahn, L. H., Brooks, J. R., Charity-Parker, B., Inniss-Thompson, M., Gumudavelly, D., ... & Anyiwo, N. (2023). "The talk" tells the story: A qualitative investigation of parents' racial socialization competency with black adolescents. *Journal of Adolescent Research, 38*(3), 562–588.

Anderson, R. E., McKenny, M. C., & Stevenson, H. C. (2019). EMBR ace: Developing a racial socialization intervention to reduce racial stress and enhance racial coping among Black parents and adolescents. *Family Process, 58*(1), 53–67.

Anderson, R. E., & Stevenson, H. C. (2019). RECASTing racial stress and trauma: Theorizing the healing potential of racial socialization in families. *American Psychologist, 74*(1), 63–75. doi: 10.1037/amp0000392.

Asante, M. K. (2001). The ideology of racial hierarchy and the construction of the European slave trade. *Black Renaissance/Renaissance Noire, 3*(3), 133–148.

Avent, J. R., & Cashwell, C. S. (2015). The Black church: Theology and implications for counseling African Americans. *The Professional Counselor, 5*(1), 81–90.

Barnes, E. F., Williams, J. M., & Barnes, F. R. (2014). Assessing and exploring racial identity development in therapy: Strategies to use with Black consumers. *Journal of Applied Rehabilitation Counseling, 45*(1), 11–17.

Baxter, K., Medlock, M. M., & Griffith, E. E. (2019). Hope, resilience, and African-American spirituality. In M. M. Medlock., D. Shtasel., N. T. Trinh., & D. R. Williams (Eds.) *Racism and Psychiatry: Contemporary Issues and Interventions*, pp. 141–156. Humana Press.

Bell-Tolliver, L., & Wilkerson, P. (2011). The use of spirituality and kinship as contributors to successful therapy outcomes with African American families. *Journal of Religion & Spirituality in Social Work: Social Thought*, *30*(1), 48-70. https://doi.org/10.1080/15426432.2011.542723

Black, L. L., Johnson, R., & VanHoose, L. (2015). The relationship between perceived racism/discrimination and health among Black American women: A review of the literature from 2003 to 2013. *Journal of Racial and Ethnic Health Disparities*, *2*, 11–20.

Blassingame, W.-S., N. N., Au, J., Mekawi, Y., Lewis, C. B., Ferdinand, N. L., Wilson, T. E., Dunn, S. E., & Kaslow, N. J. (2023). Racial identity profiles and indicators of well-being in suicidal African American women. *Journal of African American Studies*, *27*(4), 359–376.doi: 10.1007/s12111-023-09638-1.

Boyd-Franklin, N. (2010). Incorporating spirituality and religion into the treatment of African American clients. *The Counseling Psychologist*, *38*(7), 976–1000. doi: p10.1177/0011000010374881.

Boyd-Franklin, N. (2013). *Black families in therapy: Understanding the African American experience*. New York, NY: Guilford Publications.

Boykin, A. W. (1983). The academic performance of Afro-American children. In J. Spence (Ed.), *Achievement and achievement motives* (pp. 321–371). San Fransisco: Freeman.

Boykin, A. W., Jagers, R. J., Ellison, C. M., & Albury, A. (1997). Communalism: Conceptualization and measurement of an afrocultural social orientation. *Journal of Black Studies*, *27*(3), 409–418.

Brown, T. L., Phillips, C. M., Abdullah, T., Vinson, E., & Robertson, J. (2011). Dispositional versus situational coping: Are the coping strategies African Americans use different for general versus racism-related stressors? *Journal of Black Psychology*, *37*(3), 311–335.

Byrd, C. M., & Legette, K. B. (2022). School ethnic–racial socialization and adolescent ethnic–racial identity. *Cultural Diversity and Ethnic Minority Psychology*, *28*(2), 205–216. doi: 10.1037/cdp0000449.

Carter, R. T. (1995). *The influence of race and racial identity in psychotherapy: Toward a racially inclusive model*. Hoboken, NY: John Wiley & Sons.

Carter, R. T., & Pieterse, A. L. (2005). Race: A social and psychological analysis of the term and its meaning. In R. T. Carter (Ed.), *Handbook of racial-cultural psychology and counseling, Vol. 1. Theory and research* (pp. 41–63). John Wiley & Sons, Inc.

Challenger, C. D., Duquette, K., & Pascascio, D. (2020). "Black boys: Invisible to visible": A psychoeducational group fostering self-efficacy, empowerment, and sense of belonging for African American boys. *The Journal for Specialists in Group Work*, *45*(3), 257–271.

Coard, S. I., Foy-Watson, S., Zimmer, C., & Wallace, A. (2007). Considering culturally relevant parenting practices in intervention development and adaptation: A randomized controlled trial of the Black Parenting Strengths and Strategies (BPSS) Program. *The Counseling Psychologist*, *35*, 797–820.

Columbus, O. (2014). African cultural values and inter-communal relations: The case with Nigeria. *Developing Country Studies*, *4*(24), 208–217.

Constantine, M. G., Alleyne, V. L., Wallace, B. C., & Franklin-Jackson, D. C. (2006). Africentric cultural values: Their relation to positive mental health in African American adolescent girls. *The Journal of Black Psychology, 32*(2), 141–154. doi: 10.1177/0095798406286801.

Cooper-Patrick, L., Gallo, J. J., Powe, N. R., Steinwachs, D. M., Eaton, W. W., & Ford, D. E. (1999). Mental health service utilization by African Americans and Whites: The Baltimore epidemiologic catchment area follow-up. *Medical Care, 37*(10), 1034–1045.

Cuevas, A. G., O'Brien, K., & Saha, S. (2016). African American experiences in healthcare: "I always feel like I'm getting skipped over". *Health Psychology, 35*(9), 987–995.

Curry, M. C. (2020). *Making the gods in New York: The Yoruba religion in the African American community*. London: Routledge.

Dodson, H. (2002) *Jubilee: The emergence of African-American Culture*. Washington. D.C.: National Geographic.

Ernest, J. (Ed.). (2014). *The Oxford handbook of the African American slave narrative*. Oxford: Oxford University Press.

Escott, P. D. (1979). *Slavery remembered: A record of twentieth-century slave narratives*. UNC Press Books.

Forsyth, J., & Carter, R. T. (2012). The relationship between racial identity status attitudes, racism-related coping, and mental health among Black Americans. *Cultural Diversity & Ethnic Minority Psychology, 18*(2), 128–140. https://doi.org/10.1037/a0027660

Gibson, B., Robbins, E., & Rochat, P. (2015). White bias in 3–7-year-old children across cultures. *Journal of Cognition and Culture, 15*(3–4), 344–373.

Grayman-Simpson, N., & Mattis, J. S. (2017). Communalism Scale 2015 cultural validity study. *Journal of Pan African Studies, 10*(3), 163–172.

Greer, T. M. (2011). Coping strategies as moderators of the relation between individual race-related stress and mental health symptoms for African American women. *Psychology of Women Quarterly, 35*(2), 215–226.

Greer, T. M., & Cavalhieri, K. E. (2019). The role of coping strategies in understanding the effects of institutional racism on mental health outcomes for African American men. *Journal of Black Psychology, 45*(5), 405–433. doi: 10.1177/0095798419868105.

Grills, C. N., Aird, E. G., & Rowe, D. (2016). Breathe, baby, breathe: Clearing the way for the emotional emancipation of Black people. *Cultural Studies? Critical Methodologies, 16*, 333–343. doi: 10.1177/1532708616634839.

Grills, C., Cooke, D., Douglas, J., Subica, A., Villanueva, S., & Hudson, B. (2016). Culture, racial socialization, and positive African American youth development. *Journal of Black Psychology, 42*(4), 343–373.

Haeny, A. M., Holmes, S. C., & Williams, M. T. (2021). Applying anti-racism to clinical care and research. *JAMA Psychiatry, 78*(11), 1187–1188.

Harrell, S. P. (2000). A multidimensional conceptualization of racism-related stress: Implications for the well-being of people of color. *American Journal of Orthopsychiatry, 70*(1), 42–57. https://doi.org/10.1037/h0087722

Hayward, R. D., & Krause, N. (2015). Religion and strategies for coping with racial discrimination among African Americans and Caribbean Blacks. *International Journal of Stress Management, 22*(1), 70–91. doi: 10.1037/a0038637.

Hodge, D. R. (2004). Spirituality and people with mental illness: Developing spiritual competency in assessment and intervention. *Families in Society, 85*(1), 36–44. doi: 10.1606/1044-3894.257.

Hughes, Kiecolt, K. J., Keith, V. M., & Demo, D. H. (2015). Racial identity and well-being among African Americans. *Social Psychology Quarterly, 78*(1), 25–48. doi: 10.1177/0190272514554043.

Jacob, G., Faber, S. C., Faber, N., Bartlett, A., Ouimet, A. J., & Williams, M. T. (2023). A Systematic Review of Black People Coping With Racism: Approaches, Analysis, and Empowerment. *Perspectives on Psychological Science, 18*(2), 392–415. https://doi.org/10.1177/17456916221100509

Jones, J. M. (2004). TRIOS: A model for coping with the universal context of racism. In G. Philogène (Ed.), *Racial identity in context: The legacy of Kenneth B. Clark* (pp. 161–190). Washington DC: American Psychological Association. doi: 10.1037/10812-010.

Jones, S. C., Simon, C. B., Yadeta, K., Patterson, A., & Anderson, R. E. (2023). When resilience is not enough: Imagining novel approaches to supporting Black youth navigating racism. *Development and psychopathology, 35*(5), 2132–2140. doi:10.1017/S0954579423000986

Jones, S. C., Anderson, R. E., & Metzger, I. W. (2020). "Standing in the gap": The continued importance of culturally competent therapeutic interventions for black youth. *Evidence-Based Practice in Child and Adolescent Mental Health, 5*(3), 327–339. doi: 10.1080/23794925.2020.1796546.

Jones, S. C., Anderson, R. E., & Stevenson, H. C. (2021). Not the same old song and dance: Viewing racial socialization through a family systems lens to resist racial trauma. *Adversity and Resilience Science, 2,* 225–233.

Kerney, M. A., Hargons, C. N., Peterson, R., Cannon, B., Stevens-Watkins, D., Burnett, C., & Higgins-Hord, L. (2024). "The State of Your Psyche": Black Conceptualizations of Mental Health. The Counseling Psychologist, 52(4), 522-550. https://doi.org/10.1177/00110000241230556

Kingsman, J. (2021). Rites of passage programs for adolescent boys in schools: A scoping review. *Boyhood Studies, 14*(2), 90–115.

LaFave, S. E., Suen, J. J., Seau, Q., Bergman, A., Fisher, M. C., Thorpe Jr, R. J., & Szanton, S. L. (2022). Racism and older Black Americans' health: A systematic review. *Journal of Urban Health, 99*(1), 28–54.

Lateef, H., Gale, A., Parker, M., & Frempong, M. K. (2024). Measuring Afrocentrism: A review of existing instruments. *Social Work Research, 48*(1), 50–60. doi: 10.1093/swr/svad023.

Lateef, H., Nartey, P. B., Amoako, E. O., & Lateef, J. S. (2022). A systematic review of African-centered therapeutic interventions with Black American adults. *Clinical Social Work Journal, 50,* 256–264.

Lazarus, R. S., & Folkman, S. (1984). *Stress, appraisal, and coping.* New York, NY: Springer.

Lewis, J. A., Cameron, R. P., Kim-Ju, G. M., & Meyers, L. S. (2020). Examining the association between racial identity attitudes and coping with racism-related stress. *Journal of Multicultural Counseling and Development, 48*(2), 108–119. DOI: 10.1002/jmcd.12169

Lewis, F. B., Boutrin, M. C., Dalrymple, L., & McNeill, L. H. (2018). The influence of Black identity on wellbeing and health behaviors. *Journal of Racial and Ethnic Health Disparities, 5,* 671–681.

Mattis, J. S., & Grayman-Simpson, N. A. (2013). Faith and the sacred in African American life. In K. I. Pargament, J. J. Exline, & J. W. Jones (Eds.), *APA handbook of psychology, religion, and spirituality (Vol. 1): Context, theory, and research* (pp. 547–564). American Psychological Association. https://doi.org/10.1037/14045-030

Mbiti, J. S. (1990). *African religions and philosophy* (2nd ed.). Portsmouth, NH: Heinemann.

McClain, Beasley, S. T., Jones, B., Awosogba, O., Jackson, S., & Cokley, K. (2016). An examination of the impact of racial and ethnic identity, impostor feelings, and minority status stress on the mental health of Black college students. *Journal of Multicultural Counseling and Development, 44*(2), 101–117. doi: 10.1002/jmcd.12040.

Metzger, I. W., Anderson, R. E., Are, F., & Ritchwood, T. (2021). Healing interpersonal and racial trauma: Integrating racial socialization into trauma-focused cognitive behavioral therapy for African American youth. *Child Maltreatment, 26*(1), 17–27.

Miller, D., & McDaniel, D. (2021). Trauma and education among young Black males: Exploring African-centered rites of passage programming as a protective factor. In *Trauma and Mental Health Social Work With Urban Populations* (pp. 155–165). London: Routledge.

Myers, J. E., Sweeney, T. J., & Witmer, J. M. (2000). The wheel of wellness counseling for wellness: A holistic model for treatment planning. *Journal of Counseling and Development, 78*(3), 251–266. doi: 10.1002/j.1556-6676.2000.tb01906.x.

Neblett Jr, E. W., Terzian, M., & Harriott, V. (2010). From racial discrimination to substance use: The buffering effects of racial socialization. *Child Development Perspectives, 4*(2), 131–137.

Oliver, W. (1989). Black males and social problems: Prevention through Afrocentric socialization. *Journal of Black Studies, 20*(1), 15–39.

Parham, T. A., & Parham, W. D. (2002). Understanding African American mental health: The necessity of new conceptual paradigms. In T. A. Parham (Ed.), *Counseling persons of African descent: Raising the bar of practitioner competence* (pp. 25–37). Thousand Oaks, CA: Sage Publications, Inc. doi: 10.4135/9781452229119.n3.

Parham, T. A., White, J. L., & Ajamu, A. (2015). *Psychology of Blacks: Centering our perspectives in the African consciousness.* Boston, MA: Prentice Hall.

Pierre, M. R., & Mahalik, J. R. (2005). Examining African self-consciousness and Black racial identity as predictors of Black men's psychological well-being. *Cultural Diversity & Ethnic Minority Psychology, 11*(1), 28–40. doi: 10.1037/1099-9809.11.1.28.

Pieterse, A. L., Miller, M. J. (2009). Current considerations in the assessment of adults: A review and extension of culturally inclusive models. In J. Ponterotto, L. A. Suzuki, C. Alexander, & J. M. Cases (Eds.). *Handbook of multicultural counseling* (3rd ed.) (pp. 649–666). Thousand Oaks, CA: Sage Publications.

Pieterse, A. L., Todd, N. R., Neville, H. A., & Carter, R. T. (2012). Perceived racism and mental health among Black American adults: A meta-analytic review. *Journal of Counseling Psychology, 59*(1), 1–9. doi: 10.1037/a0026208.

Planey, A. M., Smith, S. M., Moore, S., & Walker, T. D. (2019). Barriers and facilitators to mental health help-seeking among African American youth and their families: A systematic review study. *Children and Youth Services Review, 101*, 190–200. https://doi.org/10.1016/j.childyouth.2019.04.001

Queener, J. E., & Martin, J. K. (2001). Providing Culturally Relevant Mental Health Services: Collaboration between Psychology and the African American Church. *Journal of Black Psychology, 27*(1), 112–122. https://doi.org/10.1177/0095798401027001007

Pollock, A. (2021). *Sickening: Anti-Black racism and health disparities in the United States*. Minneapolis: University of Minnesota Press.

Rowland, M. L., & Isaac-Savage, E. P. (2014). The Black church: Promoting health, fighting disparities. *New Directions for Adult and Continuing Education, 2014*(142), 15–24.

Seaton, E. K., & Iida, M. (2019). Racial discrimination and racial identity: Daily moderation among Black youth. *American Psychologist, 74*(1), 117–127. doi: 10.1037/amp0000367.

Shahid, N. N., Nelson, T., & Cardemil, E. V. (2018). Lift every voice: Exploring the stressors and coping mechanisms of Black college women attending predominantly White institutions. *Journal of Black Psychology, 44*(1), 3–24.

Snowden, L. R. (1999). African American service use for mental health problems. *Journal of Community Psychology, 27*(3), 303–313.

Stephen, S. (2023). Congruent functioning: the continuing resonance of Rogers' theory. *Person-Centered & Experiential Psychotherapies, 22*(4), 397–416. https://doi.org/10.1080/14779757.2022.2164334

Stephens, M. L., Carter-Francique, A. R., & McClain, T. J. (2020). The Black church, an agency for learning, informal religious adult education, and human capital development: A qualitative inquiry into rural African American primary caregiving grandmothers' experiences. *New Horizons in Adult Education and Human Resource Development, 32*(4), 37–49.

Stevenson, H. C. (Ed.). (2003). *Playing with anger: Teaching coping skills to African American boys through athletics and culture*. Westport, CT: Greenwood Publishing Group.

Stoute, B. J. (2020). Racism: A challenge for the therapeutic dyad. *American Journal of Psychotherapy, 73*(3), 69–71. doi: 10.1176/appi.psychotherapy.20200043.

Torres, A. (2023). The history of ethnic minority psychological associations in the United States. *North American Journal of Psychology, 25* (1), 87–98.

Turner, N., Hastings, J. F., & Neighbors, H. W. (2019). Mental health care treatment seeking among African Americans and Caribbean Blacks: What is the role of religiosity/spirituality? *Aging & mental health, 23*(7), 905–911. doi: 10.1080/13607863.2018.1453484.

Turner, E. A., Malone, C. M., & Douglas, C. (2019). Barriers to mental health treatment for African Americans: Applying a model of treatment initiation to reduce disparities. In M. T. Williams, D. C. Rosen, & J. W. Kanter (Eds.), *Eliminating race-based mental health disparities: Promoting equity and culturally responsive care across settings* (pp. 27–42). Oakland, CA: Context Press/New Harbinger Publications.

Twenge, J. M., & Crocker, J. (2002). Race and self-esteem: Meta-analyses comparing Whites, Blacks, Hispanics, Asians, and American Indians and comment on Gray-Little and Hafdahl (2000). *Psychological Bulletin, 128*(3), 371–408. doi: 10.1037/0033-2909.128.3.371.

Vickery, A. E. (2016). "I worry about my community": African American women utilizing communal notions of citizenship in the social studies classroom. *International Journal of Multicultural Education, 18*(1), 28–44.

Umaña-Taylor, A. J., & Hill, N. E. (2020). Ethnic–racial socialization in the family: A decade's advance on precursors and outcomes. *Journal of Marriage and Family, 82*(1), 244–271.

University of Pittsburgh School of Education Race and Early Childhood Collaborative. (2016). Positive racial identity development in early education: Understanding PRIDE in Pittsburgh. Pittsburgh: University of Pittsburgh.

Utsey, S. O., Gernat, C. A., & Bolden, M. A. (2003). Teaching racial identity development and racism awareness: Training in professional psychology programs. In M. Bravo., G. Bernal., J. E. Trible., A. K. Burlew., F.T.L. Leong (Eds.) *Handbook of racial & ethnic minority psychology* (pp. 147–166). Thousand Oaks, CA: SAGE Publications, Inc.

Utsey, S. O., Stanard, P., & Hook, J. N. (2008). Understanding the role of cultural factors in relation to suicide among African Americans: Implications for research and practice. In F. T. L. Leong & M. M. Leach (Eds.), *Suicide among racial and ethnic minority groups: Theory, research, and practice* (pp. 57–79). Routledge/Taylor & Francis Group. New York, NY.

Wallace, C. M., McGee, Z. T., Malone-Colon, L., & Boykin, A. W. (2018). The impact of culture-based protective factors on reducing rates of violence among African American adolescent and young adult males. *Journal of Social Issues, 74*(3), 635–651.

Wang, M.-T., Henry, D. A., Smith, L. V., Huguley, J. P., & Guo, J. (2020). Parental ethnic-racial socialization practices and children of color's psychosocial and behavioral adjustment: A systematic review and meta-analysis. *American Psychologist, 75*(1), 1–22. doi: 10.1037/amp0000464.

Wang, M. T., Smith, L. V., Miller-Cotto, D., & Huguley, J. P. (2020b). Parental ethnic-racial socialization and children of color's academic success: A meta-analytic review. *Child Development, 91*(3), e528–e544.

Williams-Butler, A., Dorsey, M., Lateef, H., Howard, T., Amoako, E. O., & Nortey, P. (2024). Black girl well-being: A scoping review of culturally and gender responsive interventions. *Research on Social Work Practice, 34*(1), 54–69.

Williams, D., & Williams-Morris, R. (2000). Racism and mental health: The African American experience. *Ethnicity & Health, 5*(3–4), 243–268.

Wilson, D., & Williams, V. (2013). Ubuntu: Development and framework of a specific model of positive mental health. *Psychology Journal, 10*(2), 1–21.

Yip, T. (2021, October). Ethnic/Racial Identity and Discrimination: Implications for Adolescent and Young Adult Development. In *68th Annual Meeting*. AACAP. *Journal of the American Academy of Child & Adolescent Psychiatry, 60*(10), S132.

Zapolski, T. C. B., Beutlich, M. R., Fisher, S., & Barnes-Najor, J. (2019). Collective ethnic-racial identity and health outcomes among African American youth: Examination of promotive and protective effects. *Cultural Diversity & Ethnic Minority Psychology, 25*(3), 388–396. doi: 10.1037/cdp0000258.

Chapter 10

Applications of Black American Cultural Strengths in Counseling and Psychotherapy

A Case Illustration

In order to conceptualize the application of Black American cultural strengths, this chapter presents a case example outlining the distinctions between a standard approach to counseling interventions and an approach that is informed by the cultural strengths outlined in the prior chapters. Note, the case vignette reflects material commonly associated with counseling and psychotherapy treatments, and does not reflect an actual clinical case.

The client, TD is a 53-year-old Black American female with two adult children – a 28-year-old daughter and a 25-year old son – both of whom are living in other parts of the country. The client presents to counseling with multiple life stressors. She is currently finalizing a divorce which has been largely free of acrimony. The client and her husband have been separated for many years. The client reports having lost many of her personal belongings after a fire in her apartment two years ago and had to exit from the ground floor unit by climbing through a window. She indicates that she is still recovering both materially and emotionally from that event. The client is currently experiencing what she describes as racial harassment at work and believes her immediate supervisor displays racial bias. At intake she reports a history of depression and anxiety which was treated with medication several years ago, however she is not currently on psychotropic medication. The client works as an administrative assistant in a very large dental practice and reports being the only Black administrative assistant – out of 10 staff. She believes she has been denied promotion opportunities and reports finding a noose drawn on the bathroom wall which was terribly upsetting. She states that gets on well with other staff in general, but often feels like an outsider. Finally, she indicates experiencing some distance with her children which upsets her, however she is trying to "let them go in order for them to live their lives." She also reports feeling isolated, has withdrawn from her circle of friends and also stopped attending her church. She reports some members of her church have reached out to her, however she feels that they are just doing their duty and questions if they are really interested in her.

DOI: 10.4324/9781003083221-11

Typically in counseling and psychotherapy, a case conceptualization is utilized to inform the treatment approach. While this might be a formal document guiding a treatment team or an informal framework utilized by an individual practitioner, the ultimate goal remains the same: to provide a way to understand the client's presenting concerns and to inform how to respond to their needs in an efficacious manner. Case conceptualization is understood to involve

> coming to an understanding about what troubles the patient, including what causes the symptoms and/or distress and what contributes to the patient's vulnerability to struggle in this particular way. Case conceptualization has been described as a working hypothesis about what causes, precipitates, and maintains a person's psychological, interpersonal, and behavioral difficulties.
>
> (Betan & Binder, 2010, p. 143)

From the earliest psychotherapy literature that drew attention to race as an important factor in counseling and psychotherapy, consistent patterns have identified factors that inhibit greater utilization of counseling and psychotherapy among Black American clients. These include a lack of understanding by the therapist of racial factors that impact the client's well-being, and Eurocentric approaches to psychological theory, assessment, practice and research, cultural mistrust, lack of cultural competence, racism in mental health care, and lack of critical consciousness among providers (Carter, 1995; Mays, 1985; Harrison, 1975; Thompson et al., 2004; Priest, 1991; Taylor & Kuo, 2019; Whaley, 2001; Lee & Boykins, 2022). On the other hand, factors that facilitate effective counseling with Black Americans have also received extensive attention in the literature (Cook & Wiley, 2000; Franklin et al., 1993; Grimmet & Locke, 2009; Queener & Martin, 2001); however, they have not been routinely implemented partly due to the lack of integration of race-related and culturally relevant variables for Black Americans in the training and practice of mental health practitioners (Bartholomew et al., 2023; Durrah et al., 2022; Galán et al., 2021; Neville et a;., 2021; Wilcox et al., 2024; Williams, Holmes, Zare, Haeny, & Faber, 2023). Carrol and Jamison (2011) have noted that "African centered psychological theorists are concerned with the development of models that accurately describe the reality of African descended peoples and prescribe culturally relevant solutions to our lived conditions" (p. 53). As such, in conceptualizing the case of TD, we review factors associated with effective counseling and psychotherapy with Black Americans and draw on many of the cultural values that we have identified as strengths. These include: integrating religious and spiritual values and utilizing the Black American church (Boyd-Franklin & Lockwood, 2009: Coombs et al., 2022); attending to within-group variation and not treating Black Americans as a monolithic group (Carter, 1995; Carter 2025; Hypolite, 2020; Kincaid, 1969); integrating Afrocentric values and practices (Lateef et al., 2022; Shannon et al., 2024); drawing on communal experiences to foster connection (Gamby et al., 2021; Boyd-Franklin & Bry, 2012; Grier-Reed et al., 2018); incorporating expressive arts to facilitate expression of racialized events (McGann, 2006; Karcher, 2017); facilitating active racism-related coping, critical consciousness, and resistance (Chioneso et al., 2020; Jacob et al., 2023; Wallace, 2004; Williams et al., 2023; Mosley et al., 2021); and using storytelling and narrative practices as culturally consistent practice (Fabius, 2016; Maree & DuToit, 2011; Vereen et al., 2013; McNeil-Young et al., 2023).

Case Conceptualization

There is literature that addresses the application of a cultural conceptualization to Black American clients. One of the first approaches to incorporating culture in psychotherapy with Black Americans is NTU psychotherapy (Phillips, 1990). NTU, based on the Bantu principle of unity, seeks to integrate the following core principles in the psychotherapy process: "harmony, balance, interconnectedness, authenticity, and cultural awareness" (p. 55). Additionally, understanding that Black Americans might hold a worldview that to varying degrees incorporates/rejects both Eurocentrism and Afrocentrism is important to entering the client's experience. As such, Morris (2001) suggests the following when working with Black American clients: be willing to adopt flexible roles; be sensitive to cultural idiosyncrasies, and be willing to discuss racial differences; include the church and the extended family in the assessment process; use a problem-solving approach that focuses on the client's everyday experiences; and focus not on deficits but on the client's social, emotional, and cultural strengths (p. 570). Recognizing Black Americans, strengths is central to another model of counseling and psychotherapy, this time outlined for use with Black American women. The HERS model (Moore & Madison-Colomore, 2005) highlights the need to focus on history, empowerment, rapport, and spirituality when working with Black American women. In regard to using a cultural strengths approach, the HERS model emphasizes both opportunities for empowerment and utilizing aspects of the Black experience that have proved to be empowering such as the incorporation of spirituality, which as previously noted is a definite cultural strength of the Black American experience (Baxter et al., 2019). In addition to being a source of strength and a coping mechanism, spirituality has also been viewed as having a protective factor, buffering against the psychological harm of racism

The Case of TD – Standard Case Conceptualization

A practitioner engaging the case of TD from a standard counseling and psychotherapy lens would most likely identify the following areas for further enquiry and possibly the focus of psychotherapeutic intervention:

1 Adjustment disorder with mixed anxiety and depression

   a The presence of significant life stressors including the ending of her marriage.
   b The prior history of depression and anxiety.

    c The distance from her children and her growing isolation – e.g., having stopped attending church.

    d The stress she is encountering at work – failure to advance and overt acts of racial discrimination

2 Posttraumatic stress

    a The apartment fire and subsequent loss of personal belongings plus the immediate threat to her life causing her to evacuate the apartment through a bathroom window.

Employing a standard therapeutic approach, the focus of the work would be to attend to the intrapsychic discomfort and pain associated with multiple losses she has experienced and the post traumatic symptoms related to her apartment fire. Given that adjustment disorder is characterized as a sub-clinical disorder, treatment options range from standard cognitive behavioral intervention for stress reduction, relaxation techniques, and improved coping efficacy; engagement of structured self-help tools such as bibliotherapy and psychoeducation for life-skills; use of brief psychodynamic therapy to facilitate insight into thoughts, feelings and reactions to the stressor; and mindfulness and attachment-based compassion therapy, which have all been found to be efficacious to varying degrees (Ben-Itzhak et al., 2012; Collado-Navaro, et al., 2021; O'Donnel, Agathos, Metcalf, Gibson, & Lau, 2019). With regard to TD's experience of posttraumatic stress, suggested psychotherapeutic interventions include cognitive and trauma-focused cognitive behavioral therapy (CBT-T), mindfulness and relaxation techniques, prolonged exposure and eye movement desensitization and reprocessing (EMDR), emotional debriefing, self-help materials, supportive counseling, psychoeducation, and psychodynamic therapy. The goal is to reduce intrusive thoughts, increase a sense of safety, and manage affective and behavioral re-activation in response to thoughts and memories about the traumatic event (Forneris et al., 2013; Jericho et al., 2022; Lewis et al., 2020)

The Case of TD – Black Cultural Strengths Conceptualization

Engaging the case of TD from a Black cultural strengths perspective allows the therapist greater access to the experience of TD, especially from the perspective of being a Black female living in a racialized and gendered society (Lewis, 2023). Indeed, there is evidence to suggest that the effects of trauma are attenuated by experiences of racial discrimination among Black women (Mekawi et al., 2021). As such, employing a trauma lens to understand TD's experience would include experiences of trauma associated with her belonging to racial and cultural groups that have been historically and generationally marginalized and victimized within American society (Heberle et al., 2020; Williams et al., 2018).

Africentric Psychology and Philosophy. Prior to outlining the case conceptualization from a cultural strengths perspective, a very brief overview of African Psychology/Philosophy is offered within which to locate and center the cultural strengths-based conceptualization. Within this paradigm, spirituality is a fundamental Africentric dimension, which relates to the belief in the relationship between transcendent forces/energies and human life/living. Spirituality is not separated from aspects of life, but it is a philosophical approach to living life with reference to a Supreme Being. Collectivism is an approach to living that values interdependence and cooperation. As such, competition is minimized, harmony is emphasized, interpersonal relationships are viewed as a source of well-being, and one's well-being is interwoven with the well-being of others. Time orientation is cyclical rather than linear and incorporates an emphasis on past, present, and future. There is therefore a fluidity and elasticity with time orientation, and it is not as boundaried as is the Western notion of time. Orality refers to the manner of receiving and transferring knowledge. Orality has a generational component and was utilized in the transmission of knowledge from one generation to the other. Verbal communication is seen as the preferred mode. Maat is a dynamic principle that guides understanding of balance and harmony and is driven by seven cardinal virtues or assets: truth, justice, propriety, compassion, balance, reciprocity, and order (Belgrave & Allison, 2018; Kalonji, 2014) Research evidence suggests that for Black Americans engaging an Afriocentric worldview facilitates personal and collective thriving and the experience of more positive emotions (Parker et al., 2024)

Cultural Strengths-Based Conceptualization. Given the core experience of connectivity and community with the Black experience, understanding the psychological distress that TD is reporting from the perspective of connectivity and community is critical. Recall that the Black cultural strengths we have outlined all hinge on the experience of and sense of connection with the larger cultural group, be it racial identity, racial socialization, spirituality, communalism, and racism-related coping. A review of TD's case highlights areas of significant disconnection from family (children and husband), in her work setting where she is ostracized and marginalized and experiences racial harassment, a withdrawal from her church community resulting in both spiritual and communal disconnection, and a disconnection from self due to the trauma associated with her apartment fire and the threat to her life. The disconnections most likely have engendered feelings of fear and shame, resulting in isolation and withdrawal.

In order to respond to TD's emotional distress and psychological symptoms, the following approach is suggested:

1 Provide a culturally and racially informed trauma case conceptualization that captures the experience of disconnection and being severed from cultural-communal resources. Examine the extent to which TD resonates with the conceptualization. In the process, explore what meaning TD has attached

to the dissolution of her marriage, and the distance she experiences in relation to her children. It is important to keep in mind that for Black families,
kinship often extends to individuals who might not be part of the core nuclear
and extended families and is also found through intergenerational communal
connections. Help TD identify other ways in which she can experience family
and work through any possible impediments such as shame or guilt.

2   Conduct an assessment of racial identity and racial socialization process/
practice to assist her in understanding her racial experience and the manner
in which the racially informed trauma conceptualization provides a useful
explanatory model. Allow TD to outline how she learned about her racial
group membership, themes associated with being a Black woman, stories of
socialization with regard to gender and race, and examine areas of intersectionality (e.g., the client refraining from displaying or expressing any anger
associated with the experience of racial harassment for fear of fulfilling the
stereotype of the Angry Black Woman, a noted gendered racial microaggres-
sion experienced/identified by Black women; Lewis et al., 2016).

3   Allow the therapeutic relationship to facilitate the beginning of the experience
of being connected with another. Note that the role of the therapist in this facilitation is critical and includes within the therapist a recognition and integration
of their own experience as a racial being in a racialized society (i.e., critical
consciousness and racial awareness; Sanchez & Davis, 2010; Shin, 2015).

4   Utilize narrative approaches that allow TD to describe the various life stressors she has and is experiencing centering her words, thoughts, and feelings.
Connect TD's words, thoughts, and feelings to her state of being disconnected from cultural, communal, spiritual, and interpersonal identities. Identify themes of disconnection, individual, cultural, and social isolation, and
trauma informed narratives as you are drawn into TD's story. Identify themes
of strength, improvisation, coping, and creativity that might be lost on the
client as it emerges in her narrative.

5   Facilitate agency through identifying elements of racism-related coping that
TD has employed. Provide psycho-education associated with racism-related
coping, helping TD identify strategies that have been adaptive or maladaptive, and provide experiential awareness through the implementation of active
coping such as helping TD write a letter of complaint to human resources
identifying racial harassment in the workplace.

6   Explore TDs experience of disconnection from her spiritual community,
including a focus on the loss of both external supports (community) and internal calm (sense of congruency) that has resulted from being disconnected
from her spiritual community. Propose accompanying the client back to her
church congregation to facilitate re-entry and engagement.

The focus on Black cultural strengths will lead the therapist to re-examine some
core tenets in counseling and psychotherapy, including the need to take the

counseling out of the consulting room, the nature of dual relationships, and the parameters informing the counseling relationship in regard to the intrapsychic versus contextual emphasis. As Morris (2001) notes, in "traditional mental health settings, professional roles are relatively prescribed," however "given the utilization pattern of African Americans in mental health settings...To meet the client's sociocultural and emotional needs, the service provider may need to be a clinician, adviser, advocate, facilitator, consultant, educator, and social intervener" (p. 570).

Furthermore the focus on Black cultural strengths is consistent with an emerging literature that encourages therapists to consider structures of oppression associated with psychological distress referred to as structural competence (Wilcox et al., 2024), and to approach facilitating well-being through the tenets of liberation which has been described as "a perspective shift from individual to collective well-being and incorporates a consciousness about social injustices, which lays the foundation for individual and institutional transformation" (Neville et al., 2021; p. 1251). Additionally, utilizing a Black cultural strengths approach is also consistent with literature on African-centered therapeutic interventions which notes that African-centered and culturally congruent therapeutic interventions have been found to be associated with positive outcomes in self-concept, cultural identity, and emotion coping skills (Lateef et al., 2022). It could be that the efficacy of African-centered interventions is related to the very principles on which African-centered approaches are built – principles that are consistent with the Black cultural strengths we have outlined including values of community, spirituality, resilience, and orality. In addition, efficacy is also thought to reflect the attention to the impacts of systemic racism, a focus that is absent in standard approaches to counseling and psychotherapy, which deemphasize context and systemic oppression and make the individual intrapsychic process of primary importance (Ingle, 2021).

For TD, the need to navigate the intersection of race and gender has most likely been a central aspect of her life experience, both with and without her awareness. As noted by Jones and colleagues (2020), racism-related stress impacts Black Americans across the lifespan and therefore coping strategies have also been implemented across the lifespan. Focusing on adaptive coping processes that are associated with great health and well-being, Jones et al. document family support, racial socialization, positive racial identity, awareness of racism, and protesting and activism. Working with TD to explicitly outline the coping strategies she has utilized, examining these strategies from an adaptive and maladaptive perspective, and providing psychoeducation on the utility of both individual level (mindfulness, spirituality) and communal level (social support, community engagement, collective resistance) is another approach to outline the cultural strengths that TD might have employed over her lifespan while possibly not identifying it as such. In order to operationalize the application of the cultural strengths within the therapeutic process, a set of questions are offered to inform the practitioner.

Spirituality

A simple and effective spiritual assessment has been offered by Hodge (2004 p. 38), which includes the following questions:

1 I was wondering if you consider spirituality or religion to be a personal strength?
2 In what ways does your spirituality help you cope with the difficulties you encounter?
3 Are there certain spiritual beliefs and practices that you find particularly helpful in dealing with problems?
4 Are there aspects of your spiritual or religious experience that are directly associated with your racial or cultural group?
5 How do your church or spiritual practices provide you a sense of community?
6 What resources exist in your church community that might be helpful to you?
7 What are some spiritual needs that might be helpful for us to focus on in our work together?
8 Would it be helpful for me to speak with members of your spiritual or church community?

In TD's case, it would be important to develop an understanding of her spiritual and religious history in general, as well as her experience with her current church. While exploring ways to help her reconnect to her church community is likely an important intervention, it is also essential to develop an understanding of why it is that she has retreated from her church community in what seems to be a moment of significant emotional upheaval and need. Is her church, a traditionally Black church or is it a mixed-race church? To what extent does the racial make-up of her church influence her recent disconnection? Has she disconnected because it is difficult for her to present as someone who is in need of support? To what extent may her tendency to isolate when she is feeling vulnerable relate to a sense that she needs to adhere to the stereotype of a strong Black (super)woman? To what extent might her tendency to isolate be related instead to aspects of her church community that reflect an instinct toward safety and self-preservation on her part? Understanding this context for her behavior will inform the appropriate intervention, which could range from assisting her in identifying and/or developing her own individualized spiritual practices that she can incorporate into her routine to exploring ways to reconnect with her church community, or finding a new church or spiritual community that is better suited to her needs.

Individual spiritual practices may include a range of activities from reading the bible, listening to scripture or religious music, journaling, engaging in meditation and/or prayer, cathartic activities such as singing or dancing, or even seeking out Black wellness and healing practitioners (e.g., of Reiki, acupuncture, breath work, mindfulness, or meditation) who she can work with one on one or in a group. If she feels that the church is a good fit, appropriate interventions may include: assisting her in exploring the possibility of participating more regularly in church activities such as bible study or other events or ministries; exploring the church as a space where she can connect more deeply with the spirit of her ancestors and community to tap into their collective strength, even if she is not yet ready to connect with individuals in the community; discussing different members of the church who she might approach, such as a pastor or deacon or other congregation members; and exploring and rehearsing ways that she might approach them for support.

Racial Identity

A simple and effective racial identity assessment could include the following questions:

1   I am interested in hearing more about your experience as a Black American and in which ways being Black is important to you.
2   What are your most memorable experiences about what it means to be Black, both positive and negative?
3   What did these experiences communicate to you about race in America?
4   In counseling we refer to how someone thinks and feels about their race as their racial identity. What do you think about when you think of your racial identity?
5   What are some important experiences that have influenced your racial identity?
6   How does your racial identity help you deal with challenges you encounter?
7   Do you see your racial identity as a source of strength?
8   Are there areas in which you would like to grow or change in your racial identity?

In TD's case, it would be essential to get a deeper understanding of which aspects of her racial identity are positive and healthy and in what ways she may have internalized negative ideas about Blackness and herself as a Black woman that could potentially be undermining her ability to function in a way that is healthy and conducive to positive self-esteem and healthy coping. A strong and positive racial identity is the foundation for most of the other Black cultural strengths discussed in this book, including one' ability to establish a supportive community, recognize and cope with racial discrimination, resist the internalization of negative racial messages and stereotypes, and have a sense of self-efficacy in the face of life's challenges.

TD's racial identity will influence her openness to certain types of interventions, the way that she interprets and understands the experiences she has been having at work, as well as which coping strategies will be most effective for her. As such, collecting a thorough history of the evolution of her racial identity over time through her developmental experiences across her lifespan will help her to better understand the lens through which she views the world and her current life experiences and circumstances. It is important to note that racial identity is dynamic and can be influenced by the settings in which one operates, with certain environments making the cognitions, affect, and behaviors associated with certain racial identity statuses more or less salient. If it is determined that TD struggles with maintaining a positive racial identity across the various settings where she operates, intervening to assist TD in developing, shoring up, and/or maintaining a healthy positive racial identity may entail the therapist engaging in a process akin to racial socialization.

Racial Socialization

A simple and effective assessment of racial socialization would include the following inquiries:

1   In counseling, we refer to messages or lessons you have learned about your racial group and how to deal with racism as racial socialization. I would like to discuss your experience of racial socialization.
2   Can you recall some of the earliest memories you have about being a Black person?
3   What messages were communicated to you through these experiences about being Black in America?
4   Who communicated these messages to you – parents, adults, teachers, etc.?
5   How did these lessons/messages leave you feeling about being Black?
6   What have these messages/lessons taught you about how to respond to racism?
7   Please tell me what you learned about the strengths of Black people and the history of Black Americans.
8   How have messages about being Black and Black culture been a positive source in your life?

Depending on her family background and circumstances, and educational context, TD may or may not have had access to the positive racial socialization messages and information about the socioracial historical context necessary to develop a strong, healthy, positive racial identity. Or perhaps, despite her family's best intentions, it is possible and likely that she was exposed to myriad and pervasive sources of negative messages and stereotypes about Black people in American society, which promote a deficit view of Black people and culture. Given the high rates of implicit bias in favor of Whiteness and against Blackness found even among Black people, it is possible that she continues to struggle with internalized racism. As such, it would be important to get a complete sense of the racial/ethnic composition of her family, neighborhood, community, schools, and workplaces, and to understand what racial socialization messages were communicated to her, both explicitly and implicitly, by people in positions of power and influence, by the media, and by things she observed and experienced. It is essential to understand what formative racial experiences she had over the course of her life and how these experiences continue to influence her view of herself and of the Black community.

Depending on the extent to which TD has had positive or negative racial socialization experiences, the therapist's role may entail being a source of corrective healthy racial re-socialization or reinforcement and validation of positive racial socialization. This may include validating the impact of negative experiences and normalizing the internalization of negative bias; critical consciousness raising; educating; unpacking and challenging negative perceptions, biases, or assumptions; and working to enhance a sense of racial pride and connection. An important source of positive racial socialization messages is engagement and participation in communities of like-minded Black people.

Communalism

An inquiry into the client's experience of communalism can be facilitated by the following framing and accompanying questions:

1 In counseling, we understand that people are often connected to larger groups based on many factors including their racial group. I'd like to ask you a few questions to better understand your experiences of being connected to other Black folk.
2 How connected do you feel to other Black people?
3 Do you feel that you are part of a larger Black community?
4 How does this connection help to deal with challenges in your life?
5 What types of challenges are easier to manage because you are part of a larger community?
6 Do you see patterns or cultural ways of doing things in the Black community that you believe are a strength?
7 In what ways do you feel connected to your ancestors?
8 Knowing what your ancestors had to experience coming to America as slaves, how does it impact your experience of either feeling powerful or weak?

Given TD's current level of isolation, as well as the research supporting the centrality of communalism to well-being among Black Americans, helping her to find ways to re/establish a deeper connection to the Black community would likely be beneficial, if not essential to improving her mental health. This could entail establishing and/or enhancing a sense of spiritual connection to ancestors and members of the Black community at large that came before her, as well as seeking out instrumental ways to increase her connection to her living family and kin and other members of the Black community in her day-to-day life. TD could be encouraged to share and explore her family history and perhaps establish practices oriented toward honoring her ancestors. As mentioned previously, this could mean engaging more deeply in church services or activities as a way to connect with the positive intergenerational communal energy of the space. Another way might be preparing a simple ancestor altar or other place in her home where she can collect photographs and items connected to her ancestors or other members of the Black community that inspire a sense of peace and strength, and where she can engage in a practice of quiet meditation or expression of honor and gratitude.

Re/establishing or extending community could entail seeking out Black professional associations or alumni organizations and beginning to participate in associated meetings or gatherings. The therapist could assist her in seeking out healing spaces for Black people and or People of Color. One example is the Association of Black Psychologists' Sawubona Healing Circles, which are virtual supportive, culturally affirming, and safe spaces for people of African descent focused on using culturally grounded healing strategies to help community members deal with racial trauma and stress. The therapist could also assist TD in exploring ways to engage more intentionally with her circle of friends and with her immediate and extended family.

Racism-Related Coping

An exploration of the client's strategies for coping with racism can be facilitated through the following framing and questions:

1 I was wondering if you could describe some experiences of racism that you have had.
2 How do you see racism impact the larger society?
3 How has your life been impacted by racism in the society at large? We refer to this as institutional or cultural racism.
4 In counseling we refer to the ways that Black Americans manage, cope, and resist racism, as racism-related coping. What are ways that you cope with racism?
5 Are there resources in the Black community that have or could help you cope with racism?
6 How does coping with racism impact your self-esteem?
7 What are the ways in which you cope with racism on your own?
8 What are ways in which you cope with racism by being part of the larger Black community?

Since TD is actively dealing with ongoing workplace racial harassment and discrimination, it is essential that the therapist assist her in finding adaptive ways to cope with and manage these experiences. This would include exploring in depth and processing the specific experiences she has had and the people involved, as well as the various factors such as her racial identity that may be influencing her appraisal of the situation and the types of coping strategies she has been using.

Given that research has suggested that finding ways to be active and develop a sense of agency in the face of experiences of racial discrimination are generally associated with better mental health outcomes, it may be helpful to guide TD through a process of researching options that are available to her, and related policies and procedures in her workplace as well as via formal channels such as the Equal Employment Opportunity Commission or the Human Rights Commission in her city or state. She will likely need support in exploring and evaluating the pros and cons of, as well as her willingness to engage in any sort of action against her employer, however small, as engaging in these sorts of actions can be an extremely difficult, daunting, protracted, stressful, and lonely process. An alternative to individual action is collective action which can take the form of finding ways to participate in or support movements such as Black Lives Matter or volunteering in other civic engagement initiatives. Research has also provided support for mindfulness as a means of reducing anxious arousal associated with racial discrimination. As such, assisting TD in developing mindfulness practices may help her to manage anxiety associated with her current experiences as well as help her to experience reduced hypervigilance in future encounters. Finally, encouraging her to seek out and participate in Black, BIPOC, or People of Color mindfulness meditation groups or Sanghas, which are available in-person in many cities or virtually, could provide significant benefits through providing a space for collective healing, while also helping to build community.

Beyond the Talking Cure – Culture as Liberation

Psychotherapy, the hallmark of psychological interventions for distress and healing, has been referred to as the talking cure, an approach to relief of psychological distress that relies primarily on verbal communication (Marx et al., 2017). At this point in time, talk therapy remains the most widely used non-pharmacological treatment in mental health care, irrespective of the availability of a range of therapeutic interventions that utilize the use of movement and touch (Bonitz, 2008 Hayes, 2013; Phelan, 2009), ecosystems, animals (Jones et al., 2019; Wolsko & Hoyt, 2012), and specific spiritual- and religious-based healing practices (Colbert et al., 2009; Hays & Aranda, 2016). Given the scope of practice in mental health care, it is helpful to consider the utility of moving therapeutic interventions for Black Americans outside the traditional "50-minute therapeutic hour" (see Goodman et al., 2013). The application of Black cultural strengths to psychotherapy with Black American clients could be enhanced by the idea of the practitioner taking psychotherapy to the client as opposed to the expectation that the client comes to the practitioner. As such, we would encourage practitioners to think broadly when reflecting on therapeutic approaches to work with Black Americans. For example: utilizing community spaces, or spaces for communal gathering to engage mental health care; re-imagining group therapy as a place for communal healing; allowing for collaboration between the clinician and the client as to the parameters of practice (where will me meet, how long will we meet for, what will the focus of the work be); extending the work beyond intra-psychic aspects of the client's experiences; engaging the client as a collaborator in advocating for their material, psychosocial, and spiritual needs; and utiliz-ing the community as an agent of resistance. All of these approaches allow the practitioner to draw more heavily on Black cultural strengths in the areas of communalism, spirituality, racism-related coping, racial-socialization, and racial identity and are consistent with the hope expressed by Akinyela (2002) when stating "it is my hope that African centered therapy could provide African indi-viduals and families a space to talk about their lives, to make sense of their rela-tionships, free from the interpretations and judgments of dominant Eurocentric culture" (p. 41).

Radical healing has been offered as a framework within which to engage mental health care with Black Americans and as a path to recover from racial trauma (French et al., 2020; Jean et al., 2023). Radical healing encompasses five domains, namely: (a) collectivism, (b) critical consciousness, (c) radical hope, (d) strength and resistance, and (e) cultural authenticity and self-knowledge, and is understood to provide a "culturally relevant heuristic for exploring oppres-sion and liberation among Black queer people" (Mosley et al., 2023, p. 293). It is clear that the elements of cultural strengths that we have addressed in this volume provide a complimentary set of values and skills that can be easily applied within the radical healing framework. The process of reclaiming iden-tity and restoring connection, and aspects of the psychological experience of Black Americans that are directly related to the ongoing experience of racial oppression are approaches that could also facilitate the healing of TD in regard to her loss of status in her community, the loss of connection within her fam-ily, the loss of avenues to express her spirituality, and the inability to cope with racial stressors at her place of work. The practitioner who recognizes the losses not as personal deficits or indeed as evidence of psychopathology but as natu-ral responses to traumatic losses is the type of practitioner that would facilitate a greater utilization of the talking cure for Black Americans. Furthermore, the practitioner who incorporates cultural strengths as part of the radical healing process, who is willing to engage therapeutic services outside of the traditional "50-minute" hour, and who acknowledges their own subjectivities as a racial being, is the practitioner that will facilitate not only greater utilization but also most likely more effective outcomes for Black Americans engaging counseling, psychotherapy, and other aspects of mental health care and treatment.

References

Akinyela, M. (2002). De-colonizing our lives: Divining a post-colonial therapy. *Interna-tional Journal of Narrative Therapy & Community Work, 2002*(2), 32–43.

Bartholomew, T. T., Pérez-Rojas, A. E., Bledman, R., Joy, E. E., & Robbins, K. A. (2023). "How could I not bring it up?": A multiple case study of therapists' comfort when

Black clients discuss anti-Black racism in sessions. *Psychotherapy, 60*(1), 63–75. doi: 10.1037/pst0000404.

Baxter, K., Medlock, M. M., & Griffith, E. E. (2019). Hope, resilience, and African-American spirituality. *Racism and Psychiatry: Contemporary Issues and Interventions*, Oct 4: 141–156.

Belgrave, F. Z., & Allison, K. W. (2018). African *American psychology: From Africa to America*. Los Angels: Sage Publications.

Ben-Itzhak, S., Bluvstein, I., Schreiber, S., Aharonov-Zaig, I., Maor, M., Lipnik, R., & Bloch, M. (2012). The effectiveness of brief versus intermediate duration psychodynamic *psychotherapy* in the treatment of adjustment disorder. *Journal of Contemporary* Psychotherapy, 42, 249–256.

Betan, E. J., & Binder, J. L. (2010). Clinical expertise in psychotherapy: How expert therapists use theory in generating case conceptualizations and interventions. *Journal of Contemporary Psychotherapy, 40*, 141–152.

Bonitz, V. (2008). Use of physical touch in the "talking cure": A journey to the outskirts of psychotherapy. *Psychotherapy: Theory, Research, Practice, Training, 45*(3), 391–404.

Boyd-Franklin, N., & Bry, B. H. (2012). *Reaching out in family therapy: Home-based, school, and community interventions*. New York, NY: Guilford Press.

Boyd-Franklin, N., & Lockwood, T. W. (2009). Spirituality and religion: Implications for psychotherapy with African American families. In F. Walsh (Ed.), *Spiritual resources in family therapy* (2nd ed.) (pp. 141–155). New York, NY: Guilford Press.

Carroll, K. K., & Jamison, D. F. (2011). African-centered psychology, education and the liberation of African minds: Notes on the psycho-cultural justification for reparations. *Race, Gender & Class, 18*(1–2), 52–72.

Carter, R. T. (1995). *The influence of race and racial identity in psychotherapy: Toward a racially inclusive model*. Hoboken, NJ: John Wiley & Sons.

Chioneso, N. A., Hunter, C. D., Gobin, R. L., McNeil Smith, S., Mendenhall, R., & Neville, H. A. (2020). Community healing and resistance through storytelling: A framework to address racial trauma in Africana communities. *Journal of Black Psychology, 46*(2–3), 95–121. https://doi.org/10.1177/0095798420929468

Colbert, L. K., Jefferson, J. L., Gallo, R., & Davis, R. (2009). A study of religiosity and psychological well-being among African Americans: Implications for counseling and psychotherapeutic processes. *Journal of Religion and Health, 48*, 278–289.

Collado-Navarro, C., Navarro-Gil, M., Pérez-Aranda, A., López-del-Hoyo, Y., Garcia-Campayo, J., & Montero-Marin, J. (2021). Effectiveness of mindfulness-based stress reduction and attachment-based compassion therapy for the treatment of depressive, anxious, and adjustment disorders in mental health settings: A randomized controlled trial. *Depression and Anxiety, 38*(11), 1138–1151. https://doi.org/10.1002/da.23198

Coombs, A., Joshua, A., Flowers, M., Wisdom, J., Crayton, L. S. S., Frazier, K., & Hankerson, S. H. (2022). Mental health perspectives among black Americans receiving services from a church-affiliated mental health clinic. *Psychiatric Services, 73*(1), 77–82.

Cook, D. A., & Wiley, C. Y. (2000). Psychotherapy with members of African American Churches and spiritual traditions. In P. S. Richards & A. E. Bergin (Eds.), *Handbook of psychotherapy and religious diversity* (pp. 369–396). American Psychological Association, Washington, D.C. doi: 10.1037/10347-015

Durrah, E., Hall, A. H., & Vajda, A. J. (2022). The Importance of Culturally Responsive and Afrocentric Theoretical Frameworks-A Call for More Inclusive Curriculum in

Counselor Education. In *Developing Anti-Racist Practices in the Helping Professions: Inclusive Theory, Pedagogy, and Application* (pp. 25–44). Cham: Springer International Publishing.

Fabius, C. D. (2016). Toward an integration of narrative identity, generativity, and storytelling in African American elders. *Journal of Black Studies, 47*(5), 423–434. https://doi.org/10.1177/0021934716638801

Forneris, C. A., Gartlehner, G., Brownley, K. A., Gaynes, B. N., Sonis, J., Coker-Schwimmer, E., ... & Lohr, K. N. (2013). Interventions to prevent post-traumatic stress disorder: A systematic review. *American Journal of Preventive Medicine, 44*(6), 635–650.

Franklin, A. J., Carter, R. T., & Grace, C. (1993). An integrative approach to psychotherapy with Black/African Americans: The relevance of race and culture. In G. Stricker & J. Gold (Eds.), *The comprehensive handbook of psychotherapy integration*, (pp. 465–479). New York, NY: Plenum Press.

French, B. H., Lewis, J. A., Mosley, D. V., Adames, H. Y., Chavez-Dueñas, N. Y., Chen, G. A., & Neville, H. A. (2020). Toward a psychological framework of radical healing in communities of color. *The Counseling Psychologist, 48*(1), 14–46.

Galán, C. A., Bekele, B., Boness, C., Bowdring, M., Call, C., Hails, K., ... & Yilmaz, B. (2021). A call to action for an antiracist clinical science. *Journal of Clinical Child & Adolescent Psychology, 50*(1), 12–57.

Gamby, K., Burns, D., & Forristal, K. (2021). Wellness decolonized: The history of wellness and recommendations for the counseling field. *Journal of Mental Health Counseling, 43*(3), 228–245.

Goodman, L. A., Pugach, M., Skolnik, A., & Smith, L. (2013). Poverty and mental health practice: Within and beyond the 50-minute hour. *Journal of Clinical Psychology, 69*(2), 182–190.

Grier-Reed, T., Gagner, N., & Ajayi, A. (2018). Countering a white racial frame at a predominantly white institution. *Journal Committed to Social Change on Race and Ethnicity (JCSCORE), 4*(2), 65–89.

Grimmett, M. A., & Locke, D. C. (2009). Counseling with African Americans. In C. M. Ellis, & J. Carlson (Eds.), *Cross cultural awareness and social justice in counseling* (pp. 121–146). New York: Routledge Taylor & Francis Group.

Handbook of Multicultural Counseling Competencies (2010). Edited by Jennifer A. Erickson Cornish, Barry A. Schreier, Lavita I. Nadkarni, Lynett Henderson Metzger, and Emil R. Rodolfa. Hoboken, NJ: John Wiley & Sons.

Harrison, D. K. (1975). Race as a counselor-client variable in counseling and psychotherapy: A review of the research. *The Counseling Psychologist, 5*(1), 124–133.

Hayes, J. (2013). *Soul and spirit in dance movement psychotherapy: A transpersonal approach*. London, UK: Jessica Kingsley Publishers.

Hays, K., & Aranda, M. P. (2016). Faith-based mental health interventions with African Americans: A review. *Research on Social Work Practice, 26*(7), 777–789.

Heberle, A. E., Obus, E. A., & Gray, S. A. (2020). An intersectional perspective on the intergenerational transmission of trauma and state-perpetrated violence. *Journal of Social Issues, 76*(4), 814–834.

Hodge, D. R. (2004). Spirituality and people with mental illness: Developing spiritual competency in assessment and intervention. *Families in Society, 85*(1), 36–44. https://doi.org/10.1606/1044-3894.257

Hypolite, L. I. (2020). "It just helps to know that there are people who share your experience" exploring racial identity development through a black cultural center. *Journal of Negro Education, 89*(3), 233–248.

Ingle, M. (2021). Western individualism and psychotherapy: Exploring the edges of ecological being. *Journal of Humanistic Psychology, 61*(6), 925–938. doi: 10.1177/0022167818817181.

Jacob, G., Faber, S. C., Faber, N., Bartlett, A., Ouimet, A. J., & Williams, M. T. (2023). A systematic review of black people coping with racism: Approaches, analysis, and empowerment. *Perspectives on Psychological Science, 18*(2), 392–415. https://doi.org/10.1177/17456916221100509

Jean, P. L., Lockett, G. M., Bridges, B., & Mosley, D. V. (2023). Addressing the impact of racial trauma on Black, Indigenous, and People of Color's (BIPOC) mental, emotional, and physical health through critical consciousness and radical healing: Recommendations for mental health providers. *Current Treatment Options in Psychiatry, 10*(4), 372–382. https://doi.org/10.1007/s40501-023-00304-7

Jericho, B., Luo, A., & Berle, D. (2022). Trauma-focused psychotherapies for post-traumatic stress disorder: A systematic review and network meta-analysis. *Acta Psychiatric Scandinavica, 145*(2), 132–155.

Jones, S. C. T., Anderson, R. E., Gaskin-Wasson, A. L., Sawyer, B. A., Applewhite, K., & Metzger, I. W. (2020). From "crib to coffin": Navigating coping from racism-related stress throughout the lifespan of Black Americans. *American Journal of Orthopsychiatry, 90*(2), 267–282. doi: 10.1037/ort0000430.

Jones, M. G., Rice, S. M., & Cotton, S. M. (2019). Incorporating animal-assisted therapy in mental health treatments for adolescents: A systematic review of canine assisted psychotherapy. *PloS One, 14*(1), e0210761.

Kalonji, T. (2014). The Nguzo Saba & Maat, a path for self-reconstruction and recoveredness Exploring a Kawaida paradigm for healing addiction in the Black community. *Journal of Pan African Studies, 7*(4), 195–210.

Karcher, O. P. (2017). Sociopolitical oppression, trauma, and healing: Moving toward a social justice art therapy framework. *Art Therapy, 34*(3), 123–128.

Kincaid, M. (1969). Identity and therapy in the black community. *The Personnel and Guidance Journal, 47*(9), 884–890.

Lateef, H., Nartey, P. B., Amoako, E. O., & Lateef, J. S. (2022). A systematic review of African-centered therapeutic interventions with Black American adults. *Clinical Social Work Journal, 50*(2): 1–9.

Lee, C. C., & Boykins, M. (2022). Racism as a mental health challenge: An antiracist counselling perspective. *Canadian Psychology / Psychologie canadienne, 63*(4), 471–478. doi: 10.1037/cap0000350.

Lewis, C., Roberts, N. P., Andrew, M., Starling, E., & Bisson, J. I. (2020). Psychological therapies for post-traumatic stress disorder in adults: Systematic review and meta-analysis. *European Journal of Psychotraumatology, 11*(1), 1729633.

Lewis, J. A. (2023). Contributions of Black psychology scholars to models of racism and health Applying intersectionality to center Black women. *American Psychologist, 78*(4), 576–588. doi: 10.1037/amp0001141.

Lewis, J. A., Mendenhall, R., Harwood, S. A., & Browne Huntt, M. (2016). "Ain't I a woman?" Perceived gendered racial microaggressions experienced by Black women. *The Counseling Psychologist, 44*(5), 758–780.

Maree, J. G., & Du Toit, C. M. (2011). The role of the oral tradition in counseling people of African ancestry. Ed., E.Mpofu, *Counseling People of African Ancestry*, 22–40. London, U.K.: Cambridge University Press.

Mays, V. M. (1985). The Black American and psychotherapy: The dilemma. *Psychotherapy: Theory, Research, Practice, Training, 22*(2S), 379–388.

Marx, C., Benecke, C., & Gumz, A. (2017). Talking cure models: A framework of analysis. *Frontiers in Psychology, 8*, 1589. https:// doi.org/10.3389/fpsyg.2017.01589

McGann, E. P. (2006). Color me beautiful: Racism, identity formation, and art therapy. *Journal of Emotional Abuse, 6*(2–3), 197–217.

McNeil-Young, V. A., Mosley, D. V., Bellamy, P., Lewis, A., & Hernandez, C. (2023). Storying survival: An approach to radical healing for the Black community. *Journal of Counseling Psychology, 70*(3), 276–292. doi: 10.1037/cou0000635.

Mekawi, Y., Carter, S., Brown, B., Martinez de Andino, A., Fani, N., Michopoulos, V., & Powers, A. (2021). Interpersonal trauma and posttraumatic stress disorder among black women: does racial discrimination matter? *Journal of Trauma & Dissociation, 22*(2), 154–169.

Moore, J. L., & Madison-Colmore, O. (2005). Using the HERS model in counseling African-American women. *Journal of African American Studies, 9*, 39–50.

Morris, E. F. (2001). Clinical practices with African Americans: Juxtaposition of standard clinical practices and Africentricism. *Professional Psychology: Research and Practice, 32*(6), 563–572. doi: 10.1037/0735-7028.32.6.563.

Mosley, D. V., Hargons, C. N., Meiller, C., Angyal, B., Wheeler, P., Davis, C., & Stevens-Watkins, D. (2021). Critical consciousness of anti-Black racism: A practical model to prevent and resist racial trauma. *Journal of Counseling Psychology, 68*(1), 1–16. doi: 10.1037/cou0000430.

Mosley, D. V., McNeil-Young, V., Bridges, B., Adam, S., Colson, A., Crowley, M., & Lee, L. (2021). Toward radical healing: A qualitative metasynthesis exploring oppression and liberation among Black queer people. *Psychology of Sexual Orientation and Gender Diversity, 8*(3), 292–313. doi: 10.1037/sgd0000522.

Neville, H. A., Ruedas-Gracia, N., Lee, B. A., Ogunfemi, N., Maghsoodi, A. H., Mosley, D. V., …, & Fine, M. (2021). The public psychology for liberation training model: A call to transform the discipline. *American Psychologist, 76*(8), 1248–1265. doi: 10.1037/amp0000887.

O'Donnell, M. L., Agathos, J. A., Metcalf, O., Gibson, K., & Lau, W. (2019). Adjustment disorder: Current developments and future directions. *International Journal of Environmental Research and Public Health, 16*(14), 2537.

Parker, J. S., Jackson, T., Haskins, N., Wright, D., & Avent Harris, J. (2025). Young black American's use of afrocentric and black liberation spiritual-based practices to thrive amid racism: A meta-synthesis. *Journal of Cross-Cultural Psychology, 56*(1), 83–104. https://doi.org/10.1177/00220221241292591

Phelan, J. E. (2009). Exploring the use of touch in the psychotherapeutic setting: A phenomenological review. *Psychotherapy: Theory, Research, Practice, Training, 46*(1), 97.

Phillips, F. B. (1990). NTU psychotherapy: An Afrocentric approach. *Journal of Black Psychology, 17*(1), 55–74.

Priest, R. (1991). Racism and prejudice as negative impacts on African American clients in therapy. *Journal of Counseling & Development, 70*(1), 213–215.

Queener, J. E., & Martin, J. K. (2001). Providing culturally relevant mental health services Collaboration between psychology and the African American church. *Journal of Black Psychology, 27*(1), 112–122.

Sanchez, D., & Davis III, Claytie. (2010). Becoming a racially competent therapist. In *Handbook of multicultural counseling competencies* (pp. 267–290).

Shannon, J., Green, D. A., White, D., Beauduy, G. J., Jr., & Rosser, A. (2024). A 50-year content analysis on Black males' experiences in counseling. *Journal of Counseling & Development, 102*(3), 279–291. https://doi.org/10.1002/jcad.12511

Shin, R. Q. (2015). The application of critical consciousness and intersectionallty as tools for decolonizing racial/ethnic identity development models in the fields of counseling and psychology. In R. D. Goodman & P. C. Gorski (Eds.), *Decolonizing "multicultural" counseling through social justice* (pp. 11–22). Springer Science + Business Media. https://doi.org/10.1007/978-1-4939-1283-4_2.

Taylor, R. E., & Kuo, B. C. H. (2019). Black American psychological help-seeking intention: An integrated literature review with recommendations for clinical practice. *Journal of Psychotherapy Integration, 29*(4), 325–337. doi: 10.1037/int0000131.

Thompson, V. L. S., Bazile, A., & Akbar, M. (2004). African Americans' perceptions of psychotherapy and psychotherapists. *Professional Psychology: Research and Practice, 35*(1), 19–26. doi: 10.1037/0735-7028.35.1.19.

Vereen, L. G., Hill, N. R., & Butler, S. K. (2013). The use of humor and storytelling with African American men: Innovative therapeutic strategies for success in counseling. *International Journal for the Advancement of Counselling, 35*, 57–63.

Wallace, B. C. (2005). A practical coping skills approach for racial-cultural skill acquisition. Ed., R.T. Carter, *Handbook of Racial-Cultural Counseling and Psychology: Training and Practice 2*, 97–119. John Wiley & Sons, Inc., Hoboken, New Jersey.

Whaley, A. L. (2001). Cultural mistrust: An important psychological construct for diagnosis and treatment of African Americans. *Professional Psychology: Research and Practice, 32*(6), 555.

Wilcox, M. M., Reid Marks, L., Franks, D. N., Davis, R. P., & Moss, T. (2024). Are training programs addressing anti-Black racism and white supremacy? A descriptive analysis. *The Counseling Psychologist, 52*(1), 124–157.

Williams, M. T., Holmes, S., Zare, M., Haeny, A., & Faber, S. (2023). An evidence-based approach for treating stress and trauma due to racism. *Cognitive and Behavioral Practice, 30*(4), 565–588.

Williams, M. T., Printz, D., Ching, T., & Wetterneck, C. T. (2018). Assessing PTSD in ethnic and racial minorities: Trauma and racial trauma. *Directions in Psychiatry, 38*(3), 179–196.

Wolsko, C., & Hoyt, K. (2012). Employing the restorative capacity of nature: Pathways to practicing ecotherapy among mental health professionals. *Ecopsychology, 4*(1), 10–24.

Chapter 11

Employing Black American Cultural Values

Training Guidelines for Mental Health Professionals

In this chapter, we discuss some issues and guidelines for training and teaching mental health professionals and trainees, so they can effectively use knowledge of Black cultural strengths in practice. We consider the challenges embedded in the educational landscape, both in mental health (i.e., psychology and mental health counseling) and health care (i.e., psychiatry, social work), that would need to be addressed and altered in educational practices and activities that are currently used by those who administer, structure, and train health care and mental health professionals. We also offer some recommendations for those who wish to benefit from employing and incorporating Black American cultural strengths into their teaching and training of mental health professionals.

The mental health profession has begun to alter its identity from mental health-oriented disciplines to that of health care providers, such that licensed professionals trained in mental health and counseling are becoming providers in the larger medical health care system. In the last few decades, there has been greater recognition, by some, that mental health plays a role in physical health as the role of stress, wellness, and disease prevention is seen in a broader framework of health. The new ways of providing mental health care have meant that there are expectations that mental health treatments be evidence-based, and there are also calls for more inclusive and equitable services, which has implications for People of Color in general and Black Americans in particular (Phelps, Bray, & Kearney, 2017; Washburn, 2019).

The shift from mental health to health care as the focus of psychology means that the medical model has more importance in mental health practice and there is more reliance on research evidence typical in medicine, like clinical trials, to demonstrate that treatment approaches are effective. This new trend is problematic in that the medical profession and the applied social sciences (e.g., mental health disciplines) have histories of racism and racial oppression regarding People of Color (see Carter 1995; Washington 2006).

There is little reason to believe that treatment guidelines will include knowledge and skills about racial issues, race-related stress/trauma, or Black cultural strengths. We take this position because racial-cultural considerations have not

DOI: 10.4324/9781003083221-12

been important, despite the rhetoric and aspirational policy statements in the mental health profession. It has been the practice in mental health to assume universal human principles and to not rely on group specific characteristics to guide treatment and interventions (cf, Carter & Pieterse, 2019).

In the same way that mental health professionals have difficulty with race and racism, we suspect that they have trouble with understanding and using Black cultural strengths in treatment with Black clients. The issues arise in several ways. The perspective of the client/patient suggests that s/he would be less likely to discuss his/her cultural pattens and practices with therapists of any racial group. A complication here is that many Black clients may not be aware that they are using or living according to these deeply embedded cultural values. Even if they knew, most would not disclose these details to their therapist. Most mental health professionals are not taught to see or integrate considerations of race and culture into their understanding of human development and functioning.

Most therapists have no training that would aid them in understanding that Black people have cultural strengths, nor would they have been taught to apply such knowledge if they had it. Hemmings and Evans (2018) examined professional counselors' experiences in dealing with race-based stress and trauma in their clinical work. Counselors reported working with clients who had distressing racial experiences, but these counselors had received no training to assess or treat these issues, nor were there any professional policies on race-related or cultural stress/trauma with treatment recommendations. More importantly, the policy, training, and treatment associated with race-related stress/trauma were found to be inversely related to competencies, perhaps indicating that the counselors knew they were ill equipped to deal with racism-related issues in clients (Hemmings & Evans, 2018). Even with the issues and events pertaining to how mental health care is delivered and the policy statements about attending to racial-cultural differences that have challenged mental health professionals, less has been done, as these researchers document, to include consideration of the effects of culture and racism. It remains true that most training occurs in settings where Whiteness is paramount, and learning is focused on theories of human personality and development that are presumed to be universal.

The context for our discussion is the current state of mental health training programs, which McCubbin et al. (2023) argue are grounded in White supremacy. They contend that higher education in North America is constructed and dominated by Whiteness and White supremacy. These authors offer tools and resources to help dismantle the systems and organizations that operate according to Whiteness. We suspect that professionals and trainees would need to employ the resources and tools provided in this paper to be able to connect with Black clients, such that they can recognize and effectively use their cultural strengths. Their article was written

to bring into focus the forces of sabotage that so commonly stifle well-intentioned deep structural changes within psychology [or health care].

While acknowledging this dynamic and identifying the role of Whiteness, we encourage developmental change and (...) decolonization that can be heard and authentically sustained across psychology training programs.

(p. 15)

Several recent developments should be noted before we consider their arguments. It is not often that institutions and organizations take responsibility for their past and current actions. It seemed that the 2020 murder of George Floyd sparked recognition of racism and how deeply embedded it was and continues to be in our society. This moved some organizations to address their roles in promoting and sustaining racism. For instance, in 2021, the American Pychological Association issued an apology to People of Color for not pushing back against societal racism and for taking part in systemic inequalities. The statement also claimed that the organization would seek to move toward equity. Yet, the Association of Black Psychologists rejected much of the apology stating that it was vague and non-specific about what would actually be done to combat racism.

McCubbin and colleagues (2023) state that Whiteness permeates higher education from top to bottom. It is created daily through overt action and inaction that operate to marginalize People of Color, and keep Whites in positions of power. The importance of centering Whiteness is that higher education is where psychology and related mental health programs and training are situated. For these authors, Whiteness is not simply skin-color but rather it is a social concept and racial discourse that has several dimensions. Among them are colorblindness, a commitment to remaining ignorant, operating according to White ontological expansiveness, and maintaining racial comfort.

Colorblindness means understanding inequality as anything but racism. Ignorance is grounded in a commitment to seeing human suffering as being unrelated to systemic racism, "allowing people to be racially ignorant, uphold systemic racism, and remain uninterrogated identities" (McCubbin et al., 2023, p. 15). White expansiveness refers to how, according to the principles of Whiteness, all physical spaces belong to White people. Regardless of whether the space is geographic, psychic, linguistic, economic, or other, it is or should be theirs, no matter what. Whiteness as property refers to the notion that Whiteness is a commodity, such that holders of the title have the privileges and benefits of a property holder, thus they are able to exclude and are able to limit the rights of others. Racial comfort bestows the colonizer with the ability to dehumanize the colonized. These scholars argue that the science and organizations in psychology and health care are permeated by Whiteness and White supremacy, making them pervasive in the training and education of mental health professionals. Both are intertwined and reflect a profound ignorance as reflected in the presumption and centrality of European history and standards for what is knowledge and fact.

The situation in healthcare, while different, is no less dire. Many scholars (e.g., Marcelin, Siraj, Victor, Kotadia, & Maldonado, 2019) contend that both conscious and unconscious bias are harmful in health care settings and training. Evidence shows that the professions in healthcare are dominated by White providers, with smaller numbers of People of Color, those who reflect diversity and inclusion, or members of groups who have been denied access and opportunity. For example, Blacks and Latinos comprise 13% and 18% of the general population, but only 6% and 5% of medical school graduates, and 3% and 4% of medical school faculty, respectively (Marcelin et al., 2019). Bias, whether unconscious or not, has been shown to be expressed as reflexive associations and attitudes that affect perceptions, which, in turn, influence behavior and decision-making, and therefore contribute to healthcare disparities. Bias effects decisions about admissions to medical school, patient care, and hiring at all levels, and therefore hinders opportunity as well in numerous ways. While overt racism has diminished in medical practice and training, unconscious bias is still very present and effects many outcomes. Because such bias operates outside of awareness, there is still debate about how it works and can be addressed. The discussion about medical training and practice is important for our arguments since psychiatrists, psychiatric nurses, and social workers are trained and often practice in medical settings. It is also increasingly where many psychologists and other mental health providers practice, and the medical model exerts significant pressure over the mental healthcare industry as a whole. Marcelin et al. (2019) point out that "in one systemic review on the impact of unconscious bias on healthcare delivery, there was strong evidence demonstrating the prevalence of unconscious bias... affecting clinical judgement and the behavior of physicians and nurses toward patients" (p. S64).

While other studies found moderate associations, the fact that an association between bias and clinical care exists is of note and suggests this is an area that might hamper effective treatment and healthcare delivery to People of Color. These authors note also that the research on implicit bias has been around now for decades and has revealed several important facts. One is that such bias can operate in people who openly express fair-minded beliefs and attitudes. Also, among the four million people who have been tested, the vast majority, including 75% of Blacks, show automatic White preferences, wherein they associate White people with goodness and Blacks with negative or bad characteristics. Because implicit bias is considered unintentional, mitigation of its effects needs to be intentional and must be implemented both at the individual and organizational level.

Marcelin and colleagues (2019) state that in the same way that healthcare and related professionals are required to stay up to date with techniques and procedures in their field to serve patients effectively, they should be held to the same standard in terms of the social and interpersonal aspects of healthcare. For this to occur, there need to be both leaders and an organizational focus on having an inclusive staff and a higher number of currently unrepresented group members as part of the system and organization. Professional societies that set standards and accredit such learning environments must also hold institutions and training programs accountable for these changes and for making the issue as essential as is learning the basics and proper methods to practice life-enhancing health care.

Buchanan, Perez, Prinstein, and Thurston (2021) state that psychology has a long history of promoting social justice yet has not made much progress in creating just outcomes, in particular in rooting out racism as a critical aspect of institutional practice. These authors note that racism is often defined as something individuals engage in, while its cultural and institutional aspects are largely ignored and dismissed. They argue that this in effect maintains White supremacy. To illustrate, they indicate how the rejection of research articles that are focused on People of Color and marginalized communities ignores these issues and communicates that they are devalued, as are many diversity-related issues. Buchanan et al. argue that changing racism's presence in psychology requires change in many systems, an argument made by other scholars and researchers (e.g., Marcelin et al., 2019; McCubbin et al., 2023).

Buchanan and colleagues (2021) outline ways that psychological science can be conducted such that it pushes back against racism, by changing how science is practiced and who is included and how. In essence, they argue that greater numbers of People of Color should be included in all phases of knowledge production. They suggest more research on race be published. They highlight the value of being inclusive by linking grants and funding to diversity efforts, and encouraging involvement and participation of People of Color in studies. Their recommendations extend to the manuscript review process and publication of research articles. All of these factors influence what is consumed as scientific knowledge and, as a result, impact the profession of psychology.

Much of what we have presented thus far has been from the perspective of active professionals, some of whom have been working as faculty and as clinicians for some time. It is also valuable to hear from students of Color about aspects of their experiences. Jendrusina and Martinez (2019) provide their experiences in clinical supervision as a way to give the profession insight into a mostly closed aspect of training in the mental health discipline. For the most part, a core aspect of training helping professionals involves an experienced and licensed superior providing guidance and feedback to trainees as they work with clients. Supervision can be done in various ways. One way is in a group, where each trainee reports on his/her work with clients. Based on the trainee's report, the supervisor provides guidance through questions of the trainee or by having the trainee reflect on his/her interaction with clients. Often, the trainee is asked to explore several aspects of the interaction, and perhaps consider how come s/he acted or spoke in a particular way. Another approach could be where the supervisor observes sessions in real time. Another method is where the supervisor reviews an audio recording of the trainee's session with a client prior to supervision sessions, and provides individual feedback and discusses the work based on what actually took place rather than on the trainee's report.

Usually, trainees are at advanced stages of training before they begin to work with clients, but supervision is a critical aspect of their learning process. While the number of students has become more diverse – one estimate is that some 30% of graduate students are non-White – more than 80% of supervisors are White (Jendrusina & Martinez, 2019). The authors point out that even though they were located in major cities, during the time of their training, they had some 18 supervisors, of which only 2 were People of Color. Supervisors can come from training program faculty, which is less common; most are drawn from the field of professionals practicing in agencies and private practice. So, they contend that since many clients receiving help in agencies and seeking help in private practices could come from non-White groups, all supervisors should have some competence in working across racial-cultural groups.

Jendrusina and Martinez (2019) point out that the majority of trainees in supervision encounter professionals who seldom address or deal with racial-cultural issues in the student-client or the student-supervisor interaction. They report evidence that many supervisors refuse to consider racial-cultural issues in case conceptualization or treatment approaches. In these situations, they argue that students can be left with feelings of distrust, leading students to become guarded during the supervision sessions, an outcome that can disrupt learning and is not conducive to helping students provide effective help to clients. They cite research evidence that has shown that clients who experience their therapist as being racially culturally competent tend to be more satisfied with their treatment, beyond the general counseling aspects of their treatment.

Their paper presents examples via vignettes that illustrate responsive and non-responsive supervisor-supervisee interactions that negatively and positively impacted their development as trainees of Color (one is a South Asian male and the other is a multiracial female). Their illustrations of aspects of their supervisory experiences that were good or not good are centered on race. The South Asian male recounts an interaction with a supervisor in which he (the supervisee) shared the experience of being the only Person of Color in his community, and the White supervisor responded that this was similar to his own experience, and that the only South Asian person he encountered was at the Seven-Eleven store. The trainee describes this interaction as a micro-aggression in which the supervisor emphasized the student's otherness and presented the stereotype of South Asians as workers in convenience stores, rather than acknowledging his own social position and status, in being raised in a homogenous community. The trainee talks about the ways this interaction was negative to their development and how it raised deep concerns about what could be shared in this relationship. It is clear that the supervisor was not effective in dealing with their racial differences and, as such, he was not able to provide an environment in which the trainee felt comfortable discussing or exploring such topics. Consider that this example might characterize many similar interactions, in which the trainee comes away feeling unable to bring their life and experiences into the supervisory interaction and thus, is unable to fully engage in training. This supervisory relationship is akin to what Carter (1995) described as a regressive therapeutic dyad wherein the trainee has more advanced racial identity attitudes than the supervisor. These types of therapeutic relationships can be characterized by strong affective reactions, conflict, and even power struggles.

Situations like this suggest that it would be a challenge for trainees to bring questions about how to utilize Black clients' cultural strengths in treatment, since it is likely the trainee would not learn about such methods in their training either in lectures or experiential courses. The authors provide other examples of different ways that supervisors can support trainees, and they go on to call for more diversity and accountability in training programs such that issues of race and diversity are more central to the training and preparation of mental health professionals at all levels. There are also recommendations that mental health professionals seek out continuing education to enhance their racial-cultural competency.

Thus far, our discussion has shown the ways that the health care and mental health professions are structured to promote the status quo and as such create barriers to the effort to train mental health or health care providers to treat people using their own experiences and values, such as we advocate in the case of Black Americans, who have strengths that can be used and encouraged in treatment approaches. According to McCubbin and colleagues (2023), this would mean de-centering Whiteness in higher education, and health, psychology, or mental health training programs. To do so, they suggest several tools including critical race theory, decolonization, indigenizing the academy, and employing positionality or intersectionality. They argue that these tools can help training programs move toward becoming "spaces of anti-racism, empowerment, and liberation" (McCubbin et al., 2023, p. 16).

Despite local, state, and federal efforts to ban it in educational systems, through critical race theory (CRT) educators and mental health providers can learn about the ways that racism is deeply embedded into our institutions and society. The theory can help people learn and perhaps reverse the placement of property rights above human rights, and help people examine how this belief functions in our systems of education. Lastly, CRT can help create spaces for People of Color, so that their experiences can be added and empower all people to learn what has been sidelined, and their voices can be used to disrupt color-blindness, such that the role and place of color and race in our society can be held up and understood, making it a powerful force for change. The process of decolonization begins when research and scholarship enlist community members as co-investigators and collaborators in the production of knowledge, thus empowering and advancing the knowledge and information held by communities of Color, which currently is withheld from view, but which contributes to its members' well-being. It means moving away from seeing others as "at-risk" and "in need," to a view that sees the benefits of their ways of being and knowing. Such efforts would make knowing and learning about Black life and culture a common, rather than an unusual, endeavor.

Carter (2005) describes how one graduate program taught racial-cultural competence through a series of didactic and experiential courses, combined and integrated with the non-racial-cultural oriented courses in the license-eligible mental health counseling masters and counseling psychology doctoral programs. The conceptual framework of this competence training is what he called the racially inclusive model (Carter 1995). It is based on the notion that all people are socialized as racial-cultural beings in North America, and that racial-cultural learning is an aspect of one's personality. Thus, it is only by learning and understanding the significance of these racial-cultural parts of oneself that it is possible to grasp the importance of, and ways in which, racial-cultural factors function in others.

Carter (2005) contends that racial-cultural competence supersedes helping skills in being effective as a mental health professional, a view that is not shared by many or most training programs in mental health disciplines. Moreover, there are a variety of ways to define and teach about multiculturalism or diversity, yet it seems clear that mental health providers need to develop awareness of their own racial-cultural worldview to be effective and to avoid bias. So, the self is the key to racial-cultural knowledge and skill. This means that self-exploration is the road to finding and using that key. One way to build awareness is through exploration of the meaning of various reference groups (i.e., race, ethnicity, gender, social class, religion, disability, sexual orientation) as well as the intersections between them. The courses described are based on the principles discussed. These courses are more effective if the training environment is geared to racial-cultural competence, such that all courses are culturally-focused (i.e., present content with a cultural perspective) or racially culturally specific (i.e., have specific racial-cultural content). Here it is possible that core classes, such as theories of counseling, human development, basic intervention skills training, research methods, and so on, employ a cultural-focus, by teaching about the context in which theories were developed and promulgated. This means that most would learn about the European-American context in which most models and theories of human personality and development were grounded, as well as that the assumptions about language, relationships, the meaning of health and illness, and interactions were based on these cultural beliefs, which are not shared by all people.

Racially culturally specific courses are geared toward trainees learning about cognitive, psychological, and emotional knowledge and experiences that people encountered. Such classes help the student understand the varied expressions of race and culture, that each person has a race and culture, that most are affected by race and racism as well as the other "isms," and that the effects impact everyone, not just targets of the "isms."

Training for African-Centered Approaches

Given the manner in which racial oppression has shaped the lives of Black Americans, we suggest that beyond training approaches that decenter

Whiteness, promote racial-cultural competence and the development of racial self-awareness, examine unconscious bias, and integrate race and culture within clinical supervision, there is a need for instruction that specifically incorporates Black cultural strengths and an understanding of the socio-political context that informs the lived experience of Black Americans. As such, the training of mental health practitioners should include an integration of African-centered perspectives into the therapy process at the level of both case conceptualization and intervention. As Lateef et al., (2022) notes:

> The evidence demonstrated by the majority of examined studies suggested that African-centered approaches may be effective in informing interventions for Black American adult clients. Noteworthy, the reviewed findings suggest that African-centered approaches to inform intervention may be particularly helpful to support Black adult clients in areas related to emotional coping and depressive symptomology. This finding is consistent with previous research supporting that an African-centered worldview may serve a protective function in the context of Black American adults' stress experiences and psychological health.
>
> (p. 262)

The remainder of this chapter therefore will highlight training approaches at both the content and instructional level including addressing the centrality of racism, elements and examples of African-Centered approaches, and integrating a recognition of racial socialization and racial identity. We also provide examples of materials practitioners can utilize for continuing education associated with Black cultural strengths and African-Centered approaches to counseling and interventions for mental health.

Centrality of Racism

As we have previously noted, a defining aspect of the experience of Black Americans is the manner in which racial oppression has and continues to shape their lived reality (Alexander, 2010; Frederickson, 1988; Hannah-Jones, 2021). We have also contended that cultural strengths reflect both historical aspects of cultural patterns that pre-dated enslavement and forced relocation to the Americas (e.g., spirituality, communalism), as well as cultural strengths that emerged from the experience of racial oppression (patterns of racial socialization and racial identity). In order to effectively apply cultural strengths to the experience of Black Americans, the mental health practitioner therefore needs to have a knowledge of, and an appreciation for the nature of anti-Black racism within the United States. As such, training in mental health practice should include specific instruction on the definition, development, and maintenance of anti-Black racism, as well as therapeutic interventions such as healing circles that seek to ameliorate and restore health in the face of ongoing racial oppression (see Turner et al., 2019). Cénat and colleagues (2024) have reviewed and provide an outline of current approaches to anti-racism training in the field of applied psychology. For mental health clinicians, anti-racist training is noted to include the following areas: understanding the social and historical context of mental health problems; developing awareness of self-identity and privilege; recognizing oppressive behaviors; developing anti-racist competence; and incorporating alternative approaches such as recognizing trauma as a social and cultural phenomenon, as opposed to the traditional scientific approaches, which view it from an intrapsychic, individual perspective (Cénat et al., 2024). The outcome of anti-racist training can be summed up in the following definition of anti-racism offered by Williams and colleagues (2022):

> Being anti-racist means actively combatting systemic in-group preferences, and structural injustices, wherever they may appear. This means working to counter racial prejudice, systemic racism, and the oppression of racialized groups. This includes conscious efforts and deliberate actions to provide equal opportunities for all people on both an individual and a systemic level. It is necessary to center and prioritize the voices of people who are racialized. It requires a life-time philosophy of humility, acknowledging personal privileges, confronting acts as well as systems of racial discrimination, and working to change personal racial biases.
>
> (p. 9)

We understand that anti-racism can be learned, and that anti-racism includes a knowledge base and an accompanying set of behaviors and skills that can consist of both internal (e.g., awareness of privilege, educating self on racism, not making assumptions) and external strategies (e.g., interrupting racist jokes, joining a racial justice organization, etc.), as described by Rozas and Miller (2009). We also believe that the ability to engage in anti-racist behaviors hinges on one's ability to commit to anti-racism as a way of life, and that anti-racism is ultimately about who we are before it's about what we do.

Integrating Africentric Perspectives in Training – Pedagogy

There is now a recognition by professional associations such as the American Psychological Association and the American Psychiatric Association of their collusion with scientific racism. As such, scholars and practitioners are increasingly calling for psychology to be more inclusive and are encouraging actively challenging Eurocentric dominance in the field, a phenomenon currently being referred to as the "Decolonizing" of psychology (Bhatia, 2020; Jamison, & Carroll, 2014; Malherbe et al., 2021). Accordingly, the need to incorporate

African-Centered approaches into the training of mental health clinicians is also receiving increased attention in the mental health literature. Awosogba et al. (2023) suggest that African-centered approaches should be foundational in the training of American mental health clinicians. The authors demand that contributions of Africentric scholars be given equal weight as other schools of thought in the training of psychologists, arguing that such diversification of pedagogy benefits all of psychology through the promotion of critical thinking and more expansive approaches to understanding the human condition. Furthermore, Awosogba and colleagues suggest that Africentric approaches be included in foundational courses and assigned in courses emphasizing race and culture, such as multicultural or cross-cultural psychology. The notable African-centered theorists identified by Awosogba et al. (2023) include Wade Nobles, Linda James Myers, Na'im Akbar, and Cheryl Tawede Grills. To this list, we would add John Henrik Clark, Amos Wilson, Franz Fanon, and James Jones. By including the contributions of these scholars, African-centered approaches will not only be more accessible, but also increased familiarity should widen the available pool of practitioners equipped to effectively work with Black Americans. As noted by Asowoga et al. "To ignore Africentric perspectives would leave the profession vulnerable to perpetuate erroneous conceptualization, examination, and treatment of Black persons, contributing to mental health inequity for Black Americans" (p. 465).

Suggestions for Continuing Education

Recent data coming from the American Psychological Association and the American Counseling Association suggests that demographic changes are slowly occurring within the mental health profession, however White practitioners continue to dominate the profession (American Psychological Association, 2022). Additionally, while including African-centered perspectives in current training models is important, we recognize that a large and significant precentage of current practitioners have been trained under conditions in which Eurocentric models were treated as normative, universal, and authoritative. As such, there is a need to explore other avenues by which current mental health practitioners can engage material that will begin equipping them to work more effectively with Black Americans through incorporating a strength-based approach and incorporating the cultural values that have been articulated in this volume.

In a disturbing yet intuitive finding, Price et al. (2022) report that psychotherapy efficacy in Black youth participating in randomized clinical trials is lower in states with higher levels of cultural racism. This finding, in addition to the presence of clinician discomfort when responding to client reports of anti-Black racism (Bartholomew et al., 2023) suggest that there is an urgent need for therapists who possess the requisite knowledge and skills to work effectively with Black Americans. Furthermore, these data suggest that the noted reluctance of Black Americans to engage counseling and psychotherapy should not be viewed as a deficit, but as an appropriate hesitancy to engage treatment that might be at best culturally insensitive and at worst dehumanizing.

At this juncture we would like to offer an important reminder that is germane to a discussion of improving the ability of practitioners to engage Black Americans in counseling and psychotherapy. There is fortunately a large body of literature that identifies the important role of such race-related variables as racial identity (see Hoggard et al., 2017; Worrell et al., 2023) and racial socialization (see Anderson & Stevenson, 2019; Reynolds & Gonzalez-Blacken, 2017) among Black Americans. What we have learned from this literature is simply that Black Americans are not a monolith. The heterogeneity that exists among Black Americans in regard to their understanding of themselves as racial beings at both the individual and collective level, and the extent to which they have internalized both negative and positive messages associated with their racial group, has implications for a range of life experiences, including perceptions of racial discrimination, engagement in anti-racism activities, differential religious and spiritual orientations, and levels of psychological well-being and distress (Cokley, 2005; Carter, 1995, 2025; Hughes et al., 2015; Pieterse & Carter, 2010). As such, as we encourage practitioners to gain more familiarity with African-centered perspectives, we also stress the need to understand and value the within-group variables that exist as highlighted in the racial identity and racial socialization literature.

With that said, we now draw attention to various opportunities for ongoing education for mental health practitioners. Table 11.1 outlines resources that could serve as an introduction to both the literature on Black American psychology and accompanying approaches to the provision of culturally congruent and African-centered interventions. These suggestions are by no means exhaustive; however, they do provide an overview of culturally consistent approaches to the provision of mental health care (see Boyd-Franklin, 2013), and illustrate approaches that are more specifically shaped by African-centered approaches (see Lateef et al., 2022; Turner, 2019).

Additional approaches to engaging education on culturally congruent approaches to working with Black Americans include participating in continuing educational opportunities and attending conferences. The newly created African American Behavioral Health Center of Excellence is supported by the Department of Health and Human Services and is housed at Morehouse School of Medicine. The center provides training and research opportunities designed to create more equitable behavioral health care for the Black American population (see https://africanamericanbehavioralhealth.org/). Recent trainings have included such topics as *Cultivating Emotional Wellness and Racial Healing for African American Students*; *Healing History Learning Community*; and *Addressing Disparities in Access and Utilization of Behavioral Health Services Among African American Communities.*

The Association of Black Psychologists (ABPsi) annual convention provides an opportunity for mental health practitioners to engage cutting edge research and discussion on contemporary treatment approaches designed to provide culturally congruent services to Black Americans (Obasi et al., 2012). Additionally, engaging in the many community building activities provides participants an

Table 11.1 Resource List

Resource	Description	Reference
Counseling Intervention for African Americans	Community-based model for Healing and Resilience that incorporates relationships, identity, spirituality and Active Expressions of cultural congruence and authenticity	Turner, E. A., Harrell, S. P., & Bryant-Davis, T. (2022). Black love, activism, and community (BLAC): The BLAC model of healing and resilience. *Journal of Black Psychology, 48*(3–4), 547–568.
Review	Provides a description of the current status and historical development of the Association of Black Psychologists (ABPSi)	Obasi, E. M., Speight, S. L., Rowe, D. M., Clark, L. O., & Turner-Essel, L. (2012). The Association of Black Psychologists: An Organization Dedicated to Social Justice. *The Counseling Psychologist, 40*(5), 656–674. doi: 10.1177/0011000012450417
Certification in African/Black Psychology (CABP)	A certification process that indicates proficiency in the application of African-centered psychology and establishes qualifications to provide culturally congruent services to populations of Black/African ancestry	Association of Black Psychologists (ABPsi) https://abpsi.org/cabp/
Healing Intervention: Sawubona Healing Circle (SHC)	Collaboration between the Black Family Summit and ABPSi to develop a community-based intervention designed to offer healing and restoration in the face of ongoing anti-Black traumas and stressors	https://abpsi.org/sawubona/ Auguste, E., Lodge, T., Carrenard, N., Onwong'a, J. R., Zollicoffer, A., Collins, D., & London, L. (2024). Seeing One Another: The Creation of the Sawubona Healing Circles. *Journal of Black Psychology, 0*(0). doi: 10.1177/00957984241250227

(Continued)

Table 11.1 (Continued)

Resource	Description	Reference
Racial Socialization Intervention	Empirically Supported Intervention that integrates racial socialization as part of a manualized treatment approach For Black American adolescents and their caregivers	https://www.recastingrace.com/research/embrace Anderson, R. E., McKenny, M. C., & Stevenson, H. C. (2019). EMBR ace: Developing a racial socialization intervention to reduce racial stress and enhance racial coping among Black parents and adolescents. Family Process, 58(1), 53–67.
EASI Intervention	A 12-week theory-based mentoring intervention that incorporates Nguzo Saba (the seven principles), namely unity; self-determination; collective work and responsibility; cooperative economics; purpose; creativity; and faith.	Washington, G., Caldwell, L. D., Watson, J., & Lindsey, L. (2017). African American rites of passage interventions: A vehicle for utilizing African American male elders. Journal of Human Behavior in the Social Environment, 27(1–2), 100–109. doi: 10.1080/10911359.2016. 1266858
Book	Describes Mental health Interventions that integrate race-related stress, Afro-centric perspectives, and the impact of scientific racism in medicine and psychology	Turner, E. A. (2019). Mental health among African Americans: Innovations in research and practice. Lanham, Maryland: Rowman & Littlefield Publishing.
Book	Describes an empowerment-based multi-systemic approach for working with Black Americans at all socio-economic levels	Boyd-Franklin, N. (2013). Black families in therapy: Understanding the African American experience. New York, NY: Guilford Publications.
Book	Presents an overview of the principles and applications of Black American psychology	Belgrave, F. Z., & Allison, K. W. (2018). African American psychology: From Africa to America. Thousand Oaks, CA: Sage Publications.
Book	Provides an overview of African-centered perspectives on the psychology of Black and African Americans	Parham, T. A., Ajamu, A., & White, J. L. (2015). Psychology of Blacks: Centering our perspectives in the African consciousness. East Sussex, England, UK: Psychology Press.

opportunity to experience many of the cultural values outlined in this volume including communalism, spirituality, racial socialization, and racism-related coping (Woodyard & Gadson, 2018). One finds these values imbued through presentations and social gatherings that occur during the convention and reflect the ongoing work and mission of the association, which is "concerned with the liberation of the African mind, empowerment of the African character, and enlivenment and illumination of the African spirit" (Grills, 2013, p. 278). Furthermore, active participation in the Association provides additional opportunities to both learn and experience Black cultural values associated with a strength-based approach to the mental health of Black Americans (Grills et al., 2018).

Finally, most licensing boards and credentialing agencies require some form of ongoing or continuing education credits for mental health professionals to maintain licensure in their respective jurisdictions (Niemeyer et al., 2010). The Continuing Education (CE) program has been viewed by some as an important avenue for instruction on aspects of mental health practice consistent with racial and cultural competence for more seasoned practitioners (Delphin & Rowe, 2008); however, the efficacy of such programs has yet to be clearly established (Chu et al., 2022). Even a cursory search of the internet will reveal many opportunities for continuing education associated with serving Black populations, addressing the impact of racism, and engaging African-centered therapeutic approaches. The challenge of course is to ensure that all practitioners can display some baseline level of clinical competence with regard to working with Black American populations. Although the resources and training approaches we have reviewed in this chapter provide some direction, the challenge of systemic change remains elusive, and begs the need for ongoing imagining associated with the training and education of mental health providers with the goal of ensuring congruent care and equitable mental health care for Black American populations, which we attempt to do in the next and concluding chapter.

References

Alexander, M. (2010). *The new Jim Crow: Mass incarceration in the age of colorblindness*. New York: New Press.

American Psychological Association. (2022). Demographics of U.S. Psychology Workforce [Interactive data tool]. Retrieved January 31, 2025 from https://www.apa.org/workforce/data-tools/demographics.

Anderson, R. E., & Stevenson, H. C. (2019). RECASTing racial stress and trauma: Theorizing the healing potential of racial socialization in families. *American Psychologist, 74*(1), 63–75. doi: 10.1037/amp0000392.

Awosogba, O. O. R., Jackson, S. M., Onwong'a, J. R., Cokley, K. O., Holman, A., & McClain, S. E. (2023). Contributions of African-centered (Africentric) psychology: A call for inclusion in APA-accredited graduate psychology program curriculum. *American Psychologist, 78*(4), 457–468. doi: 10.1037/amp0001164.

Bartholomew, T. T., Pérez-Rojas, A. E., Bledman, R., Joy, E. E., & Robbins, K. A. (2023). "How could I not bring it up?": A multiple case study of therapists' comfort when

Black clients discuss anti-Black racism in sessions. *Psychotherapy, 60*(1), 63–75. https://doi.org/10.1037/pst0000404

Bhatia, S. (2020). Decolonizing psychology: Power, citizenship and identity. *Psychoanalysis, Self and Context, 15*(3), 257–266.

Boyd-Franklin, N. (2013). *Black families in therapy: Understanding the African American experience.* New York, NY: Guilford Publications.

Buchanan, N. T., Perez, M., Prinstein, M. J., & Thurston, I. B. (2021). Upending racism in psychological science: Strategies to change how science is conducted, reported, reviewed, and disseminated. *American Psychologist, 76*(7), 1097–1112. doi: 10.1037/amp0000905.

Carter, R. T. (1995). *The influence of race and racial identity in psychotherapy: Toward a racially inclusive model* (Vol. 183). New York. NY.: John Wiley & Sons.

Carter, R. T. (2005). Teaching racial-cultural counseling competence: A racially inclusive model. In R. T. Carter (Ed.), *Handbook of racial-cultural psychology and counseling.* Volume II. Hoboken, NJ: Wiley & Sons.

Carter, R. T., & Pieterse, A. L. (2019). *Measuring the effects of racism: Guidelines for the assessment and treatment of race-based traumatic stress injury.* Columbia University Press. New York, NY.

Cénat JM, Broussard C, Jacob G, Kogan C, Corace K, Ukwu G, Onesi O, Furyk SE, Bekarkhanechi FM, Williams M, Chomienne MH, Grenier J, Labelle PR. Antiracist training programs for mental health professionals: A scoping review. (2024) *Clinical Psychology Review.* Mar, 108, 102373. doi: 10.1016/j.cpr.2023.102373.

Chu, W., Wippold, G., & Becker, K. D. (2022). A systematic review of cultural competence trainings for mental health providers. *Professional Psychology: Research and Practice, 53*(4), 362–371. https://dx.doi.org/10.1037/pro0000469

Cokley, K. O. (2005). Racial(ized) Identity, Ethnic Identity, and Afrocentric Values: Conceptual and Methodological Challenges in Understanding African American Identity. *Journal of Counseling Psychology, 52*(4), 517–526. https://doi.org/10.1037/0022-0167.52.4.517

Delphin, M. E., & Rowe, M. (2008). Continuing education in cultural competence for community mental health practitioners. *Professional Psychology: Research and Practice, 39*(2), 182–191. https://doi.org/10.1037/0735-7028.39.2.182

Frederickson, G. M. (1988). The Arrogance of Race: Historical Perspectives on Slavery. *Racism and Social Inequality.* Middletown, CT: Wesleyan University Press.

Grills, C. (2013). The context, perspective, and mission of ABPsi: Past and present. *Journal of Black Psychology, 39*(3), 276–283. doi: 10.1177/0095798413480685.

Grills, C., Nobles, W. W., & Hill, C. (2018). African, Black, neither or both? Models and strategies developed and implemented by the association of Black psychologists. *Journal of Black Psychology, 44*(8), 791–826. doi: 10.1177/0095798418813660.

Hannah-Jones, N. (2021). *The 1619 project: A new American origin story.* New York, N.Y: Random House.

Hemmings, C., & Evans, A. M. (2018). Identifying and treating race-based trauma in counseling. *Journal of Multicultural Counseling and Development, 46*(1), 20–39.

Hoggard, L. S., Jones, S. C. T., & Sellers, R. M. (2017). Racial cues and racial identity implications for how African Americans experience and respond to racial discrimination. *Journal of Black Psychology, 43*(4), 409-432. doi: 10.1177/0095798416651033.

Hughes, M., Kiecolt, K. J., Keith, V. M., & Demo, D. H. (2015). Racial identity and well-being among African Americans. *Social Psychology Quarterly, 78*(1), 25–48.

Jamison, D. F., & Carroll, K. K. (2014). A critical review and analysis of the state, scope and direction of African-centered psychology from 2000–2010. *The Western Journal of Black Studies, 38* (2), 98–107.

Jendrusina, A. A. & Martinez, J. H. (2019). Hello from the other side: Student of color perspectives in supervision. *Training and Education in Professional Psychology, 13*(1), 160–166.

Kapten, S. W. (2021). *Becoming an African-Centered psychologist: A phenomenological study of African-centered wisdom and practice* (Doctoral dissertation, The New School).

Lateef, H., Nartey, P. B., Amoako, E. O., & Lateef, J. S. (2022). A systematic review of African-centered therapeutic interventions with Black American adults. *Clinical Social Work Journal, 50*, 256–264. https://doi.org/10.1007/s10615-021-00825-9

Malherbe, N., Ratele, K., Adams, G., Reddy, G., & Suffla, S. (2021). A decolonial Africa (n)-centered psychology of antiracism. *Review of General Psychology, 25*(4), 437–450.

Marcelin, J. R., Siraj, D. W., Victor, R., Kotadia, S., & Maldonado, Y. A. (2019). The impact of unconscious bias in healthcare: How to recognize and mitigate it. *The Journal of Infectious Disease, 220*, S62–S73.

McCubbin, L. D., Alex, R. M., Bergkamp, J., Malone, C. M., Wang, C. D. C., & Reynolds, A. L., (2023). Returning the colonizer's gaze: Critiquing Whiteness in our training programs. *Training and Education in Professional Psychology, 17*, 14–21.

Neimeyer, G. J., Taylor, J. M., & Philip, D. (2010). Continuing education in psychology: Patterns of participation and perceived outcomes among mandated and nonmandated psychologists. *Professional Psychology: Research and Practice, 41*(5), 435–441. doi: 10.1037/a0021120.

Obasi, E. M., Speight, S. L., Rowe, D. M., Clark, L. O., & Turner-Essel, L. (2012). The Association of Black Psychologists: An Organization Dedicated to Social Justice. *The Counseling Psychologist, 40*(5), 656–674. https://doi.org/10.1177/0011000012450417

Phelps, R., Bray, J. H., & Kearney, L. K. (2017). A quarter century of psychological practice in mental health and health care: 1990–2016. *American Psychologist, 72*(8), 822–836. doi: 10.1037/amp0000192.

Pieterse, A. L., & Carter, R. T. (2010). The role of racial identity in perceived racism and psychological stress among Black American adults: Exploring traditional and alternative approaches. *Journal of Applied Social Psychology, 40*(5), 1028–1053.

Price, M. A., Weisz, J. R., McKetta, S., Hollinsaid, N. L., Lattanner, M. R., Reid, A. E., & Hatzenbuehler, M. L. (2022). Meta-analysis: Are psychotherapies less effective for black youth in communities with higher levels of anti-black racism? *Journal of the American Academy of Child & Adolescent Psychiatry, 61*(6), 754–763.

Reynolds, J. E., & Gonzales-Backen, M. A. (2017). Ethnic-racial socialization and the mental health of African Americans: A critical review. *Journal of Family Theory & Review, 9*(2), 182–200. doi: 10.1111/jftr.12192

Rozas, L. W., & Miller, J. (2009). Discourses for social justice education: The web of racism and the web of resistance. *Journal of Ethnic & Cultural Diversity in Social Work, 18*(1–2), 24–39.

Turner, E. A. (2019). *Mental health among African Americans: Innovations in research and practice*. Lanham, MD: Rowman & Littlefield.

Washburn, J. J. (2019). Master's level providers in health service psychology: An idea that has come and passed, and now must come again. *Training and Education in Professional Psychology, 13*(2), 92–99. doi: 10.1037/tep0000228.

Washington, H. A. (2006). *Medical apartheid: The dark history of medical experimentation on Black Americans from colonial times to the present*. New York, N.Y: Doubleday Books.

Williams, M. T., Faber, S. C., & Duniya, C. (2022). Being an anti-racist clinician. *The Cognitive Behaviour Therapist, 2022*(15), e19. doi: 10.1017/S1754470X22000162.

Woodyard, O. T., & Gadson, C. A. (2018). Emerging Black scholars: Critical Reflections on the impact of the association of Black psychologists. *Journal of Black Psychology, 44*(8), 772–790. doi: 10.1177/0095798418813237.

Worrell, F. C., Vandiver, B. J., & Fhagen, P. E. (2023). Nigrescence theory from 1971 to 2021: The critical contributions of William E. Cross, Jr. *American Psychologist, 78*(4), 389–400. doi: 10.1037/amp0001052.

Chapter 12

Emerging Issues for Mental Health Policy and Services for Black Americans

The past few years have garnered an increased focus on the mental health needs of Black Americans, partly in response to the heightened awareness of the role of systemic racism as a result of the COVID-19 pandemic and the highly visible police murder of George Floyd. With notable apologies by the American Psychological Association (2021) and the American Psychiatric Association (2021) for their historical involvement in the mistreatment of Black Americans, there have also been increased publications identifying the need for psychology and allied professions to be more intentional in combating and dismantling racism in all domains of mental health practice including research, clinical intervention, prevention, policy, and training/education (Gregory & Clark, 2021; Legha & Miranda, 2020; Mayes & Byrd, 2022; Pieterse, Lewis, & Miller, 2023; Pieterse & Kim, 2024; Schouler-Ocak et al., 2021; Wilcox, 2023; Wilcox et al., 2024; Buchanan et al., 2021; Stern et al., 2022; Roberts et al., 2020; Roberts, 2024; Rodriguez-Seijas et al., 2024; Williams et al., 2022).

Collectively, these papers call for a reduction in the dominance of Eurocentric perspectives in theory building and research practices, centering the experiences of Black Americans and their understanding and experience of mental illness, abandoning scientific practices that obscure the experience of racism, and promoting greater racial diversity in both representation and practice in the field. There have, however, been some voices questioning the validity, integrity, and operationalization of purported shifts in professional sentiment, claiming that professional psychology gate-keeping bodies such as licensure examinations continue to reflect "linguistic bias and systemic racism," which has an adverse impact on racial and ethnic diversification in professional psychology, namely limiting the number of potential psychologists of Color (Callahan et al., 2021). Taking up the role of defending the need for more culturally congruent services for Black Americans the Association of Black Psychologists has issued a commitment to

> continue its 53-year commitment made by its founding members, to the liberation of the African mind, the empowerment of the African Character,

DOI: 10.4324/9781003083221-13

and the enlivenment and illumination of the African Spirit. ABPsi continues to forge ahead in the reclamation and application of hundreds of years of African deep thought and sacred science – African/Black Psychology, while always countering the APA's destructiveness, revisionist history, and attempts at creating a new narrative. Most importantly, the ABPsi will continue our teaching, research, counseling, advocacy (for our graduate students and "our way" of practices), and other work, singularly and unapologetically addressing the restoration of wellness to African persons, families, and communities worldwide.

(Association of Black Psychologists, 2021)

As we pull back from focusing on the application of cultural strengths in the psychotherapy/counseling context, we acknowledge that the mental health industry is situated in and governed by the very structures that have maintained anti-Black racism for centuries. Therefore, in considering policy-related changes that would facilitate the implementation of Black cultural strengths, we will focus on three areas: (1) the need for a major paradigm shift moving from a deficit-based perspective of understanding the Black American experience to a strength-based approach to both conceptualization and intervention; (2) the need for an interrogation of the manner in which capitalism shapes health care and contributes to the reification of society's racist structure, thereby creating and maintaining health inequities that exist across racial lines; (3) the need to focus on representation and participation by Black American mental health practitioners both in regard to numerical increase but also an enhance their ability to influence and shape the field at the level of credentialing; and (4) the need for greater efforts at the level of prevention.

Shifting the Paradigm

There is an enduring belief in the deficiency of Black Americans. Tracing it's roots back to the colonial era when perceived physical and psychological deficiencies were noted as a rationale for enslavement de (Maharaj, Bhatt, & Gentile, 2021), perceptions of deficiency are now often exhibited through implicit bias associated with the use of more serious mental illness diagnoses for Black individuals and lower expectations of compliance with treatment and recovery (Londono et al., 2021; Heberlein, Chen, & Trinh, 2019). Indeed, Cogburn and colleagues (2024) have noted:

Anti-Blackness has been situated as the fundamental counterpart to White supremacy. Thus, as White supremacy culture often functions as an invisible guide for social norms and values, Blackness is both visibly and invisibly situated as the derivative or deviation from those norms.

(p. 58)

It is clear that the application of Black cultural strengths to the understanding of mental illness among Black Americans would serve as a deterrent to the deficit-based approaches that continue to inform current practice. Although there has been a shift from the sense of inherent Black racial inferiority that characterized much of 19th-century pseudo-scientific racism (Winston, 2020; Fairchild, 1991), the notion that Black Americans are "damaged" as a result of social disadvantage provides a different entry to the same set of implicit assumptions associated with inequities in mental health care. Although the literature supports the negative mental health effects of such factors as poverty and racial discrimination, the response is often to focus on the intra-psychic patterns rather than focus on the systemic structures that account for and in fact shape the psychological distress. Stated another way, the focus tends to be on the individual's "illness" rather than on the social pathology that causes and informs the psychological distress. Furthermore, Cogburn and colleagues indicate that the categories of psychiatric diagnosis and psychological distress that are common to the nomenclature of mental health have rarely included an "analysis of the systems that produce illness and compromise mental health" (p. 56). It is encouraging to observe attempts to apply Afrocentric principles in an approach to the delivery of health care. Gebremikael and colleagues (2022) describe the application of Ubuntu (I am because we are), and Nguzo Saba (the seven principles of unity; self-determination; collectivism work; co-operative economics; collective purpose; and faith in humankind) as a guiding approach to empowering Black Canadians and providing an anti-colonial and anti-racism approach to health Care. We do however acknowledge that there are significant economic and ideological forces that challenge these approaches.

Racial Capitalism and Mental Health

We understand that mental health care as an industry is closely aligned to the market-driven principles that have underscored and informed the development of the racial hierarchy within the United States. Leong (2012) introduced the term "racial capitalism" to refer to the historical and deep-rooted practice of the creation of inequities between different groups of people perpetuating a system of privilege. Liu, Liu, and Shin (2023) further emphasize this perspective in suggesting that a purpose of racism in the US was to acquire land and thereby maintain economic inequity that consequently placed limits on the lives of Black and Indigenous people. Industry is often based on a set of principles that reward the accumulation of wealth and allow those with wealth (power) to set the parameters for practice (Zeira, 2022). Mental health care is not immune in this endeavor. In fact, Spector (2014) has argued that "strategies to eliminate racist oppression must include the personal but must confront the structural power and class relationships that reinforce racist oppression" (p. 116).

Drawing on Pieterse and Gale (2023), we note that at present mental health care in the United States occurs within the context of a federally recognized mental health crisis (The White House, 2023), and that the mental healthcare system has historically proven inadequate to meet the needs of communities of Color specifically (American Psychiatric Association, 2017; Mensah et al., 2021) or contributed to ongoing racial injustices in health care (Roberts & Trejo, 2022). Additionally, mental healthcare systems that are focused on maximizing profit tend to support and reward behaviors that prioritize those elements of organizational functioning, such as maximizing individual provider caseloads and organizational efficiency metrics such as timeliness of case notes/reports and treatment plans based on early diagnosis and manualized therapy, that increase the likelihood of insurance reimbursement (Greene, 2023; Mauch, 2011). In an important review of the nexus between neoliberal economic policies and mental health, Zeira (2022) suggests that policies that eliminate restrictions on the market and curtail government regulation have resulted in significant increases in income inequality, decreases in government-run social services, higher rates of incarceration, and a more expensive and ineffective health care system. Furthermore, data suggests that market-driven countries such as the United States that prioritize individualism and competition also display significantly higher rates of mental distress, especially in relation to anxiety and depression. It seems fair to conclude that neoliberal capitalism is both associated with higher rates of psychological distress and increased limitations in the delivery of effective mental health care. As Black Americans are disproportionately and more negatively impacted by growing income inequality, it is important to consider the application of Black cultural strengths in mental health care against the backdrop of pervasive systematic inequalities that are racialized, and are associated with mental health functioning among Black Americans. In an interesting paradox, it is important to note that some authors argue that structural racism presents an additional cost to health care systems.

As such, ensuring appropriate, effective, and equitable mental health care for Black Americans, and anti-racist approaches to mental health care becomes critical (see Legha, 2020). Anti-racism in mental health treatment occurs at both the individual level (the nature of the clinical interactions between clinician and patient – including assessment, diagnosis and treatment strategies) – and the structural level. Fortunately, the current clinical literature is replete with examples and approaches to reduce racist encounters at the clinical/therapeutic level and engage an anti-racist approach to clinical care. In general, strategies include clinical racial self-awareness and examination of implicit bias, knowledge of how racism operates in society including the history of racism in psychology and psychiatry, engaging patients as collaborators in their own health, being attentive to and understanding how culture frames the client's experience, engaging cultural humility, engaging ongoing education and building racial justice allyships, slowing down the diagnostic process, and considering systemic factors that impact mental health (see Cénat, 2020; Lee & Boykins, 2022; Legha, 2023; Miller & Garran, 2017; Miller et al., 2018; Mosley et al., 2021; Williams et al., 2022).

Although individual anti-racist measures by practitioners have been noted to be associated with improved engagement by clients of Color and greater treatment efficacy (Meyer & Zane, 2013; Hassen et al., 2021), the literature on anti-racism and treatment outcomes is emerging and has yet to be fully developed. Fortunately, there is in existence a growing framework (see Gilbert & Roe, 2023) and accompanying set of research tools designed to assess the efficacy of anti-racism initiatives at both the individual and institutional level. To illustrate, the Anti-racism Behavioral Inventory (ARBI; Pieterse et al., 2016) is a self-report measure to assess an individual's level of awareness of racism and their participation in behaviors that support anti-racism at both the individual and institutional levels. Wang, Gomes, Rosa, Copeland, and Santana (2024) report a review of training-related diversity, equity, and inclusion initiatives with the majority being directed at anti-racism training. The authors describe a range of training approaches, however they indicate significant limitations associated with the actual interventions (e.g., the majority were single session trainings) and research methodologies (e.g., lack of longitudinal studies). Additionally, the emergence of empirically supported novel approaches to deliver anti-racism instruction to mental health professionals is another encouraging development in the field (Brown et al., 2024). In sum, there is evidence of a greater interest in assessing the efficacy of anti-racism approaches within the health care setting which has important implications for the implementation of more culturally congruent and racially equitable mental health care for Black Americans (See Talley, Shoyinka, & Minkoff, 2021).

Addressing Structural Anti-Black Racism in Mental Health Care

In order to increase the efficacy of the application of Black cultural strengths in mental health care, there is an urgent need to address the structures in which mental health care exists and the credentialling requirements that inform mental health practice. There is a tension that exists between practitioner implementation of anti-racist care and the institutions in which care exists. Pieterse and Gale (2023) note the limits of anti-racist clinical practice without accompanying organizational commitment and regulatory mandates. After conducting a review of anti-racist interventions within health care systems, Hassan et al. (2021) identify the following strategies associated with long-term organization change: (1) incorporating and sharing explicit anti-racism language; (2) establishing leadership buy-in and commitment; (3) investing in dedicated funding and resources including engaging a sufficient level of expertise; (4) using a multi-level, long term approach including the creation of racial equity policies and procedures that inform hiring, retention, and promotion; (5) requiring mandatory anti-racism training and education linking this work to broader systems of power, hierarchy, and dominance; and (6) building in opportunities for ongoing assessment, re-evaluation, and revision of efforts as informed by data. They conclude by suggesting that "one of the key components in creating systems-level change to dismantle racism is to increase infrastructure, accountability, and monitoring" (p. 12).

"These socio-political causes of mental distress have affected so many and can only be achieved by widespread governmental interventions that help people instead of profit margins" (Zeira, 2023, pp. 211–212). We therefore suggest that mental health practitioners should be engaging political advocacy and joining movements that are more likely to elect political leadership invested in utilizing government as a tool for social good instead of as an engine for profit. Given the close relationship between racial categorization and social class oppression within the United States (Spector, 2014), we view political movements that challenge neoliberal policies to be an important part of anti-racist approaches to equitable mental health care for Black Americans. As noted by White (2002),

> Devising prevention efforts that focus on solely behavior, culture and value systems will not eliminate health disparities.... Because inequality, racism, sexism, and class-related phenomena profoundly and collectively affect risk behavior, each of these must be addressed to [...] eliminate health disparities associated with race and ethnicity in the United States.
>
> (p. 311)

Finally, there have been advances in the measurement of structural racism which also allows for the examination of mental health care benefits associated with reductions in structural racism. In research focused on the unmet mental health needs of a sample of Black American adults, Alang (2019) noted that two of the five categories identified by participants referenced structural factors including cost of care/insurance and accessibility factors. Hardeman and colleagues (2022) have identified several approaches to greater precision in the measurement of structural racism including the use of latent variable modeling, and the more accurate identification of factors that could be utilized as proxies for structural racism, including establishing sets of exposures such as measured inequities in political participation, employment, education, and judicial treatment that could be associated with various health and mental health outcomes.

Professional Credentialling as a Tool for Combating Anti-Black Racism

In a blistering response to the American Psychological Association's offer of an apology to Black, Indigenous and other people of Color, the Association of Black Psychologist identified what they view as a significant impediment to greater equity in mental health care for Black Americans:

> Oppression is a corollary of racism, white supremacy, and its subsequent hoarding of power. To even begin to make good on its promises, the APA

must empower the survivors of its ongoing terrorism. They may accomplish this by abdicating their unjustifiable claim to be the arbiter of universal human functioning and by granting full authority to the Association of Black Psychologists, the Hispanic Psychological Association, the Society of Indian Psychologists, the Association of Asian American Psychologists, and other Ethnic centered Associations to establish their own independent and separate codes of ethics, licensing, certification and education and training.

(ABPsi, 2021)

There continues to be significant disproportionality in racial representation in mental health care. To illustrate, recent data from clinical and counseling psychology doctoral training programs as well as predoctoral internship programs suggest that Black trainees continue to be disproportionately underrepresented in comparison to census data. Callahan and colleagues (2018) report data indicating a significant racial disparity in the ranks of professional psychologists with active psychologists being 83.6% White and 5.3% Black. Furthermore, Black students account for only 7.2% of all doctoral-level trainees. When turning attention to predoctoral internships, Dimmick and Callahan (2022) report continued disproportionate underrepresentation of Black trainees. Racial representation for Black individuals is further complicated by the reported higher rate of failure among Black applicants when undertaking the national psychology licensure exam, the EPPP. Sharpless (2019, 2021) reports consistent findings of failure at a rate of 38% (NY) and 23% (CT) across two Northeast states in the United States compared to failure rates of White applicants at 12.5% (NY) and 5.5% (CT).

These data suggest significant structural impediments to increasing the number of Black mental health professionals within the United States. Of note, even though Black professionals are present with greater levels of frequency in the discipline of social work, there is also data to suggest racial bias in social work licensure exams due to disproportionate passing rates and examinee reports of racial bias (Walker & Bruhn, 2024; Ricciardelli et al., 2024). It is also important to note that while Black professionals are represented at higher rates within the social work profession, given the breadth of practice within social work, there is also a need to increase Black representation among Licensed Clinical Social Workers (LCSW), the group or practitioners more likely to provide direct psychotherapeutic services to Black Americans (Hirsch, DeCarlo, Lewis, & Walker, 2024).

In addition to these systemic barriers, there appears to be curricular challenges that limit the ability to prepare psychologists to work effectively with Black populations. A study of 343 early career psychologists and current psychology trainees on the need for diversity science, including instruction in critical race theory and anti-racism, evidenced high-factor loadings on a measure designed to assess perceived curricular needs in psychology training (Yarrington et al., 2023).

In thinking about how to combat structural racism and the limits to racial diversity that it represents, we draw on Reynolds' (2022) suggestion that licensure boards can play a pivotal role in reducing racial disproportionality by adopting anti-racist approaches. Although the focus of Reynold's comments pertains to medical boards, we believe they have due applicability to licensing and regulatory boards within the mental health disciplines. The following suggestions/inventory is offered by Reynolds (2022, p. 39).

1 Are members of racial and ethnic minority groups represented on the regulatory board?
2 Are members of racial and ethnic minority groups represented among staff and investigators of the regulatory board?
3 Does the board require ongoing training about diversity, cultural competence, and implicit bias for board members, staff, and investigators?
4 Does the board require ongoing training about diversity, cultural competence, and implicit bias as a requirement for licensees?
5 Do the board's mission statement and website embrace fairness and justice toward ethnic and racial minorities and their issues?
6 Do the board's regulations, policies, and procedures consider the needs of racial and ethnic minority groups?
7 Does the board influence lawmakers to enact legislation that addresses racial and ethnic minority needs?
8 Are there mechanisms in place to measure disciplinary disparity outcomes and the effectiveness of efforts to achieve fair outcomes?

Prioritizing African-Centered Perspectives and the Application of Black Cultural Strengths

We have purposefully focused on the phenomenon of structural racism as an active impediment to providing culturally congruent and effective mental health care for Black Americans. We have established that one important aspect of cultural congruence is the application of Black cultural strengths in counseling and psychotherapy. In addition, we have articulated barriers to the consistent application of cultural strengths due to racist structures that limit representation of Black mental health professionals, as well as curricular requirements that do not integrate African-centered approaches to mental health care.

In conclusion, we would like to revisit the utilization of mental health care by Black Americans and propose an approach to rethinking said underutilization from a cultural strengths perspective. There continues to be research suggesting that Black Americans underutilize mental health care and also experience persistent unmet mental health needs (Armstrong et al., 2022; Gaston et al., 2016; Lu et al., 2021; Thomeer, Moody, & Yahirun, 2023). Reviewing research associated with potential barriers to mental health care experienced by Black Americans,

Summers, Abrams and Harris (2021) identify the following: "stigma, institutional discrimination, religious beliefs, cultural distrust of healthcare and mental health systems, lack of healthcare insurance, mental health illiteracy, and lack of representation among practitioners" (p. 13) as significant barriers to health care for Black Americans. Without disputing the data, we wish to offer an alternative explanation, which simply is to say that as long as racism persists in mental health care – the underutilization of the mental health care system by Black Americans should not be viewed as an unwillingness to seek our care, rather it should be viewed as an adaptive response to a system that has systematically dehumanized the suffering of Black Americans, pathologized their response to racial oppression, and failed in providing culturally appropriate care. Additionally, reframing underutilization as "obstructed use" (Burkett, 2017) highlights the role of structural and historical barriers rooted in racism, and shifts the focus from the perceived problematic behavior of Black Americans' help-seeking to the real and credible barriers that continue to impede access and utilization. The four areas of "obstruction" identified by Burkett include "historical trauma, environmental toxicity, culturally bound economic insecurity, and cultural mistrust" (p. 827), therefore any attempt to increase participation by Black Americans in mental health care has to address these barriers at both interpersonal and structural levels. Finally, the mental health care industry is not the only vehicle for mental health care and psychological support for Black Americans experiencing mental health challenges. The St. Louis Bridges program (Hong et al., 2024) is a prime example of a collaboration between the health care industry and community partners to provide mental health care to Black Americans who might be experiencing some hesitancy in accessing standard mental health care services. A central aspect of the Bridges program is the utilization of church-based wellness coordinators – this is akin to the notion of bringing services to the people as opposed to providing instruction as to where people should go to receive services. The Bridge program is also a reminder that Black Americans might be more likely to access informal sources of support and assistance when it comes to their mental health with informal sources identified as faith-based programs, family and friendship networks, mentoring programs, self-help support groups, and online support (Curry, Lipscomb, Ashley, & McCarty-Caplan, 2022; Jones et al., 2020; Nguyen et al., 2016; Planey et al., 2019; Taylor et al., 2013; Ward & Besson, 2013).

In sum, there is data to suggest that Black Americans are willing to engage standard mental health care, see benefit in these services, and appreciate opportunities to focus on their emotional and psychological needs (Meyer, & Zane, 2013). Additionally, the lack of cultural sensitivity in mental health care, historical trauma, and ongoing experiences of interpersonal and institutional racism suggest that the infusion of cultural strengths in both the conceptualization and treatment of mental needs for Black Americans remains a pressing reality. The reminder by Curry et al. (2022) suggests that if we build it, they will come: "The results suggested that African American men were willing to embark on conversations about their mental health...reporting that these experiences yielded them significant psychological, emotional, and social well-being" (p. 66).

Concluding Thoughts

In this volume, we have offered the integration of Black American cultural values as an important aspect of providing strength-based mental health care to Black Americans. Cultural strengths counter the deficit narrative applied to Black Americans, increase the interest in and utilization of mental health support, and provide a layer of protection against the adverse psychological outcomes associated with the experience of racial oppression (Jones, 2004, 2020; Jones & Neblett, 2017). Community cultural wealth has been identified as the "array of knowledges, skills, abilities, and networks possessed and utilized by Communities of Color to survive and resist racism and other forms of oppression" (Acevedo & Solozarno, 2023, p. 1473). Mental health providers are therefore encouraged to approach their work with Black Americans from a starting point that recognizes the cultural capital that exists within the Black community, and to utilize this wealth in the service of supporting the mental health of Black Americans.

The integration of the cultural strengths we have outlined constitutes an anti-racist approach to mental health practice (Fani et al., 2022). We recognize that efforts to promote anti-racist practice do not only lie with clinicians but also require a systemic and institutional shift. To illustrate, an anti-racist approach to mental health care entails organizing and advocating for changes in accreditation requirements (e.g., to require explicit focus on culturally informed and anti-racist practice within training curriculum), ethical standards (e.g., including engagement in anti-racism, advocacy, and social justice efforts in mental health professions' code of ethics rather than as aspirational guidelines), and jurisprudence (e.g., for new licensure to require training in anti-racism; for licensure renewal to require continuing education focused on anti-racism; Alvarez, 2022; Kirmayer & Jarvis, 2019; Rodriguez-Seijas et al., 2024).

For centuries, the lives of Black Americans have been shaped by racial oppression that has carried profound psychological effects (Rogers & Bryant-Davis, 2022; Stoute, 2021; Williams & Williams-Morris, 2000). Additionally, Black Americans have endured the impact of racist approaches to health care that also contributed to their ongoing experiences of dehumanization (Alang, 2019; Gordon-Achebe et al., 2019; Shim, 2021). The deficit narrative that has accompanied the racial oppression of Black Americans has represented a significant impediment to both the mental health and mental health care of Black Americans. As such, we are hopeful that the cultural strengths outlined in this volume can be effective instruments in blunting the ongoing effects of racism and providing additional clinical tools in the provision of mental health and healing for Black Americans.

References

Acevedo, N., & Solorzano, D. G. (2023). An overview of community cultural wealth: Toward a protective factor against racism. *Urban Education, 58*(7), 1470–1488.

Alang, S. M. (2019). Mental health care among blacks in America: Confronting racism and constructing solutions. *Health Services Research, 54*(2), 346–355.

Alvarez, K., Cervantes, P. E., Nelson, K. L., Seag, D. E., Horwitz, S. M., & Hoagwood, K. E. (2022). Structural racism, children's mental health service systems, and recommendations for policy and practice change. *Journal of the American Academy of Child & Adolescent Psychiatry, 61*(9), 1087–1105.

American Psychological Association (2021). *Apology to people of color for APA's role in promoting, perpetuating, and failing to challenge racism, racial discrimination, and human hierarchy in U.S.* Retrieved from https://www.apa.org/about/policy/racism-apology

American Psychiatric Association (2021). *APA's apology to Black, indigenous and people of color for its support of structural racism in psychiatry.* Retrieved from https://www.psychiatry.org/news-room/apa-apology-for-its-support-of-structural-racism

American Psychiatric Association (2017). Mental health disparities: Diverse populations. Washington, DC: American Psychiatric Association.

Armstrong, T. D., Pinson, V. M., Avent-Alston, L., & Buckner, D. N. (2022). Increasing mental health service utilization in Black populations during COVID-19: Clarifying clinician responsibility. *Practice Innovations, 7*(3), 188–202. doi: 10.1037/pri0000155.

Association of Black Psychologists (2021). Retrieved from https://abpsi.org/wp-content/uploads/2021/11/ABPsi-Full-Statement.pdf

Brown, T. R., Amir, H., Hirsch, D., & Jansen, M. O. (2024). Designing a novel digitally delivered antiracism intervention for mental health clinicians: Exploratory analysis of acceptability. *JMIR Human Factors, 11*(1), e52561.

Buchanan, N. T., Perez, M., Prinstein, M. J., & Thurston, I. B. (2021). Upending racism in psychological science: Strategies to change how science is conducted, reported, reviewed, and disseminated. *American Psychologist, 76*(7), 1097–1112.

Burkett, C. A. (2017). Obstructed use: Reconceptualizing the mental health (help-seeking) experiences of Black Americans. *Journal of Black Psychology, 43*(8), 813–835. doi: 10.1177/0095798417691381.

Callahan, J. L., Bell, D. J., Davila, J., Johnson, S. L., Strauman, T. J., & Yee, C. M. (2021). Inviting ASPPB to address systemic bias and racism: Reply to Turner et al. (2021). *American Psychologist, 76*(1), 167–168. doi: 10.1037/amp0000801.

Callahan, J. L., Smotherman, J. M., Dziurzynski, K. E., Love, P. K., Kilmer, E. D., Niemann, Y. F., & Ruggero, C. J. (2018). Diversity in the professional psychology training-to-workforce pipeline: Results from doctoral psychology student population data. *Training and Education in Professional Psychology, 12*(4), 273–285. doi: 10.1037/tep0000203.

Cénat, J. M. (2020). How to provide anti-racist mental health care. *The Lancet Psychiatry, 7*(11), 929–931.

Carter, R.T (2025) Recognizing the Psychological and Cultural Strengths of Black Americans: Historical, Social and Psychological Perspectives. Routledge, New York, NY.

Cogburn, C. D., Roberts, S. K., Ransome, Y., Addy, N., Hansen, H., & Jordan, A. (2024). The impact of racism on Black American mental health. *The Lancet Psychiatry, 11*(1), 56–64.

Curry, M., Lipscomb, A., Ashley, W., & McCarty-Caplan, D. (2022). Black barbershops exploring informal mental health settings within the community. *Journal of Humanities and Social Sciences Studies*, 4(1), 60–69. doi: 10.32996/jhsss.2022.4.1.6.

Dimmick, A. A., & Callahan, J. L. (2022). Racial and ethnic diversity among clinical psychology doctoral students applying for internship. *Training and Education in Professional Psychology*, 16(4), 412–419. doi: 10.1037/tep0000382.

Fairchild, H. H. (1991). Scientific racism: The cloak of objectivity. *Journal of Social Issues*, 47(3), 101–115.

Fani, N., White, D., Marshall-Lee, E., & Hampton-Anderson, J. (2022). Antiracist practice in psychiatry: principles and recommendations. *Focus*, 20(3), 270–276.

Gaston, G. B., Earl, T. R., Nisanci, A., & Glomb, B. (2016). Perception of mental health services among Black Americans. *Social Work in Mental Health*, 14(6), 676–695. doi: 10.1080/15332985.2015.1137257.

Gebremikael, L., Sicchia, S., Demi, S., & Rhoden, J. (2022). Afrocentric approaches to disrupting anti-Black racism in health care and promoting Black health in Canada. *CMAJ*, 194(42), E1448–E1450.

Gilbert, K. L., & Roe, K. M. (2023). From health disparities to an agenda for anti-racism in health promotion. *Health Promotion Practice*, 24(2), 197–200. doi:https://doi.org/10.1177/15248399221148135

Greene, E. M. (2023). The mental health industrial complex: A study in three cases. *Journal of Humanistic Psychology*, 63(1), 84–102.

Gregory, V. L., & Clary, K. L. (2021). Addressing anti-black racism: The roles of social work. *Smith College Studies in Social Work*, 92(1), 1–27. https://doi.org/10.1080/00377317.2021.2008287

Gordon-Achebe, K., Hairston, D.R., Miller, S., Legha, R., & Starks, S. (2019). Origins of racism in American medicine and psychiatry. In M. Medlock, D. Shtasel, N.H. Trinh, & D. Williams (Eds.), Racism and psychiatry: Contemporary issues and interventions (pp. 3–19). Springer International Publishing. https://doi.org/10.1007/978-3-319-90197-8_1

Hardeman, R. R., Homan, P. A., Chantarat, T., Davis, B. A., & Brown, T. H. (2022). Improving the measurement of structural racism to achieve antiracist health policy: study examines measurement of structural racism to achieve antiracist health policy. *Health Affairs*, 41(2), 179–186.

Hassen, N., Lofters, A., Michael, S., Mall, A., Pinto, A. D., & Rackal, J. (2021). Implementing anti-racism interventions in healthcare settings: A scoping review. *International Journal of Environmental Research and Public Health*, 18(6), 2993.

Heberlein, A. S., Chen, J. A., & Trinh, N. T. (2019). Implicit bias in mental health care. In J. A. Chen & N.T. Trinh (Eds.), Sociocultural issues in psychiatry: A casebook and curriculum. (pp. 1–21). Oxford University Press. https://doi.org/10.1093/med/9780190849986.003.0011

Hirsch, J., DeCarlo, M., Lewis, A., & Walker, C. (2024). Alternative pathways to social work licensure: A critical review and social equity policy analysis. *Journal of Evidence-Based Social Work*, 21(2), 177–198.

Hong, B., Scribner, S., Downs, D., Jackson-Beavers, R., Wright, T., Orson, W., ... & Poirier, R. (2024). The Saint Louis bridges program: A mental health network of more than one hundred churches and the mental health community. *Journal of the National Medical Association*, 116(1), 16–23.

Jones, J. M. (2004). TRIOS: A model for coping with the universal context of racism. In G. Philogène (Ed.), *Racial identity in context: The legacy of Kenneth B. Clark* (pp. 161–190). American Psychological Association. doi: 10.1037/10812-010.

Jones, J. M. (2020). Toward a cultural psychology of African Americans. In., Edited By D.L. Dinne, D.K. Forgays, S.A. Hayes, W.J. Lonner, *Merging past, present, and future in cross-cultural psychology* (pp. 52–62). Garland Science, London U.K.

Jones, S. C. T., Anderson, R. E., Gaskin-Wasson, A. L., Sawyer, B. A., Applewhite, K., Metzger, I. W. (2020). From "crib to coffin": Navigating coping from racism-related stress throughout the lifespan of Black Americans. *American Journal of Orthopsychiatry, 90*(2), 267–282. doi: 10.1037/ort0000430.

Jones, S. C., & Neblett, E. W. (2017). Future directions in research on racism-related stress and racial-ethnic protective factors for Black youth. *Journal of Clinical Child & Adolescent Psychology, 46*(5), 754–766.

Kirmayer, L. J., & Jarvis, G. E. (2019). Culturally responsive services as a path to equity in mental healthcare. *Healthcare Papers, 18*(2), 11–23.

Lee, C. C., & Boykins, M. (2022). Racism as a mental health challenge: An antiracist counselling perspective. *Canadian Psychology / Psychologie canadienne, 63*(4), 471–478. doi: 10.1037/cap0000350.

Legha, R. K. (2023). Getting off the racist sidelines: An antiracist approach to mental health supervision and training. *The Clinical Supervisor, 42*(2), 213–236.

Legha, R. K., & Miranda, J. (2020). An anti-racist approach to achieving mental health equity in clinical care. *Psychiatric Clinics, 43*(3), 451–469.

Leong, N. (2012). Racial capitalism. *Harvard Law Review, 126*, 2151.

Liu, W. M., Liu, R. Z., & Shin, R. Q. (2023). Understanding systemic racism: Anti-Blackness, white supremacy, racial capitalism, and the re/creation of white space and time. *Journal of Counseling Psychology, 70*(3), 244–257. doi: 10.1037/cou0000605.

Londono Tobon, A., Flores, J. M., Taylor, J. H., Johnson, I., Landeros-Weisenberger, A., Aboiralor, O., ... & Bloch, M. H. (2021). Racial implicit associations in psychiatric diagnosis, treatment, and compliance expectations. *Academic Psychiatry, 45*, 23–33.

Lu, W., Todhunter-Reid, A., Mitsdarffer, M. L., Muñoz-Laboy, M., Yoon, A. S., & Xu, L. (2021). Barriers and facilitators for mental health service use among racial/ethnic minority adolescents: a systematic review of literature. *Frontiers in Public Health, 9*, 641605.

Maharaj, A. S., Bhatt, N. V., & Gentile, J. P. (2021). Bringing it in the room: Addressing the impact of racism on the therapeutic alliance. *Innovations in Clinical Neuroscience, 18*(7–9), 39.

Mauch, D. (2011). *Reimbursement of mental health services in primary care settings.* Collingdale, PA: DIANE Publishing.

Mayes, R. D., & Byrd, J. A. (2022). An antiracist framework for evidence-informed school counseling practice. *Professional School Counseling, 26*(1a). https://doi.org/10.1177/2156759X221086740

Mensah, M., Ogbu-Nwobodo, L., & Shim, R. S. (2021). Racism and mental health equity: history repeating itself. *Psychiatric services, 72*(9), 1091–1094.

Meyer, O. L., & Zane, N. (2013). The influence of race and ethnicity in client's experiences of mental health treatment. *Journal of Community Psychology, 41*(7), 884–901. doi: 10.1002/jcop.21580

Miller, J. L., & Garran, A. M. (2017). *Racism in the United States: Implications for the helping professions*. New York, NY: Springer Publishing Company.

Miller, M. J., Keum, B. T., Thai, C. J., Lu, Y., Truong, N. N., Huh, G. A., Li, X., Yeung, J. G., & Ahn, L. H. (2018). Practice recommendations for addressing racism: A content analysis of the counseling psychology literature. *Journal of Counseling Psychology, 65*(6), 669–680. doi: 10.1037/cou0000306.

Mosley, D. V., Hargons, C. N., Meiller, C., Angyal, B., Wheeler, P., Davis, C., & Stevens-Watkins, D. (2021). Critical consciousness of anti-Black racism: A practical model to prevent and resist racial trauma. *Journal of Counseling Psychology, 68*(1), 1–16. doi: 10.1037/cou0000430.Nguyen, A. W., Chatters, L. M., Taylor, R. J., & Mouzon, D. M. (2016). Social support from family and friends and subjective well-being of older African Americans. *Journal of Happiness Studies, 17*, 959–979.

Pieterse, A. L., & Gale, M. M. (2023). There are no sidelines: a reaction to Legha's "getting off the racist sidelines: an antiracist approach to mental health supervision and training". *The Clinical Supervisor, 42*(2), 263–279.

Pieterse, A. L., & Kim, B. S. K. (2024). Introduction to the special issue: Dismantling anti-black racism and counseling psychology. *The Counseling Psychologist, 52*(4), 514–521. https://doi.org/10.1177/00110000241237530

Pieterse, A. L., Lewis, J. A., & Miller, M. J. (2023). Dismantling and eradicating anti-Blackness and systemic racism. *Journal of Counseling Psychology, 70*(3), 235–243. doi: 10.1037/cou0000660.

Pieterse, A. L., Utsey, S. O., & Miller, M. J. (2016). Development and initial validation of the anti-racism behavioral inventory (ARBI). *Counselling Psychology Quarterly, 29*(4), 356–381.

Planey, A. M., Smith, S. M., Moore, S., & Walker, T. D. (2019). Barriers and facilitators to mental health help-seeking among African American youth and their families: A systematic review study. *Children and Youth Services Review, 101*, 190–200.

Reynolds, N. T. (2022). The role of regulatory boards in combating racism and promoting diversity. *Journal of Medical Regulation, 108*(1), 32–44.

Ricciardelli, L., Mcgarity, S. V., Mbao, M., Erbetta, K., Herzog, J., & Knierem, M. (2024). Racial disparity in social work professional licensure exam pass rates: Examining institutional characteristics and state licensure policy as predictors. *Journal of Evidence-Based Social Work, 21*(2), 199–213.

Roberts, K. M., & Trejo, A. N. (2022). Provider, heal thy system: An examination of institutionally racist healthcare regulatory practices and structures. *Contemporary Family Therapy, 44*(1), 4–15.

Roberts, R. (2020). Psychology estranged: Mind, culture, and capitalism. In *The Routledge international handbook of global therapeutic cultures* (pp. 372–384). Routledge.

Roberts, S. O. (2024). Dealing with diversity in psychology: Science and ideology. *Perspectives on Psychological Science, 19*(3), 590–601.

Roberts, S. O., Bareket-Shavit, C., Dollins, F. A., Goldie, P. D., & Mortenson, E. (2020). Racial inequality in psychological research: Trends of the past and recommendations for the future. *Perspectives on Psychological Science, 15*(6), 1295–1309.

Rodriguez-Seijas, C., McClendon, J., Wendt, D. C., Novacek, D. M., Ebalu, T., Hallion, L. S., ... & Mekawi, Y. (2024). The next generation of clinical-psychological science: moving toward anti-racism. *Clinical Psychological Science, 12*(3), 526–546.

Rogers, G., & Bryant-Davis, T. (2022). Historical and contemporary racial trauma among Black Americans: Black wellness matters. In R. Geffner, J. W. White, L. K. Hamberger, A. Rosenbaum, V. Vaughan-Eden, & V. I. Vieth (Eds.), Handbook of interpersonal violence and abuse across the lifespan: A project of the National Partnership to End Interpersonal Violence across the Lifespan (NPEIV) (pp. 165–199). Springer Nature Switzerland AG. https://doi.org/10.1007/978-3-319-89999-2_338

Schouler-Ocak, M., Bhugra, D., Kastrup, M. C., Dom, G., Heinz, A., Küey, L., & Gorwood, P. (2021). Racism and mental health and the role of mental health professionals. *European Psychiatry, 64*(1), e42.

Sharpless, B. A. (2019). Are demographic variables associated with performance on the examination for professional practice in psychology (EPPP)? *The Journal of Psychology, 153*(2), 161–172.

Sharpless, B. A. (2021). Pass rates on the examination for professional practice in psychology (EPPP) according to demographic variables: A partial replication. *Training and Education in Professional Psychology, 15*(1), 18–22. doi: 10.1037/tep0000301.

Shim, R. S. (2021). Dismantling structural racism in psychiatry: A path to mental health equity. *American Journal of Psychiatry, 178*(7), 592–598.

Spector, A. (2014). Racism and capitalism—crisis and resistance: exploring the dynamic between class oppression and racial oppression. *Humanity & Society, 38*(2), 116–131.

Stern, J. A., Barbarin, O., & Cassidy, J. (2022). Attachment perspectives on race, prejudice, and anti-racism: Introduction to the Special Issue. *Attachment & Human Development, 24*(3), 253–259.

Stoute, B. J. (2021). Black rage: The psychic adaptation to the trauma of oppression. *Journal of the American Psychoanalytic Association, 69*(2), 259–290.

Summers, L. M., Abrams, L. P., & Harris, H. L. (2021). Identifying barriers and access to mental health care for African Americans. In M. A. Adekson (Ed.). *African Americans and Mental Health: Practical and Strategic Solutions to Barriers, Needs, and Challenges* (pp. 13–21). Berlin, Germany: Springer.

Talley, R. M., Shoyinka, S., & Minkoff, K. (2021). The Self-assessment for Modification of Anti-Racism Tool (SMART): Addressing structural racism in community behavioral health. *Community Mental Health Journal, 57*(6), 1208–1213.

Taylor, R. J., Chatters, L. M., Woodward, A. T., & Brown, E. (2013). Racial and ethnic differences in extended family, friendship, fictive kin, and congregational informal support networks. *Family Relations, 62*(4), 609–624.

The White House (2023). A Proclamation on National Mental Health Awareness Month, 2023. Retrieved from https://www.whitehouse.gov/briefing-room/presidential-actions/2023/04/28/a-proclamation-on-national-mental-health-awareness-month-2023/

Thomeer, M. B., Moody, M. D., & Yahirun, J. (2023). Racial and ethnic disparities in mental health and mental health care during the COVID-19 pandemic. *Journal of Racial and Ethnic Health Disparities, 10* (2), 961–976.

Walker, M., & Bruhn, C. (2024). Perspectives of African American social workers regarding clinical licensure. *Journal of Evidence-Based Social Work, 21*(2), 145–161.

Wang, M. L., Gomes, A., Rosa, M., Copeland, P., & Santana, V. J. (2024). A systematic review of diversity, equity, and inclusion and antiracism training studies: Findings and future directions. *Translational Behavioral Medicine, 14*(3), 156–171.

Ward, E. C., & Besson, D. D. (2013). African American men's beliefs about mental illness, perceptions of stigma, and help-seeking barriers. *The Counseling Psychologist*, *41*(3), 359–391.

White, R. T. (2002). Reconceptualizing HIV infection among poor Black adolescent females: An urban poverty paradigm. *Health Promotion Practice*, *3*(2), 302–312. doi: 10.1177/152483990200300224.

Wilcox, M. M. (2023). Oppression is not "culture": The need to center systemic and structural determinants to address anti-Black racism and racial trauma in psychotherapy. *Psychotherapy*, *60*(1), 76–85. doi: 10.1037/pst0000446.

Wilcox, M. M., Reid Marks, L., Franks, D. N., Davis, R. P., & Moss, T. (2024). Are training programs addressing anti-Black racism and white supremacy? A descriptive analysis. *The Counseling Psychologist*, *52*(1), 124–157.

Williams, D. R., & Williams-Morris, R. (2000). Racism and mental health: The African American experience. *Ethnicity & health*, *5*(3–4), 243–268. https://doi.org/10.10 80/713667453

Williams, M. T., Faber, S. C., & Duniya, C. (2022). Being an anti-racist clinician. *The Cognitive Behaviour Therapist*, *15*, e19.

Winston, A. S. (2020). Why mainstream research will not end scientific racism in psychology. *Theory & Psychology*, *30*(3), 425–430. doi: 10.1177/0959354320925176.

Yarrington JS, Montgomery C, Joyner KJ, O'Connor MF, Wolitzky-Taylor K. (2023 Oct). Evaluating training needs in clinical psychology doctoral programs. *Journal Clinical Psychology*, *79*(10), 2304–2316. doi: 10.1002/jclp.23549. Epub 2023 Jun 13. PMID: 37310160; PMCID: PMC10701694.

Zeira, A. (2022). Mental health challenges related to neoliberal capitalism in the United States. *Community Mental Health Journal*, *58*(2), 205–212. https://doi.org/10.1007/ s10597-021-00840-7

Index

Note: Page numbers followed by "n" denote endnotes.